Longitudinal research on individual development

Longitudinal research is an essential element in the investigation of human development over time, with considerable advantages over more widely used cross-sectional research designs. This book examines the scope for longitudinal studies in a range of developmental fields, emphasising the advantages of this approach for the investigation of causal mechanisms and processes and the dynamics of development over the life-span. It also discusses methodological issues.

Drawing on the final conference in the European Science Foundation's network dealing with longitudinal research on individual development, this is a valuable reference work for behavioural and developmental scientists. The distinguished contributors review normal and disordered development in the emotional, cognitive and social domains, including valuable discussions of gene–environment interactions, the maturation of the human brain, and issues relating to aging.

As a source of information and ideas this volume, the concluding work in this series, will be of interest to practitioners and research workers in developmental disciplines at any stage of the life-cycle.

T0243056

Longitudinal research on individual development

Present status and future perspectives

Edited by

DAVID MAGNUSSON

Department of Psychology, University of Stockholm

and

PAUL CASAER

Department of Paediatrics, University of Leuven

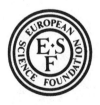

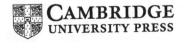

CAMBRIDGE UNIVERSITY PRESS
Cambridge, New York, Melbourne, Madrid, Cape Town, Singapore, São Paulo

Cambridge University Press
The Edinburgh Building, Cambridge CB2 2RU, UK

Published in the United States of America by Cambridge University Press, New York

www.cambridge.org
Information on this title: www.cambridge.org/9780521434782

First published 1993
This digitally printed first paperback version 2006

A catalogue record for this publication is available from the British Library

Library of Congress Cataloguing in Publication data
Longitudinal research on individual development / edited by David
Magnusson and Paul Casaer.
p.   cm. -- (European Network on Longitudinal Studies on Individual
Development ; 8)
Based on papers presented at a conference of the European Science
Foundation Network on Longitudinal Studies on Individual Development
held in Budapest, Hungary in March 1991.
Includes bibliographical references and index.
ISBN 0-521-43478-5
1. Developmental psychology--Longitudinal studies--Congresses.
2. Individual differences--Longitudinal studies--Congresses.
3. Psychology, Pathological--Longitudinal studies--Congresses.
4. Psychology--Methodology--Congresses. I. Magnusson, David.
II. Casaer, Paul Jules Maria.
BF712.5.L66   1933
155--dc20   93-18120   CIP

ISBN-13 978-0-521-43478-2 hardback
ISBN-10 0-521-43478-5 hardback

ISBN-13 978-0-521-03453-1 paperback
ISBN-10 0-521-03453-1 paperback

Contents

Principal contributors

Professor David Magnusson
Department of Psychology, Stockholm University, S-106 91 Stockholm, Sweden

Professor Sandra Scarr
Department of Psychology, University of Virginia, Gilmer Hall, Charlottesville, VA 22901, USA

Professor Dr Paul Casaer
Department of Pediatrics, University of Leuven, Herestraat 49, B-3000 Leuven, Belgium

Professor Dr Verne S. Caviness, Jr.
Pediatric Neurology Service, Massachusetts General Hospital, Fruit Street, Boston 02114, USA

Professor Dr Franz E. Weinert and co-author Professor Dr Wolfgang Schneider
Max Planck Institute for Psychological Research, Leopoldstrasse 24, D-8000 München 40, Germany

Professor Norman Garmezy
Department of Psychology, University of Minnesota, Elliott Hall, 75 East River Road, Minneapolis, Minnesota 55455, USA

Professor Michael Rutter
MRC Child Psychiatry Unit, Institute of Psychiatry, De Crespigny Park, London SE5 8AF, UK

Dr Andreas Kruse
University of Heidelberg, Department of Gerontology, Akademienstrasse 3, D-6900, Germany

Dr Ulman Lindenberger, and Professor Dr Paul Baltes
Max Planck Institute for Human Development and Education, Lentzeallee 94, D-1000 Berlin 33, Germany

Professor Dr Jochen Brandstädter
Department of Psychology, University of Trier, PO Box 3825, D-5500 Trier, Germany

Professor Lars R. Bergman
Department of Psychology, Stockholm University, S-106 91 Stockholm, Sweden

Foreword

The main task for the European Network on Longitudinal Studies on Individual Development (ENLS), initiated in 1985 under the auspices of the European Science Foundation, has been to discuss appropriate models for a developmental perspective on individual functioning in all its aspects and to analyse and discuss the consequences of such models for the application of a longitudinal design for research on this issue.

The history of systematically planned and performed studies of individual development dates back to the 1920s. One of the best-known longitudinal studies was implemented by Terman and his associates at Stanford in 1921 and followed the development of more than 1500 gifted individuals from early school years through adult life. The reports from this project cover a period of more than 50 years (see e.g. Sears, 1977). Two longitudinal studies initiated in 1928, the Berkeley Growth Study led by Nancy Bailey and the Guidance Study led by Jean W. Macfarlane, both implemented at the Institute of Human Development at Berkeley, and the Oakland Growth Study (the Adolescent Growth Study) initiated by Harold E. Jones and Herbert Stoltz in 1931, were pioneering works with the general purpose of studying a broad range of biological, behavioural, cognitive, motivational, emotional and social aspects of individual functioning. In spite of the fact that these studies were theoretically and methodologically well planned and carried out and also were concerned with central developmental issues, they did not stimulate many other researchers to follow. For a long time only a few well-planned studies appeared on the scene. During the last decades the initiation of longitudinal studies has increased, particularly in Europe. The interest in longitudinal research has been promoted by strong arguments presented by Baltes and Nesselroade (1979), Block (1971), Cairns, (1979), Gruenberg and Le Resche (1981), Livson and Peskin (1980), McCall (1977), Robins (1966), Rutter (1981), and Wohlwill (1973), among many others.

Why then was it motivated to establish a scientific network in order to stimulate and support longitudinal research and why is a discussion still needed about the motives for a longitudinal strategy for the study of individual development? There are at least two main reasons.

First, even if the number of longitudinal studies being implemented is increasing, the number does not reflect to any reasonable extent the need for such studies. An overview of the main journals presenting research on developmental issues clearly shows that the dominating number of empirical studies reported have been performed applying a cross-sectional design. This approach is often adopted even in cases where a longitudinal design would be the appropriate one with reference to the nature of the problem and the structures and processes involved.

Secondly, theoretical articles arguing against longitudinal research are still being published. These arguments have caused much debate, in spite of the fact that they suffer from a lack of insightful analysis of the phenomena which are the core object of interest in longitudinal research. This debate has, unfortunately, contributed to hesitation among funding agencies.

With reference to the importance of longitudinal research as a basis for the identification of the factors involved in the development of individual life courses and for understanding the process by which they operate, the conclusion is that there is still a need for a discussion about the theoretical basis for a longitudinal design and about the problems which have to be solved in the design and the ways this can be done.

Central substantive and methodological topics of relevance for a discussion about the application of a longitudinal research strategy in research on individual development have been dealt with in a series of workshops. The volumes emanating from the workshops demonstrate, with numerous illustrations, the importance and necessity of a longitudinal research design in this domain. These problems have been dealt with in other volumes in the series (Baltes & Baltes, 1990; Kalverboer, Hopkins & Geuze, 1993; Magnusson & Bergman, 1990; Magnusson, Bergman, Rudinger & Törestad, 1991; Rutter, 1988; Rutter & Casaer, 1991; de Ribaupierre, 1989).

This volume is the last in the series of ENLS volumes. It is my hope, and that of my colleagues in the coordination committee, that this volume and the preceding ones will contribute to more effective research in the future in the important area of scientific investigation that individual development constitutes.

David Magnusson
Chairman of the coordination committee of ENLS

REFERENCES

Baltes, P. B. & Baltes, M. (1990). *Successful aging: perspectives from the behavioural sciences.* Cambridge: Cambridge University Press.

Baltes, P. B. & Nesselroade, J. R. (1979). History and rationale of longitudinal research. In J.R. Nesselroade and P. B. Baltes (eds.), *Longitudinal research in the study of behavior and development.* New York: Academic Press.

Block, J. (1971). *Lives through time.* Berkeley. C.A.: Bancroft Books.

Cairns, R. B. (1979). *Social development: the origins and plasticity of interchanges.* San Francisco: W. H. Freeman & Co.

de Ribaupierre, A. (1989). *Transition mechanisms in child development*. Cambridge: Cambridge University Press.

Gruenberg, E. M. & Le Resch, L. (1981). Reaction: the future of longitudinal studies. In S.A. Mednick and A.E. Baert (eds.), *Prospective longitudinal research: an empirical basis for the primary prevention of psychosocial disorders*, pp. 319–325. Oxford: Oxford Medical Publications.

Kalverboer, A., Hopkins, B. & Geuze, R. (1993). *Motor development in early and later childhood: longitudinal approaches*. Cambridge: Cambridge University Press.

Livson, N. & Peskin, H. (1980). Perspectives on adolescence from longitudinal research. In J. Adelson (ed.), *Handbook of adolescent psychology*. New York: Wiley.

McCall, R. B. (1977). Challenges to a science of developmental psychology. *Child Development*, **48**, 333–44.

Magnusson, D. & Bergman, L. R. (1990). *Data quality in longitudinal research*. Cambridge: Cambridge University Press.

Magnusson, D., Bergman, L. R. Rudinger, G. & Törestad, B. (1991). *Problems and methods for longitudinal research: stability and change*. Cambridge: Cambridge University Press.

Robins, L. N. (1966). *Deviant children grow up: a sociological and psychiatric study of sociopathic personality*. Baltimore: Williams and Wilkens. Reprinted Robert E. Krieger: Huntington, NY. (1974).

Rutter, M. (1981). Longitudinal studies: a psychiatric perspective. In S. A. Mednick and A. E. Baert (eds.). *Prospective longitudinal research: an empirical basis for the primary prevention of psychosical disorders*. Oxford: Oxford University Press.

Rutter, M. (1988). *Studies of psychosocial risk: the power of longitudinal data*. Cambridge: Cambridge University Press.

Rutter, M. & Caesar, P. (1991). *Biological risk factors for psychosocial disorders*. Cambridge: Cambridge University Press.

Sears, R. R. (1977). Sources of life satisfactions of the Terman gifted men. *American Psychologist*, **32**, 119–28.

Wohlwill, J. F. (1973). *The study of behavioral development*. London: Academic Press.

Preface

In March 1991 the ESF Network on Longitudinal Studies on Individual Development completed its five-year existence with a summing-up conference in Budapest, Hungary.

The conference was built round poster sessions which were interspersed with state-of-the-art lectures by prominent scholars in various important areas. In order to make the present volume, which in the main emanates from this conference, cover the various research domains as adequately as possible, some additional scholars were invited to write chapters with respect to some of the more comprehensive fields.

In this introduction, we will try to summarize some pivotal issues in each of the chapters and also make attempts at highlighting the holistic and dynamic facets of human development. This is one important and recurrent theme in all chapters, although naturally formulated in different ways by the various contributors.

In Chapter 1, Magnusson presents a number of arguments in favour of more concentrated efforts being devoted to longitudinal research for the study of the intricate processes that mould individuals' future lives. He emphasizes the importance of rendering research on human ontogeny more vigorous by complementing the more traditional variable-oriented approaches with studies that focus on persons as the central unit of analysis. Magnusson purports that humans can be seen from a general systems theory, and also that each individual is a self-organizing system. The latter concept implies that subsystems, physiological and psychological, interact and organize in ways to optimize the functioning of the whole organism. Incidentally, the word 'organ' means 'tool' in Greek and 'organism' refers to an 'ordered structure' of interacting mechanisms. Outcomes of single individuals' life-span development cannot be predicted with any high degree of accuracy but, all the same are characterized by a lawful continuity and thus are intelligible in retrospect.

Weinert and Schneider give an extensive overview of the research concerning emotional, cognitive, and social development in Chapter 5. Among the things they stress is the fact that cross-sectional studies tend to be overly variable-oriented, a risk easier to detect and understand when the same individuals are followed up across time and, simultaneously, several variables are included. They also turn the reader's attention to another essential fact, which is that change measures in cross-sectional studies, by definition, are always based on separate groups of subjects of different ages. Furthermore, they discuss the distinction between the concepts of continuity and discontinuity vs. stability and change. The notion of stability (or change) is most often used to characterize rank orders of individuals across time with respect to some specific variable. For example, if the rank order from a certain age to a later age remains largely unaltered, stability of that specific variable, e.g. a trait is postulated.

Continuity, on the other hand, means that a developmental sequence is characterized by an uninterrupted process that goes through continual states in an unbroken whole. The authors underline that stability and continuity are two separate concepts, thereby making an important and, often overlooked, point. Most longitudinal study focuses on the stability issue. Weinert and Schneider emphasize that developmental continuity for a certain group of individuals might occur despite a substantial lack of stability as to inter-individual differences. Not taking this reminder of theirs seriously could imply that single individuals' more or less diverging life trajectories might remain undetected. If, and when, this happens the dynamics of human development and the holistic perspective are lost which will render the acquirement of deeper knowledge of inter-individual continuity difficult.

After that, two chapters on human aging follow. In Chapter 8, Kruse, Lindenberger, and Baltes (as in fact did Weinert and Schneider) emphasize that all types of repeated measures studies have their proper place, but should ideally be twinned with real-time longitudinal research.

The authors stress that short-term (or 'microgenetic') studies, historically spaced cohort-sequential and quasiexperimental research, and their developmental simulation approaches are all needed to isolate and identify the interacting factors that can be given the summary label 'causal processes'. Kruse et al. also argue that long-term studies are needed to understand the boundary conditions of human potentials in elderly people. Aging and old age, the authors state, are not concepts that indicate fixed reality. There is always change, both inter- and intra-individually. One example of the constant flux is the fact that getting older seems to be a source of inter-individual differences in cognitive functioning.

As do other contributors to the volume, Kruse et al. stress the importance of paying regard to the fact that few human experiences, like life events and changes across age in different aspects, occur universally for all people. Such non-shared events will have additive effects and can eventually result in substantial interindividual variation over the years.

Brandstädter, in Chapter 9, presents action theory as one possible and theoretical framework for studying the process of aging. This theory looks upon development as a process construed from both social and personal perspectives in various action contexts over the life-time. Developmental regularity to a large extent depends upon actions. Action theory sees human beings as active, purposeful agents who try to control and influence the outcomes of their lives. However, as Brandtstädter emphasizes, in the life-long process of attempting to optimize one's life conditions, the single individual is heavily influenced by largely uncontrollable biological, physical, and social facts in the dynamics of development. The difficulties in finding coherence and consequence in research on individual development is, according to the author, likely to be occasioned by lack of theoretical insight rather than mirroring development as a truly haphazard phenomenon.

The volume contains two chapters about developmental psychopathology. In Chapter 6, Garmezy, starting from a historical perspective on research in the area, discusses developmental and clinical aspects of vulnerability for psychopathological states, and, among other things, poses the question as to why some apparent at-risk individuals fail to manifest disorders in contrast to others who do. When posing research questions in this area, both typical and atypical developmental patterns are of interest. What common and uncommon patterning of behavioural and biological factors characterize at-risk persons and which are the precipitating events propelling individuals into disorders of various kinds? Garmezy strongly suggests a change of focus from the traditional one on people with an already diagnosed disorder to include also those who do not, sometimes unexpectedly and contra-intuitively, develop psychiatric disorders. Like most manifestations of human functioning or dysfunctioning disorders, or their absence, are also-multi-determined. One example of this, which Garmezy presents, is the complex causal processes that are involved in poverty and malnutrition. These phenomena are inter-related and will very often result in circular patterns of long-term and short-term stressors.

Rutter, in Chapter 7, following up Garmezy, discusses the limitations of stage theories when studying psychopathology and the need to take into consideration inter-individual differences, and continuities and discontinuities in individual development; and, as a consequence, the obvious fact that human beings take different and diverging paths through life. Obtaining such a goal implies utilizing longitudinal approaches. Only longitudinal data can detect and map heterogeneity within the domain of, for example, research on the development of conduct disorders.

When discussing individuals' differential susceptibility to psychological disorders, Rutter provides striking and illustrative examples of the complexities of the many factors that in interplay lie behind individual functioning in various aspects. Some conditions have been labelled 'protective', because they are supposed to mitigate the negative influences of, say, adverse childhood environments. Such protective factors can, as Rutter indicates, be related to prior as well as future circumstances at the time of exposure to risks. Often controlled exposure to the risk factor is necessary for resistance to develop.

Chapters 3 and 4 concern brain development. In Chapter 3 Casaer describes the perinatal development of the brain. He discusses its histogenesis in terms of an increased number of brain cells and their inward–outward migration to their final destinations where cell differentiation takes place. Important for the development of the child, in all areas, is the gradual myelinization of axons. One of the points that Casaer accentuates is that it is no longer meaningful to differentiate between what has been labelled structural and metabolic disturbances because both are manifestations of the same underlying programming error. Both types of disturbances should rather be seen as interactive in nature and, consequently, not as independent variables between which no interdependency exists. The brain and the environment are continually in interplay with external factors, such as social ones. As a consequence of this fact, the brain is in a constant change at different levels and not at all invariable across time.

In Chapter 8, Caviness, Filipek, and Kennedy subscribe to a cognitive science model in which the brain is seen as a computational map. As a tool for studying the function of the brain, they present the magnetic resonance technique which provides a basis for morphological analyses.

The different disorders of the brain generally imply the degrading of neural tissues in two main ways. First, there are specifically acting disruptive disorders, including tumors, ischemia and the like. Secondly, there exist more diffuse disturbances, resulting in various forms of dysfunctioning because of the destruction of a huge number of neurons.

In Chapter 2, Scarr maintains that only longitudinal analyses can provide us with a true picture of the interactive role of genes and environmental factors in development: in shaping both typical human development and inter-individual variation, manifesting themselves within a wide range of 'normal' to pronouncedly aberrant behaviors.

As a background to her presentation on genes and environments in individual development, Scarr discusses the reciprocal character of parent–child influences. Children do have an impact on their caregivers as, of course, parents, in turn, affect their offspring. Interestingly, it has been shown that there is rather more variation *within* families than *between* families with respect to various aspects of human functioning such as intelligence, psychopathology, and personality traits. Couched somewhat differently, it may not matter whether children have *different* parents provided they are supportive and willing to take on the role of caregiver.

A central aspect of Scarr's theory is that what matters are genotype–environment correlations rather than some kind of gene–environment interplay. Genotypes drive individuals so that they construct and create their own experiences. This implies that different normal environments are created by both parents' as well as by their offspring's characteristics. Differential environmental conditions *per se*, consequently, do not constitute the determinants of the child's phenotype.

In Chapter 10, Bergman, from a methodological standpoint, argues for the importance of longitudinal studies. He discusses the complex phenomenon of 'change', and pleads for better thought-out matching of problems with methods. He also describes the person-oriented approach, which, by using various statistical techniques, is designed to help avoid some of the apparent pitfalls of a purely variable-oriented view on individual functioning and development. Bergman discusses the importance of using appropriate methods when approaching a specific research question. There are two simple guidelines to follow: the method must help answer the researched problem, and the method must also help produce dependable results. The reasons why these seemingly truistic rules all too often are not followed are many and simple: practical reasons such as easy accessibility; prestigious causes, that is, the methods considered sophisticated and refined; and, last but not least, pure lack of knowledge of the diversity of available methods.

Through most chapters runs a theme that has the following message: human development is multi-faceted and multi-determined, and what makes individuals take diverging or parallel paths through life is almost impossible to predict in advance. What is actually possible is to gain an understanding of how and why an individual's life took the course it finally did. We must not believe that we can 'disentangle' the diverse factors and mechanisms that govern people's lives. Development is a process that, in itself, is entangled and intertwined.

David Magnusson, Stockholm, and Paul Casaer, Leuven, Autumn 1992

1 Human ontogeny: a longitudinal perspective

DAVID MAGNUSSON

INTRODUCTION

Development, in its most general form, refers to any process of progressive change. In biology, development refers to progressive changes in size, shape, and/or function during the life-span of an organism. Research on human ontogeny covers this process from conception to death. Two concepts are central to this definition. The first one is the concept of *change*, in size, shape and/or function. The second one is the concept of time. The definition implies that development is not synonymous with time. Time is not equivalent to development, but development always has a time dimension. Consequently, processes that go on without change, within existing structures, do not constitute development. Thus, developmental models must be distinguished from models that are restricted to current perspectives which analyse and explain why individuals function as they do in terms of their current psychological and biological dispositions.

Individual development has long been an important area of research in biology, education, medicine, psychology, sociology, and related disciplines. There are several reasons for this interest.

Knowledge about the development process; which factors operate, and how, is of scientific interest in itself. Such knowledge contributes to our understanding of individual functioning in a variety of respects that change over time and that can be seen developmentally throughout the whole life-cycle. How elderly persons function is not only determined by the fact of being old in age, but is an outcome of their life-history. Understanding the aetiology and moderating factors of senile dementia requires a process orientation, and understanding the conditions of 'life quality' at old age requires knowledge about life precursors of 'successful aging' (Baltes & Baltes, 1990).

Knowledge about the structures and processes involved in the course of individual development, and how they operate, has far-reaching implications in many applied fields. It is fundamental to the understanding and explanation of the background of physical illnesses (e.g. cancer), mental illnesses (e.g. schizophrenia) and behavioural disorders and maladjustment (e.g. criminal behaviour and alcohol abuse). Such understanding is the basis for the develop-

1

ment of effective medical and psychological treatment and for the planning and implementation of measures in the social and physical environments in order to prevent and cure illness and maladaption. Methods for the treatment and prevention of maladjustment and illness are needed at all stages of the life-cycle, from conception to death.

INDIVIDUAL DEVELOPMENT AS A DYNAMIC PROCESS

Any effective discussion of a substantive problem must be based on, and implemented with, an analysis of the character of the phenomena to be studied. In this case, the total space of phenomena of interest for study includes the individual and the environment. Together these form the total system of structures and processes that must be considered for a full understanding and explanation of individual development (Lerner, 1991). (A 'structure' is here defined as a functional organization of biological or mental elements, and a 'process' as activated structures in operation over time.)

What are, then, the main characteristics of the ways individuals function and develop that have consequences for the choice of appropriate strategies and designs in developmental research?

A basic proposition for the following discussion is the view that an individual functions and develops as a total, integrated whole, and that individual functioning, both in a current and in a developmental perspective can be characterized, at a general level, as a dynamic, multi-determined, stochastic process (cf. Cairns, 1986; Magnusson, 1988, 1990). This formulation implies two key principles for individual functioning; The first is that totalities function and develop. The second principle is that psychological and biological factors in the individual, and social and physical factors in the environment, are in a continuous process of reciprocal interaction.

A holistic perspective

As is the case with many central ideas in developmental research, the holistic view on individual functioning and development has very old roots. It is reflected, for example, in the old assumption of the four basic temperaments, in related typologies, and in the discussion of an idiographic versus a nomothetical approach to empirical research. James (1890) eloquently expounded the individual as a whole, and Dewey (1896) warned against the danger of atomistic psychology, which he saw growing out of the Wundt school of experimental psychology. In developmental research, the renewed interest in a holistic view is reflected in the contributions by Block (1971), Cairns (1983), Fogel and Thelen (1987), Gustafson and Magnusson (1991), Magnusson (1988), Sameroff (1983), Sroufe (1979), Wapner & Kaplan (1983), and Wolff (1981), among others.

A holistic approach to individual functioning has been strengthened by the development of powerful theories and models for dynamic, complex processes. The holistic dynamic processes of individual development have certain elements in common with dynamic, non-linear, complex processes, which are the object of interest in *general systems theory* (Bertalanffy, 1968; Laszlo, 1972, Miller, 1978), *chaos theory* (cf. Crutchfield et al., 1986, Gleick, 1987) and *catastrophe theory* (cf. Zeeman, 1976). The presentation of these theories has had a tremendous influence on theory development over many scientific domains. It has influenced empirical research and the development of measurement models and statistics in fields concerned with dynamic, non-linear, complex processes such as meteorology, biology, chemistry, and ecology. Chaos theory has been regarded as one of the most powerful theories in this century and has been applied in many scientific disciplines (Hall, 1991). Attempts have even been made to apply chaos theory to the functioning of the brain (cf. Basar, 1990). However, these theories have had less impact than they deserve on disciplines concerned with human functioning, such as economics, education, psychology, and sociology.

For our discussion about appropriate strategies in research on individual development, one main characteristic of individual functioning must be kept in mind: the individual is not only a passive receiver of stimulation from the environment to which he/she reacts; he/she is also an active, purposeful agent in the person–environment interaction process. This is emphasized, for example, in action theory (see Chapter 9 by Brandtstädter; Strelau, 1983; Brushlinskii, 1987). The individual's inner and outer life is guided by the functioning of the perceptual–cognitive system (including world views and self-perceptions) with attached emotions, motives, needs, values, and goals. It can be briefly summarized as the integrating mental system. By selecting and interpreting information from the external world, and transforming this information into internal and external actions, the mental system plays a crucial role both in the process of interaction between mental and physiological factors within the individual, and in the process of interaction between the individual and his/her environment. Not only does the mental system permit the organism to shape its effective environment, it provides a rapid and reversible strategy for organisms to adapt to changing environments. The mental system serves as a leading edge for adaptation in ontogeny in that it mobilizes neurobiological and physiological modifications and environmental changes. However, it should be observed that the slower acting forces of maturation can realign or cancel out short-term perceptual–cognitive–behavioural modifications when they become no longer adaptive or relevant.

Congenital factors (including genetic factors) set the stage and set the limits for the development of an individual's mediating mental system. Within the restrictions, and using the potentialities of these biological factors, the structure and functioning of an individual's mediating mental system are formed. This system changes slowly in a process of maturation and experience that takes place in the continuous, bidirectional interaction between the individual and the environment. Thus, the mediating system is a function of the individual's interaction with the environment in the course of individual development and it plays a crucial, guiding role in that interaction process at each stage of development.

A major consequence of what has just been said is that, without careful consideration, mathematical models that were developed for the treatment of data in empirical research on non-human dynamic processes, e.g. non-linear mathematics, with reference to chaos and catastrophe theories, must be applied in research on individual development processes with caution and taking careful consideration to the specific character of the human processes involved. In order to be effective in research on individual functioning, including research on human ontogeny, methods for data treatment must be developed that take into account the crucial role played by the mental mediating system in the dynamic processes of human ontogeny and in the activity of the individual as a purposeful agent.

The principle of dynamic interaction

An essential feature of individual functioning is the continuously ongoing interaction among operating factors. If a person meets a situation which is experienced as threatening or demanding, e.g. an examination or a work task, the cognitive act of interpretation of the situation stimulates, via the hypothalamus, the excretion of adrenaline which, in turn, influences other physiological processes. This cognitive–physiological interplay is accompanied by emotional states of fear and/or anxiety and/or by generally experienced arousal, which, in the next stage of the process of individual functioning, affects not only the individual's behaviour but also his/her interpretation of the sequence of changes in the situational conditions and thereby the physiological reactions in terms of autonomic activity/reactivity. Thus, the perceptual–cognitive system and the biological system of an individual are involved in a continuous loop of interaction, and the way this process functions is dependent, among other things, on the environment, particularly on the environment as it is perceived and interpreted by the individual. Across time, this interplay of biological and mental factors contributes to changes in their structure and functioning as well as in the structure and functioning of related subsystems, such as the immune system (Öhman & Magnusson, 1987).

The example illustrates interaction among operating factors at a certain level of individual functioning. Interaction is a central principle at all levels of individual functioning, from the functioning of single cells and how they organize themselves into systems to fulfil their developmental role in the total organism (cf. Edelman, 1987) to the functioning of an individual in relation to his/her environment (Cairns, 1979; Caspi, 1987; Dannefer & Perlmutter, 1990; Magnusson, 1988; Rutter, 1983).

Most of the discussion about the relevance of an interactionistic model of individual functioning has referred to empirical results demonstrating absence or presence of significant statistical interactions in experimental designs. However, the existence of interaction processes within individuals, and between the individual and the environment, does not necessarily show up in significant interactions in statistical analyses of differences. It is necessary to distinguish between lawful dynamic interaction as a principle for individual functioning and statistical interaction in experimental designs (cf. Olweus, 1977).

The concept of dynamic interaction includes seven interrelated basic principles: *multidetermination, interdependence, reciprocity, temporality, nonlinearity, and integration* (Magnusson & Törestad, 1992, 1993).

Multidetermination At all levels, activities of the system involve several underlying factors or conditions.

Interdependence The principle of interdependence implies that two operating factors are mutually dependent upon the existence of each other without necessarily influencing each other in a reciprocal way.

Reciprocity The reciprocal character of the processes involved in human ontogeny implies that the traditional assumption of a one-directional causal relation between, on the one hand, biological and environmental factors as causes and, on the other hand, mental functioning and manifest behaviour as effects, is no longer sufficient as a general model. Biological factors are both causes and results. The relation of thoughts, emotions and behaviours to physiological processes has been elucidated in much recent research. Physiological processes can be evoked by cognitive–emotional events and are maintained in a continuous interaction between mental and biological factors. The same holds for the environment; it is both a cause and an effect in the process of an individual's interaction with the environment.

In the course of development, a certain process may be triggered by factors in the environment (such as a loss of an important person), by factors in the cognitive–emotional system (such as automized thoughts about one's worthlessness), or by biological factors (such as hyperthyroidism). Changes in the individual–environment balance may then have repercussions at any other place in the total system, internally (cognitively, emotionally, physiologically) and/or externally in manifest behaviour. Sometimes it is not possible to tease out which one of several operating factors takes precedence over the other. The most common case is that a process, say an anxiety reaction, would not have had been initiated if certain situational conditions, e.g. an oral examination, and certain individual dispositions, e.g. a disposition to react with increased anxiety in that type of situation, had not been present simultaneously.

Temporality The description of individual functioning as a process or a number of interrelated processes is fundamental to the understanding and explanation of the phenomena with which we are concerned in developmental research. A process can be characterized as a continuous flow of interrelated, interdependent events. This definition introduces time as a fundamental element in any model for individual functioning. In modern models of dynamic processes, a central concept is the concept of *motion*. Key aspects of biological processes are *rhythm* and *periodicity* (Weiner, 1989). It should be emphasized that holistic, system models are not necessarily developmental, but developmental models are necessarily holistic and system oriented. The temporal perspective is important for understanding individual functioning at all levels, from micro-processes in the biological system to the individual's interaction with the environment. This has methodological and research-strategy consequences, which must be considered in developmental research.

Nonlinearity The principle of nonlinearity refers basically to the interrelations among variables operating at the individual level. The principle implies, for example, that the individual effect of hormone A on the dependent hormone B is not necessarily linear; the relation may take on any functional form. The same holds true for the interplay of a single individual with his/her environment. For example, individuals' psychological and physiological stress reactions to increasing stimulation from the environment are usually curvilinear (Hebb, 1955). The nonlinear function for the relation between two operating person-bound factors or the relation between the individual and his/her environment may differ among individuals. This circumstance has implications for the choice of appropriate designs in developmental research.

Integration At all levels of the dynamic, holistic processes, the operating parts are coordinated in their functions so as to serve the goal of the system to which they belong. This holds for parts of sub-systems at all levels as well as for the coordination of sub-systems in the functioning of the totality. Integration is the principle behind the fact that the totality is more than the sum of the parts.

Lawful organization of structures and processes

All aspects of individual functioning are basically linked to the functioning of the individual as a biological being. A basic, well-documented principle in the functioning of biological systems is their ability for *self-organization* (cf. the concept 'self-organizing systems', Nicolis & Prigogine, 1977; Prigogine & Stengers, 1985; Odum's, 1983, discussion of energy self-organization in ecology, and the presentation of models for the immune system by Farmer et al., 1987. Relevant for the discussion of this issue is also Edelman's, 1987, *Theory of*

Neuronal Group Selection and the way in which the development of the brain, both with respect to morphology and function, depends on interaction between the organism and the environment).

Within sub-systems, the operating components organize themselves in a way that maximizes the functioning of each sub-system with respect to its purpose in the total system. At a higher level, sub-systems organize themselves to fulfil their role in the functioning of the totality. Good illustrations of this principle are the functioning of the brain, along with its implications for the development and functioning of the cognitive system of an individual, and the functioning of the coronary system. In coronary research, factors and operating mechanisms involved in 'remodelling' the coronary system have become an important area of scientific study (see, e.g. Sharpe et al., 1991).

Individuals differ to some extent in the way in which operational factors are organized and function within sub-systems, such as the perceptual–cognitive–emotional system, the immune system, the coronary system, and the behavioural system. Individuals also differ in sub-system organization and function. These organizations can be described in terms of *patterns* of operating factors within sub-systems and in terms of patterns of functioning sub-systems. As emphasized by Weiner (1989), the natural pacemakers of the heart, of the stomach, and of the brain function in a patterned way.

These characteristics of the functioning of sub-systems and of the total organism form the theoretical basis for a pattern approach to the study of individual differences. In a pattern analysis, the individuals are grouped on the basis of similarities with respect to patterns of values for variables relevant to the problem under investigation (see Bergman, Chapter 10). Fundamental to the application of pattern analysis is, in most cases, that the number of biologically and psychologically possible organizations of factors within sub-systems, and of sub-systems within individuals, is limited. Thus, individuals can be grouped in homogeneous categories with characteristic patterns of values for variables which are relevant to the issue under consideration. The advantages of this approach to the study of developmental issues have been demonstrated in a number of empirical studies (see, e.g. Bergman & Magnusson, 1984*a*, *b*; Gustafson & Magnusson, 1991; Magnusson & Bergman, 1988, 1990; Pulkkinen & Trembley, in press. The approach is also being used in clinical research, e.g. by Armelius & Sundbom, 1991).

An illustration of the existence of group differences in the functioning of sub-systems can be taken from the way the coronary system functions. To study the haemodynamic effects of captopril in patients with severe heart problems, serial right heart catheterizations were performed in 51 patients who were treated over a period of 2 to 8 weeks (Packer et al., 1983). (Captopril has the effect of lowering blood pressure, among other things.) The results are summarized in Fig. 1.1.

As Fig. 1.1 shows, the patients could be grouped with respect to how they

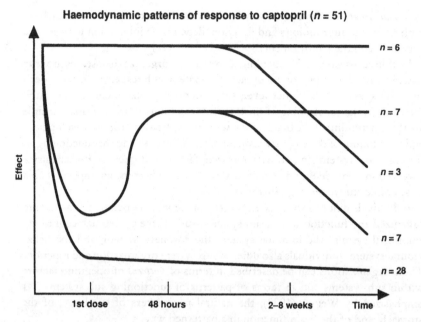

Fig. 1.1   Haemodynamic patterns of response for five different groups of individuals during long-term captopril therapy for severe chronic heart failure. (Based on data from Packer et al., 1983.)

reacted. For 28 patients, the drug had effects that were evident after 48 hours and sustained after 2 to 8 weeks. Nine patients had minimal responses initially; six of them failed to improve during long-term treatment, while three showed delayed haemodynamic benefits. In 14 patients, first doses of captopril produced marked beneficial responses. For seven of them, the responses became rapidly attenuated after 48 hours, but continued therapy for 2 to 8 weeks led to spontaneous restoration of the haemodynamic effect of first doses of the drug (i.e. three phasic response type). For the remaining seven patients, attenuation of the initial response was not reversed by prolonged captopril therapy. The authors drew the following conclusion: 'Although first dose effects of captopril are frequently sustained, the occurrence of delayed, attenuated, and triphasic responses indicates that a complex and variable relationship may exist between the early and late hemodynamic effects of vasodilator drugs in patients with severe heart problems.' (p. 803).

This study demonstrates the danger of traditional variable-oriented research in which one aspect of the holistic multidetermined integrated process is taken out of its context and regarded and treated as a nomothetical variable in statistical analyses of interindividual differences. It also shows how individuals differ in a limited number of ways in their physiological reactions.

Lawful processes of individual development

The interaction processes within given structures, and those leading to changes in the structures, take place at all levels of the integrated system. At all levels the processes are going on within organized sub-systems guided by lawful principles, and it is the task of and challenge for scientific psychological research to unveil these principles.

Sub-systems at different levels are embedded in each other and are involved in a constant dynamic, reciprocal interaction. The characteristic features of dynamic interaction, summarized above, do not apply to one sub-system at a time. One implication of this circumstance is that each sub-system must be analysed in terms of its context in the total functioning of the individual, i.e. in terms of the manner in which it affects and is affected by other sub-systems. Here Weiss's (1969) formulation, with reference to systems theory, is appropriate: 'As I have tried to illustrate in a recent article (P.W., 1967), the "more" (than the sum of parts) in the above tenet does not at all refer to any measurable quantity in the observed systems themselves; it refers solely to the necessity for the observer to supplement the sum of statements that can be made about separate parts by any such additional statements as will be needed to describe the collective behaviour of the parts, when in an organized group. In carrying out this upgrading process, he is in effect doing no more than restoring information content that has been lost on the way down in the progressive analysis of the unitary universe into abstracted elements (p. 11).'

Thus, a holistic view does not preclude systematic analyses of specific aspects of structures and processes and of specific mechanisms operating in current and developmental processes. As long as structures function in an orderly way and the processes are lawful, they are accessible to scientific analysis. The holistic view does, however, require additional propositions if the organized sub-systems are to be understood in their totality.

Changes in individual functioning across time

A central characteristic of the process of individual development is that the total system of operating factors, biological, psychological and social, changes across time as a result of maturation, experience and learning (Gottlieb, 1991). The patterning of the total system and its sub-systems is in continuous transition into new configurations across the life-span. An important consequence of the perspective applied here, with essential methodological implications, is that changes do not take place in single aspects isolated from the totality. It is the total picture of structures and processes that changes across time, partly as a result of the process itself. This implies that each system of factors (mental and biological in the individual and social and physical in the environment) changes with respect to its character per se and, as a consequence, with respect to its respective role in the total process. The extent to which different aspects of individual functioning are influenced by environmental factors in this process varies. For example, in sexual development, some features, such as gonadal structure and function, are strongly regulated by biological factors. On the other hand, other aspects of individual functioning, such as choice of peers and types of sexual relations, may be strongly open to experiential influences (Cairns, 1991).

The pace at which these changes take place varies among sub-systems and aspects of individual functioning. Generally, processes at a micro-level are characterized by shorter time perspectives than processes in systems at a macro-level. For example, the anatomical structure of the fetus changes (as a result of cell–environment context interaction) much faster than individual changes in the process of aging. This implies that the pace at which the structures in the individual and in the environment change as a result of maturation, learning and experiences varies with the character of the systems, especially the level of the sub-systems.

A methodological consequence of the different pace of the processes at different levels of the total system of structures involved is that in order to cover the essential properties of the processes, the factors involved, the character of the transition into new stages, and the mechanisms guiding the transition, the appropriate research designs differ. A longitudinal study of the development of the fetus during pregnancy covers only nine months with short-term intervals between observations, while a longitudinal study of the developmental background of adult schizophrenia or adult alcohol problems must cover decades and allows less frequent data collections per time unit (cf. Jessor, Donovan & Costa, 1991; Magnusson, 1988).

Developmental change as lawful continuity

In developmental research, much debate has been devoted to the issues of stability versus change, and continuity versus discontinuity in individual development. Characteristics of most of these studies are (a) that they deal with data for single variables, one at a time, e.g. aggressiveness, intelligence, hyperactivity, and (b) that they express temporal consistency of single variables in terms of relative stability, i.e. in terms of stable rank orders of individuals across time for the variable under consideration.

The fundamental characteristic of individual functioning as a holistic, dynamic process implies, among other things, that individuals do not develop in terms of single variables, but as total integrated systems. Individuals, not variables, function and develop. In this perspective, all changes during the life-span of an individual are characterized by lawful continuity; the functioning of an individual at a certain stage of development is lawfully related to the functioning of the individual at previous stages (Magnusson & Törestad, 1992). As described above, the perceptual–cognitive system, with its attached emotions, motives, values and goals, changes over the life time of an individual, and these changes are reflections of a continuously ongoing, dynamic process that is totally lawful. This does not imply that the functioning at each stage can be predicted from the previous stage at the individual level. As is characteristic of dynamic processes, individual development follows lawful principles, but is not necessarily predictable at all levels of the structures and processes involved.

Thus, each change in the process of human ontogeny is understandable and explainable in the light of the individual's previous life history and the functioning of the environment at the time of the change. This is true even for changes that are so abrupt that they seem to break a stable direction of development; for example, such changes that have been characterized as 'turning points' sometimes appear as a result of 'chance events' or 'significant events' (Bandura, 1982; Magnusson & Törestad, 1993; Pickles & Rutter, 1991).

From the perspective argued here, it becomes clear why, as Weinert in Chapter 5 concludes, the study of the stability of rank orders of individuals for one aspect of individual functioning after another has limited value for understanding and explaining the dynamic process of individual development. The appropriate empirical procedure would be to complement a variable approach with a person-oriented approach and study the process of individual development in terms of the patterning, over time, of factors relevant to the issue under consideration as described above (see Bergman, Chapter 10). The fact that methods for such a study are difficult and complicated does not absolve us from responsibility to develop them.

THE GOAL OF DEVELOPMENTAL RESEARCH

The overriding goal of scientific work is to formulate, as laws, the basic principles that show how and why domains of the total space of phenomena function as they do at various levels of complexity. This goal is as relevant to the study of human ontogeny as it is to the study of physics. The remarkable advances in the physical sciences and the resulting rapid development of a highly technological society have resulted in physics becoming the model for other scientific disciplines. However, other sciences have sometimes adopted the goals and values espoused by physicists, without considering whether or not the character of the phenomena involved are congruent with the model that physics provides.

A central concept supporting the search for precise laws in the framework of the Newtonian mechanistic view of nature is the concept of 'prediction'. Since the well-known claim by J. B. Watson (1913) that 'prediction and control of behavior' are the goals of scientific psychology, and with the development of technically sophisticated statistical tools to foster that claim, prediction has also been an important concept in research on individual functioning, including research on human ontogeny. The role of single variables in individual development is often gauged by how well they predict later outcomes, with success in prediction providing the ultimate goal of empirical research. From two interrelated perspectives, prediction as the ultimate goal for developmental research can be questioned. The first one is concerned with the character of human ontogeny as dynamic, complex processes, the second with the type of laws which can be found in the process of individual development.

The characteristics of the processes of individual development, as discussed above, should already make it clear that prediction of the character of the life course of an individual is not possible. The characteristic feature of dynamic, complex processes as lawful but unpredictable is also emphasized in chaos theory (Gleick, 1987).

Research on human ontogeny belongs to the 'life sciences'. Crick (1988), discussed the kinds of laws sought in different disciplines and concluded that biology is a very different kind of subject from physics: 'Physics is also different because its results can be expressed in powerful, deep and often counterintuitive general laws. There is really nothing in biology that corresponds to special and general relativity, or quantum electrodynamics, or even such simple conservation laws as those of Newtonian mechanics: the conservation of energy, of momentum, and of angular momentum. Biology has its 'laws', such as those of Mendelian genetics, but they are often only rather broad generalizations, with significant exceptions of them. The laws of physics, it is believed, are the same everywhere in the universe. This is unlikely to be true in biology. . . . What is found in biology is mechanisms, mechanisms built with chemical components and that are often modified by other, later, mechanisms added to the earlier ones. While Occam's razor is a useful tool in the physical sciences, it can be a very dangerous implement in biology (p. 138)'.

In view of this perspective and the above description of the characteristic features of individual development, the final criterion for success in our scientific endeavors is not how well we can predict later outcome in the life course of individuals, but how well we succeed in explaining and understanding the life-long processes of individual development. The scientific goal is (a) to identify the factors operating in human ontogeny and (b) to identify and understand the mechanisms by which the factors operate.

So far, the overwhelming preponderance of empirical studies has contributed to identifying operating factors in human development, while the number of studies contributing to identifying the mechanisms by which such factors work is very few. Two examples may be illustrative. A large number of empirical studies indicate that low sympathetic physiological activity/reactivity is an operating factor in the development of various kinds of antisocial behaviour. However, we still lack research showing the mechanisms by which it operates. Empirical studies performed mainly in western countries have identified urbanization as a factor related to crime frequency. What is needed then is to identify the mechanisms by which it works, to explain, among other things, why urbanization has this effect in some cultures and not in others. It works only under certain conditions and not under other ones (cf. Japan with its low crime rate and high urbanization).

A LONGITUDINAL RESEARCH STRATEGY

Methodologically, developmental issues are studied applying one of two distinctly different research strategies: cross-sectional or longitudinal.

In a cross-sectional study of a certain problem, the interrelations among the variables of interest are studied for a certain sample of individuals using data collected on one occasion in time. Often, the ideal cross-sectional design implies that chronological age of the participants is kept under control, i.e. all participants are of the same chronological age, as far as possible. When results from cross-sectional studies are used to elucidate developmental problems, inferences about individual development are drawn from successive cross-sectional studies yielding results from different samples covering different age levels. This design implies that different individuals are studied at different age levels.

The cross-sectional design is one tool for research on human functioning. In the study of many of the issues that are of importance for understanding and explaining psychosocial phenomena, a cross-sectional approach has contributed greatly and will continue to contribute. A good illustration is the recent advances in research in endocrinology, pharmacology, and neuropsychology, which have contributed much to the understanding of the interplay of biological and mental factors in individual functioning. The main advantages of a cross-sectional design are, however, linked to the study of individual functioning in a current perspective.

When the task is to identify operating factors and mechanisms in developmental change, the appropriate research strategy is a longitudinal one. Characteristic of a longitudinal study is that individuals are studied over time. Thus, data for the same individuals, referring to different points in time, form the basis for conclusions about issues relevant for understanding individual development. A longitudinal research strategy is indicated by the following interrelated considerations: (a) the dynamic, process character of the phenomena under investigation; (b) the existence of individual differences in growth rate; (c) individual differences in the age for significant events; and (d) delayed effects of prior influences. These factors become accentuated in the traditional application of linear regression models, frequently used in developmental research (see, e.g. LISREL, path analysis, and other techniques).

The dynamic process character of developmental change

A historian who claimed that he or she could understand the history of Europe at a given time merely by conducting a cross-sectional study with the aid of information from newspapers on a given day, and with the aid of means and standard deviations for various aspects of historical events, would become an object of derision. Among other things, differences among countries with respect to technological, political and cultural development invalidate such an approach even for limited purposes, for the same reason as they do in research on individual development. A meteorologist who attempted to understand meteorological processes by applying a cross-sectional design, i.e. by measuring temperature, wind velocity, humidity and other aspects of weather at different locations in Europe on a certain day, would probably trigger the same reaction.

The dynamic, temporal character of the change processes involved in individual development is in itself the self-evident reason for the need for longitudinal research. A developmental change process with its basic temporal character can never be understood by looking at a snapshot. Cross-sectional studies are not applicable to the study of the mechanisms by which factors operate in the developmental processes and for understanding the interplay between processes that operate in different time frames (e.g. maturation, and neuro-biological changes). The causal processes in the development of an individual are characterized by complex chains of events over time. Thus, only by studying the same individuals across time is it possible to understand and explain the lawful, dynamic processes of many aspects of human ontogeny and to identify causal relations in the multi-determined processes of individual development: for example, to elucidate the possible long term effects on the immune system of continuous high-level excitation of the autonomic and related physiological system. And only by studying the same individuals over time is it possible to investigate the effectiveness of measures taken to prevent illness and maladjustment and of procedures for treatment when illness and maladjustment have occurred.

Individual differences in biological growth rate

Traditionally, chronological age is used as a marker of individual development. This implies that the marker of an individual's level of development is the number of times the globe has circled the sun, since he/she was born. Yet, alternative bases for the study of individual differences ought to be considered (cf. Baltes, 1979; Horn & Donaldson, 1976; Rutter, 1989; Wohlwill, 1970).

Individual differences in growth rate, using chronological age as the marker, occur from the beginning of life throughout the whole life-span. They occur within the context of the total functioning of the individual, with respect to somatic and morphological characteristics, to perceptual–cognitive–intellectual functioning, to physical and mental capacity, and to general competence in handling the demands of the total environment, etc. Some features are apparent and important in very early infancy; other features emerge and become essential for individual functioning in adolescence, adulthood and old age.

Differences in the rate of biological maturation among individuals of the same chronological age may have profound consequences, not only for individual differences in various aspects of functioning, but also with respect to the way the environment reacts to the individual. Differences in developmental timing thereby influence individuals' social relations, as well as their capacity to meet environmental demands and to use environmental opportunities effectively.

A good illustration of the role of individual differences in developmental processes and a striking illustration of the holistic way in which individuals function is the effect of individual differences that occur when differences are manifested at menarche. In a longitudinal research programme, in which a cohort of all boys and girls in one community in Sweden were followed from the age of ten to the age of 30, a strong correlation was found between the age at menarche and different aspects of norm breaking behaviour among girls at the age of 14 to 15 (Stattin & Magnusson, 1991). For example, girls maturing very early reported much stronger alcohol use than later maturing girls. Interpreted from a cross-sectional perspective, this result indicated that a group of girls at risk for antisocial development had been identified. However, in a follow-up of the same girls at the age of 26–27, no systematic relation between age at menarche and drinking at adult age was observed. On the other hand, very early biological maturation had far-reaching consequences for education, family, own children, job status, etc. (Stattin & Magnusson, 1990). The effect could not be attributed to early maturation per se; it could be identified as the result of a net of interrelated factors, linked to biological maturation, such as self-perception and self-evaluation and, above all, the social characteristics of close friends.

This example illustrates the role of individual differences in female growth rate at a crucial age period. Other studies indicate the similar importance of individual differences in this respect among teenage boys (Andersson, Bergman & Magnusson, 1989). At the other end of the life-cycle, individual differences in biological age are considerable and conspicuous for individuals of the same chronological age.

As stated earlier, individual differences in growth rate do not appear only for biological factors such as gender characteristics, height, and weight. They also exist for cognitive, intellectual, and other aspects of individual functioning, which are usually referred to as personality factors. For example, the existence of a growth spurt in intellectual capacity and of individual differences in this respect, has been empirically demonstrated in concordance with the existence of a growth spurt for height and weight (Ljung, 1965; see also Bateson, 1978). Such individual differences in cognitive–intellectual factors and other personality factors may be an indication of a slow development which will result in a low-level adult functioning. However, it might also be an indication of a delay in components of morphological development combined with an acceleration in certain components of cognitive–perceptual development. According to one extension of the neoteny hypothesis, the end result of such a configuration is a high level of intellectual and linguistic functioning for human beings relative to

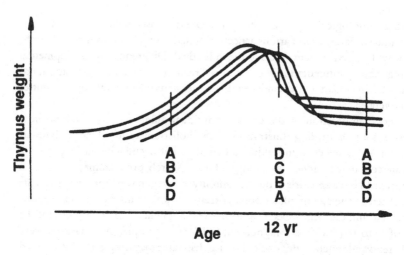

Fig. 1.2.   Fictitious curves for four individuals, A–D, with respect to thymus weight. (From Magnusson, 1988.)

other species (Cairns, 1976; Mason, 1979). Models of developmental psycho-pathology are also complicated by the existence of the 'catch up' effect which appears for some individuals in behaviours whose normal growth levels off at some point during childhood (Wenar, 1982).

For the study of individual development, the existence of individual differences in growth rate have consequences which must be considered in the choice of methodology and research strategy (see Bateson, 1978; Magnusson, 1988). Let us look at a developmental curve for a somatic variable that can be studied objectively, namely the weight of the thymus. This curve is characteristic for the lymphoid system, including lymph nodes and intestinal masses (Tanner, 1978). The typical growth curve for the weight of the thymus gland is shown in Fig. 1.2 for four hypothetical individuals, A–D, who differ with respect to biological age, as indicated by the chronological age at which the growth curve reaches its peak. (The weight of the thymus reaches its peak round 12 years of age and then declines rather rapidly to about half that weight at the age of about 20). For various chronological ages, Fig. 1.2 shows the rank orders of the individuals with respect to the weight of the thymus. It is seen, for instance, that although the rank order of individuals with respect to thymus weight varies dramatically across ages, there is perfect stability and consistency in the growth and decline of the gland once biological age instead of chronological age is taken as the reference variable.

This fact of individual differences in maturational tempo has far-reaching methodological consequences. Among other things, any cross-sectional matrix (i.e. a matrix of data for individuals of the same chronological age) for variables which reflect, or are related to, individual differences in growth rate will contain a certain variance, most of the time of unknown size, which is due to such differences. The magnitude of the variance due to individual differences in biological age introduced in the matrix depends on the kinds of variables studied and where in the developmental process the study is performed. The effect occurs, of course, independent of whether individual differences in growth rate are measured or not.

The methodological consequences of the existence of individual differences in growth rate are crucial for dealing with central issues in developmental research, such as the following: (1) in studies of the stability of single variables in terms of rank order stability; (2) in cross-sectional studies of the interrelations; among operating person and environmental factors in a current perspective; (3) in the application of factor analysis in order to identify basic factors operating in individual development; (4) in studies of early antecedents of later stages of development, e.g. in the study of the developmental background of various aspects of adult functioning.

The existence of sometimes strong individual differences in growth rate, for central factors in developmental processes, limits the applicability of a cross-sectional design in studies that control for chronological age. These differences may affect results to an extent that has not always been recognized and considered in research. A consequence of this is that *biological age* and what might be designated *functional age*, in some cases should be used as a complement to chronological age as a marker of individual development. However, to control for biological age instead of for chronological age is a remedy only under certain specified conditions. Biological and chronological factors are nested factors, since the expression of individual differences in growth rate is sometimes counteracted by societal influences which are bound to chronological age: for example, the age for beginning and ending of compulsory school education, the age for compulsory military service in some countries, the compulsory age for retirement, etc.

The occurrence of significant events

There are large individual differences in the size and type of environmental influence on the development process. Of particular interest in this connection is the occurrence of significant single events which may have profound impact on the life course of an individual. Some appear to occur randomly, but are rather a consequence of the individual's readiness for a certain type of action or reaction, such as marriage or taking on a new job, and an opportunity offered by the environment, e.g. in terms of meeting another person, receiving an offer of a new job, etc (cf. Bandura's, 1982, discussion of 'chance events'). In other cases, a significant event may be the result of deliberate action taken by the individual himself/herself or by individuals whose actions influence others. Buying a new house in a certain area with specific characteristics in terms of neighbours, opportunity for jobs, schooling, cultural and leisure-time activities and so on, instead of in an area with other characteristics, may have decisive effects on the direction of the future life course of all family members. Significant single events may occur over the whole life-span, their character depending on the readiness of the individual, mentally and physically, to act and react in relation to the opportunities and restrictions offered by the environment.

The effect of significant events is to change the direction of the life course. Sometimes this effect is not immediately visible, but grows slowly and ends up having decisive effects on the individual's life in a manner that is characteristic of the so-called 'butterfly effect' in chaos theory. For example, the choice of spouse or of occupation, both of which have profound implications for the individual, is for many individuals the result of a process in which events of that character play a decisive role, a role that was not apparent at the time of the events. In other cases, the effect is more direct and leads to what has been discussed in terms of 'turning points' (Pickles & Rutter, 1991).

Often a necessary condition for a significant event to have this dramatic effect is that the individual is in a state of disequilibrium at the time of its occurrence, and the event serves to restore the balance of the total system and give new direction to the life course. Under such conditions, significant events in individual life-cycles serve the same function as 'bifurcations' in the physical environment according to catastrophe theory.

In this connection, the existence and role of significant single events in the individual development processes are of interest for two main reasons. First, they form an important element in the life of an individual. Secondly, the fact that significant events, occasionally with profound consequences for the future life course of an individual, occur at different age levels for different individuals, has decisive consequences for effective and appropriate methodologies in the study of individual development. The important causal role of significant events, and the fact that they occur at different age levels from very early to very late in life for different individuals, invalidates a cross-sectional study of many aspects of individual development and requires a longitudinal strategy.

Delayed effects of causative agents

The effect of many causative agents is sometimes delayed, producing the so-called 'sleeper effect' (Kagan & Moss, 1962), which necessitates a follow-up of the same individuals, sometimes over very long time periods. For example, some pathogenic factors, in the individuals and in the environment, act many years before the illness manifests itself. A classic example comes from the 1946 British Birth Cohort Study. It was hypothesized that children who grew up in poor industrial areas with pollution, damp housing conditions, lack of sun, etc, would be especially susceptible to upper respiratory tract infections. When the cohort had reached the age of 16 years, such a relationship did not appear. However, at the age of 25 years the hypothesized relationship between infections and poor childhood environment was observed. Another example is from research on the long-term effects of father's interaction with his family, indicating that this influences adult criminality far more than juvenile criminality (McCord, 1991).

Conclusion

The proper use of a longitudinal research strategy presupposes planning and implementation with reference to careful analysis of the phenomena under study.[1] Longitudinal design is full of possible traps, as is demonstrated by critical analyses (Gergen, 1977; Nesselroade & Baltes, 1974; Schaie, 1965). However, misuse of a research design and misinterpretation of its results should not deter us from using it under the correct conditions. The conclusion of the discussion in this chapter should be clear: In order to understand and explain the process of human ontogeny we have to include a longitudinal strategy of empirical research in our arsenal of tools. The following citation which was formulated with reference to psychological research on individual development is valid also for research on human ontogeny in general: 'The longitudinal method is the life blood of developmental psychology; it deserves a more thorough, objective and constructive evaluation by all developmentalists' (McCall, 1977, p. 341).

WHY NOT MORE LONGITUDINAL STUDIES?

Until very recently the apparent potentiality and necessity of a longitudinal research strategy for the study of individual development has not resulted in the planning and implementation of longitudinal studies to the extent that the importance and character of the phenomena appear to demand. During recent decades, awareness of the need for such studies has grown rapidly. An important manifestation of this is the establishment by the European Science Foundation of the European Network on Longitudinal Studies on Individual Development as the first in a series of scientific networks. An indication of the recognition of a longitudinal strategy as an indispensable tool for understanding the process of individual development is the fact that in the inventory covering ongoing longitudinal research programs involving a psychosocial component, more than 500 projects are represented.

In view of the theoretical support and empirical evidence for the necessity of longitudinal research, one might well ask why it has taken such a long time for longitudinal research to become established as a general design for research on individual development. At least three interrelated factors can be identified.

One important reason is the special demands made by longitudinal research in most cases for long-term commitment, skills in planning and implementation, administrative ability, and endurance and cooperativeness of the researcher. The efforts needed in longitudinal research are considerable, and the risk of failure often high. An error in experimental work is always unpleasant, but can be 'repaired' relatively quickly. An error in a longitudinal project may result in wasted years of work, and in errors that are often irreparable.

Secondly, the scientific reward system does not favour longitudinal research. Rewards through results that answer to the questions that the researcher has put are slow to appear and uncertain, and the academic rewards in terms of scientific recognition and academic promotion are also slow and uncertain.

Thirdly, and finally, difficulties in finding the requisite, continuous financing probably make many scientists reluctant to conduct longitudinal research. This leads to special problems, particularly for long-term longitudinal research in comparison with cross-sectional research, for two reasons. (1) Continuous funding is essential. Suspending and resuming a project after a time is only possible in exceptional cases. In any event, the process can seldom be governed by the availability of funding without an adverse impact on results. (2) When grant-giving authorities evaluate the costs of different research projects, they tend, in almost every instance, to accumulate the cost of longitudinal projects in a way that differs from their approach to other types of research. A longitudinal project's need for continuity is so obvious that there is virtually no way to avoid an accumulation of project costs over the period in which the project is conducted. In evaluating costs of longitudinal research projects, funding agencies often overlook the returns that most longitudinal projects generate through spin-off effects in the form of cross-sectional studies that would otherwise have cost considerable sums to perform, apart from the yield they deliver in longitudinal elucidation of the process of individual development. Another spin-off effect is the possibility of quickly carrying out studies of new problems that arise, i.e. problems for which meaningful treatment requires longitudinal data.

Longitudinal research is based on the condition that data are collected for the same individuals over time, occasionally over a long period of time, and stored on a computer. In some countries, legal obstacles have been raised deterring effective longitudinal research. If the vital longitudinal research that is now in progress or being implemented in Europe is to continue contributing important knowledge on issues of central importance to society, e.g. the promotion of physical and mental health and life quality in general, it must be provided with optimal conditions for collecting, storing and utilizing relevant data. Technical solutions now make it possible to store and use data in ways that shield information from unauthorized access and keep it from falling into unauthorized hands.

A FINAL COMMENT

The complexity of the phenomena to be considered to understand the dynamic, multi-determined, stochastic process of individual development makes the researcher's task exceedingly difficult. However, the processes that are our concern are lawful and regular, and the scientific challenge of uncovering them is of the utmost importance (cf. Bateson, 1978). Lawfulness and regularity are characteristics of the processes at all levels of individual functioning; in the interaction of factors within sub-systems and in the interaction between sub-systems. There is nothing more mysterious or incomprehensible about the dynamic processes of individual development than there is about the subject matters of other scientific disciplines concerned with dynamic processes. What is needed to ensure progress in future research on individual development is that the dynamic, multi-determined, stochastic character of the processes involved is taken seriously as frame of reference for the specification of the problem under study and for the interpretation of results.

ACKNOWLEDGEMENTS

Valuable comments on an early version of this chapter were received from Robert B. Cairns, Joan McCord, Sigrid Gustafson, Michael Rutter, and Donald Peterson.

NOTE

1. It should be noted that a longitudinal approach includes the use of both prospective and retrospective data (see Janson, 1981; Magnusson, 1988). A longitudinal study of the criminal career can, for example, be well conducted using register data, covering the period from childhood to adulthood, and collected at adult age.

REFERENCES

Andersson, T., Bergman, L. R. & Magnusson, D. (1989). Patterns of adjustment problems and alcohol abuse in early adulthood: a prospective longitudinal study. *Development and Psychopathology*, **2**, 119–31.

Armelius, B.-A. & Sundbom, E. (1991). Hard and soft models for the assessment of personality organization by DMT. In M. Olff, G. Godaert and H. Ursin (eds.), *Quantification of human defence mechanisms*. London: Springer-Verlag.

Baltes, P. B. (1979). Life-span developmental psychology: some converging observations on history and theory. In P. B. Baltes & O. G. Brim (eds.), *Life-span development and behaviour*, vol 2. New York: Academic Press.

Baltes, P. B. & Baltes, M. (1990). *Successful aging: Perspectives from the behavioral sciences*. Cambridge: Cambridge University Press.

Bandura, A. (1982). The psychology of chance encounters and life paths. *American Psychology*, **37**, 747–55.

Basar, E. (ed.) (1990). *Chaos in brain function*. Berlin: Springer Verlag.

Bateson, P. P. G. (1978). How does behaviour develop? In P. P. G. Bateson & P. H. Klopfer (eds.), Perspectives in ecology, vol. 3: Social behaviour. New York: Plenum Press.

Bergman, L. R. This volume.

Bergman, L. R. & Magnusson, D. (1984*b*). Patterns of adjustment problems at age 10.

An empirical and methdological study. Reports from the Department of Psychology, Stockholm University, No. 615.

Bergman, L. R. & Magnusson, D. (1984a). Patterns of adjustment problems at age 13. An empirical and methodological study. Reports from the Department of Psychology, Stockholm University, No. 620.

Bertalanffy, L. von. (1968). *General system theory*. New York: Braziller.

Block, J. (1971). *Lives through time*. Berkeley. C.A.: Bancroft Books.

Brandstädter, J. This volume.

Brushlinskii, A. V. (1987). Activity, action and mind as process. *Soviet Psychology*, **4**, 59–81.

Cairns, R. B. (1976). The ontogeny and phylogeny of social behaviour. In M. E. Hahn and E. C. Simmel (eds.), *Evolution and communicative behavior* (pp. 115–139). New York: Academic Press.

Cairns, R. B. (1979). *Social development: the origins and plasticity of interchanges*. San Francisco: Freeman Cooper.

Cairns, R. B. (1983). The emergence of developmental psychology. In W. Kessen (ed.), History, theories and methods. (pp. 41–101). Vol. 1 of P. H. Mussen (ed.), *Handbook of child psychology* (4th edition). New York: Wiley.

Cairns, R. B. (1986). Phenomena lost: issues in the study of development. In J. Valsiner (ed.), *The individual subject and scientific psychology* (pp. 79–111). New York: Plenum Press.

Cairns, R. B. (1991). Multiple metaphors for a singular idea. *Developmental Psychology*, **27**, 23–6.

Caspi, A. (1987). Personality in the life course. *Journal of Personality and Social Psychology*, **53**(6), 1203–13.

Crick, F. 1988. *What mad pursuit: a personal view of scientific discovery*. New York: Basic Books.

Crutchfield, J. P., Farmer, J. D., Packard, N. H. & Shaw, R. B. (1986). Chaos. *Scientific American*, **252**, 38–49.

Dannefer, D. & Perlmutter, M. (1990). Development as a multidimensional process: individual and social constituents. *Human Development*, **33**, 108–37.

Dewey, J. (1896). The reflex arc concept in psychology. *Psychological Review*, **3**, 357–70.

Edelman, G. (1987). *Neural Darwinism: the theory of neuronal group selection*. New York: Basic Books.

Farmer, J. D., Kaufmann, A., Packard, N. H. & Perelson, A. S. (1987). Adaptive dynamic networks as models for the immune system and autocalytic sets. In S. H. Koslow, A. J. Mandell and M. F. Schlesinger (eds.), Perspectives in biological dynamics and theoretical medicine. (pp. 118–131). *Annals of New York Academy of Sciences*.

Fogel, A. & Thelen, E. (1987). Development of early expressive and communicative action: reinterpreting the evidence from a dynamic systems perspective. *Developmental Psychology*, **23**, 747–61.

Gergen, K. J. (1977). Stability, change and chance in understanding human development. In N. Datan and H. W. Reese (eds.), *Life-span developmental psychology: dialectical perspectives in experimental research*. New York: Academic Press.

Gleick, J. (1987). *Chaos: making a new science*. New York: Penguin.

Gottlieb, G. (1991). Experiential canalization of behavioural development: theory. *Developmental Psychology*, **27**, 4–13.

Gustafson, S. & Magnusson, D. (1991). Female life careers. In D. Magnusson (ed.), *Paths through life*, vol. 3. Hillsdale, N.J.: Lawrence Erlbaum Associates.

Hall, N. (ed.) (1991). *The new scientist guide to chaos*. London: Penguin Books.

Hebb, (1955). Drive and the C.N.S. (Conceptual Nervous System). *Psychological Review*, 62, 243–54.

Horn, J. L. & Donaldson, G. (1976). On the myth of intellectual decline in adulthood. *American Psychologist*, 31, 701–9.

James, W. (1890). *The principles of psychology*. New York: Holt.

Janson, C.-G. (1981). The longitudinal approach. In F. Schulsinger, S.A. Mednick, & J. Knop (eds.), *Longitudinal research: methods and uses in behavioral science*. Boston: Nijhoff.

Jessor, R., Donovan, J.E. & Costa, F. M. (1991). *Beyond adolescence: problem behavior and young adult development*. Cambridge: Cambridge University Press.

Kagan, J. & Moss, H. A. (1962). *Birth to maturity*. New York: Wiley.

Laszlo, E. (1972). *The systems view of the world*. New York: Braziller.

Lerner, R. M. (1991). Changing organism–context relations as the basic process of development: a developmental contextual perspective. *Developmental Psychology*, 27, 27–32.

Ljung, B.-O. (1965). *The adolescent spurt in mental growth*. Stockholm: Almqvist & Wiksell.

Magnusson, D. (1988). Individual development from an interactional perspective. Vol. 1. in D. Magnusson (ed.), *Paths through life*. Hillsdale, N.J.: Lawrence Erlbaum Associates.

Magnusson, D. (1990). Personality development from an interactional perspective. In L. Pervin (ed.), *Handbook of Personality*, pp. 193–222. New York: Guilford Press.

Magnusson, D., Andersson, T. & Törestad B. (in press). Methodological implications of a peephole perspective on personality. In D. Funder, C. Tomlinson-Keasey, R. Parke & K. Widaman (eds.), *Studying lives through time: approaches to personality and development*. American Psychological Association.

Magnusson, D. & Bergman, L. R. (1988). Individual and variable-based approaches to longitudinal research on early risk factors. In M. Rutter (ed.), *Studies of psychosocial risk: the power of longitudinal data* (pp. 45–61). Cambridge: Cambridge University Press.

Magnusson, D. & Bergman, L. R. (eds.) (1990). *Data quality in longitudinal research*. New York: Cambridge University Press.

Magnusson, D. & Törestad, B. (1992). The individual as an interactive agent in the environment. In W. B. Walsh, K. Craig & R. Price (eds.), *Person–environment psychology: models and perspectives*. Hillsdale, N.J.: Erlbaum.

Magnusson, D. & Törestad, B. (1993). A holistic view of personality: a model revisited. *Annual Review of Psychology*, 44, 427–51.

Mason, (1979). Ontogeny of social behaviour. In P. Marler & J. G. Vanden Bergh (eds.), *Social behavior and communication*, pp. 1–28. New York: Plenum Press.

McCall, R. B. (1977). Challenges to a science of developmental psychology. *Child Development*, 48, 333–44.

McCord, J. (1991). Family relationships, juvenile delinquency, and adult criminality. *Criminology*, 29(3), 397–417.

Miller, J. G. (1978). *Living systems*. New York: McGraw-Hill.

Nesselroade, J. R. & Baltes, P. B. (1984). Sequential strategies and the role of cohort effects in behavioural development: adolescent personality (1070–72) as a sample case. In S. A. Mednick, M. Harway & K. M. Finello (eds.), *Handbook of longitudinal research* (vol. 1, pp. 55–87).

Nicolis, G. & Prigogine, I. (1977). *Self-organization in none-equilibrium systems*. New York: Wiley Interscience.

Odum, H. T. (1983). *Systems ecology: an introduction*. New York: John Wiley & Sons.

Olweus, D. (1977). A critical analysis of the 'modern' interactionist position. In D. Magnusson & N. S. Endler (eds.), *Personality at the crossroads*. Hillsdale, N. J.: Lawrence Erlbaum Associates.

Öhman, A. & Magnusson, D. (1987). An interactional paradigm for research on psychopathology. In D. Magnusson & A. Öhman (eds.) *Psychopathology: an interactional perspective*. New York: Academic Press.

Packer, M., Medina, N., Yushak, M. & Meller, J. (1983). Hemodynamic patterns of response during long-term captopril therapy for severe chronic heart failure. *Circulation*, **68**, 803–12.

Pickles, A. & Rutter, M. (1991). Statistical and conceptual models of 'turning points' in developmental processes. In D. Magnusson, L. R. Bergman, G. Rudinger & B. Törestad (eds.), *Problems and methods in longitudinal research: stability and change*, pp. 133–166. Cambridge: Cambridge University Press.

Prigogine, I. & Stengers, I. (1985). *Order out of chaos*. New York: Bantam Books.

Pulkkinen, L. & Trembley, R. (1992). Patterns of boys' social adjustment in two cultures and at different ages: a longitudinal perspective. *International Journal of Behavioral Development*, in press.

Rutter, M. (1989). Age as an ambiguous variable in developmental research: Some epidemiological considerations from developmental psychopathology. *International Journal of Behavioral Development*, **12**, 1–34.

Rutter, M. (1983). Statistical and personal interactions: facets and perspectives. In D. Magnusson & V. Allen (eds.), *Human development: an interactional perspective*, pp. 295–319. New York: Academic Press.

Sameroff, A. J. (1983). Developmental systems: contexts and evolution. In P. H. Mussen (ed.), *Handbook of child psychology*, vol. 1. New York: Wiley.

Schaie, K. W. (1965). A general model for the study of developmental problems. *Psychological Bulletin*, **64**, 92–107.

Sharpe, N., Smith, H., Murphy, J., Greaves, S., Hart, H. & Gamble, G. (1991). Early prevention of left ventricular dysfunction after myocardial infarction with angiotensin-converting-enzyme inhibition. *Lancet*, **337**, 872–6.

Sroufe, L. A. (1979). The coherence of individual development: early care, attachment, and subsequent developmental issues. *American Psychology*, **34**, 834–41.

Stattin, H. & Magnusson, D. (1990). Pubertal maturation in female development. Vol. 2 in D. Magnusson (ed.), *Paths through life*. Hillsdale, N.J.: Lawrence Erlbaum Associates.

Stattin, H. & Magnusson, D. (1991). Stability and change in criminal behaviour up to age 30. *British Journal of Criminology*, **31**, 327–46.

Strelau, J. (1983). *Temperament-personality-activity*. New York: Academic Press.

Tanner, J. M. (1978). *Foetus into man: physical growth from conception to maturity*. London: Open Books.

Wapner, S. & Kaplan, B. (1983). *Toward a holistic developmental psychology*. Hillsdale, N.J.: Erlbaum.

Watson, J. B. (1913). Psychology as the behaviourist views it. *Psychology Review*, **20**, 158–77.

Weiner, H. (1989). The dynamics of the organism: implications of recent biological thought for psychosomatic theory and research. *Psychosomatic Medicine*, **51**, 608–35.

Weinert, F. E. & Schneider, W. This volume.

Weiss, P. A. (1969). The living system: determinism stratified. In A. Koestler & J. R. Smythies (eds.), *Beyond reductionism: new perspectives in the life sciences*. New York: MacMillan.

Wenar, Ch. (1982). Developmental psychopathology: its nature and models. *Journal of Clinical Child Psychology*, **11**, 192–201.

Wohlwill, J. F. (1970). The age variable in psychological research. *Psychological Review*, **77**, 49–64.

Wolff, P. H. (1981). Normal variation in human maturation. In K. J. Conolly & H. F. R. Prechtl (eds.), *Maturation and development: biological and psychological maturation*. London: Heinemann Medical Books.

Wundt, W. (1948). Principles of physiological psychology. In W. Dennis (ed.) *Readings in the history of psychology*. New York: Appleton-Century Crofts.

Zeeman, E. C. (1976). Catastrophe theory. *Scientific American*, **234**, 65–83.

2 Genes, experience, and development

SANDRA SCARR

OBSERVATIONS AND INFERENCES

Longitudinal research provides the most secure and believable basis for making inferences from observations about human development. When developmentalists observe changes in development and associations between parental and child behaviours, we usually make inferences about the ways in which different parental rearing techniques affect children's intellectual, social, and emotional development. Only by following development across life-spans can one study the intricate interplay of biological and social forces that shape individual lives.

Both parents and psychologists observe pervasive correlations between characteristics of parents, the environments they provide, and their children's outcomes. Both parents and psychologists make causal attributions to those correlations: they believe that differences in parental behaviours and environments *cause* differences in children's outcomes. The construction of causal inferences from the web of parent–child correlations is fraught with logical and scientific problems (Scarr, 1985). Longitudinal studies make the life course of development clearer, so that causal inferences about parental effects on their children are illuminated.

Ever since Bell's (1968) seminal paper on children's effect on their own environments, as well as vice versa, numerous studies have shown that, indeed, children do have an effect on the behaviour of their caregivers (e.g. Breitmayer & Ricciuti, 1988; Bell & Harper, 1977; Lytton, 1980; McCartney, in press). Using a variety of research designs and outcome measures, these studies have all demonstrated that, rather than being passive recipients of care, infants and children are active, influential partners in their interactions with the people around them. The notion that parental behaviours cause all observed differences among children is thus called into question.

European psychologists have for the last decade investigated the participation of young people in their own development (e.g. Magnusson, Stattin & Allen, 1985; Silbereisen & Noack, 1988). Action theory incorporates the idea that people influence in important ways the course of their development through choices across time. The theory presented here is consonant with this line of theory and inquiry.

26

Causal assumptions about the direction of effects between parental behaviour and children's outcomes have been called into question even more strongly by research over the past 20 years in the field of developmental behaviour genetics. Behavioural genetic methods are used to investigate the sources of individual variation in a population (Plomin, 1986). The focus is on what makes individuals different from one another, not on the causes of the particular mean value of a trait in a population. By studying family members with varying degrees of relatedness, estimates can be obtained of the proportion of observed variation in a population that is due to genetic variation. This estimate is referred to as heritability, and is limited to the particular population under study.

Behaviour genetic research has shown that, for a wide variety of traits, including measures of intelligence, specific cognitive abilities, personality, and psychopathology in North American and European populations, there is as much, if not more, variation within families as there is between families (Plomin, 1986). Being reared in one family, rather than another, makes few if any differences in children's personality and intellectual development. These data suggest that environments most parents provide for their children have few differential effects on the offspring. It is proposed here that each child constructs a reality from the opportunities afforded by the rearing environment, and that the constructed reality does have considerable influence on variations among children and differences in their adult outcomes.

Longitudinal studies of adoptive and biologically related families (Dunn, Plomin & Nettles, 1985; Dunn, Plomin & Daniels, 1987) and of twins (Wilson, 1983) show that, early in life, parental treatment, and differences among families, do have important effects on young children that make siblings more similar than randomly chosen youngsters. These studies also show that genetic influences on development of personality and intelligence throughout the early years are virtually the same influences that affect development of these characteristics in adulthood; in other words, the genetic correlations between earlier and later development is quite high (Plomin, 1986, Chapter 3).

Later declines in sibling similarity seen mostly to be a function of declining influences of family environments on development in later childhood, adolescence, and adulthood, as other non-familial influences (e.g. schools, peers, community opportunities) become more important in determining what experiences older children and adults have. All of these points challenge the common wisdom in developmental studies and will be explored in later sections of this chapter.

CONSTRUCTING EXPERIENCES FROM ENVIRONMENTS

The idea that people make their own environments (Scarr & McCartney, 1983) runs counter to the mainstream of developmental psychology. A large base of literature examining the relationships between familial, parental, and child characteristics has found that these characteristics are, indeed, related to each other. Developmental psychologists most often interpret these findings as evidence that the rearing conditions that parents provide for their children make differences in the children's life chances and eventual adult statuses – both socioeconomic achievements and mental health. Thus, although some developmentalists have suggested that children may affect their environments as well as vice versa (Bell, 1968), the theory that children actually construct their own environments challenges the basic tenets of much of mainstream developmental psychology.

The idea that children create their own experiences from the environments they encounter also challenges parents' beliefs about their impact on their children's development. After all, most parents invest tremendous efforts in rearing their children – efforts that involve emotional, personal and financial sacrifices for the parents. If parents can be given accurate information about how much influence they might or might not have on their children's development, it might help alleviate needless sacrifices and emotional turmoil on their part.

How people make the transitions from age to age and stage to stage in life is the most fascinating longitudinal study in all of behavioural science. Accurate information about the extent to which differences between families contribute to differences between children is particularly important for the design and implementation of timely and effective intervention programmes for at-risk children and families. Thus, although the theory that children construct their own environments challenges widely held ideas about families and children, it is important to consider and evaluate it, given available data.

MEANS AND VARIANCES

The statement that parents have few differential effects on children does *not* mean that not having parents is just as good as having parents. It may not matter much that children have different parents, but it does matter that they have parent(s) or some supportive, affectionate person who is willing to be parent-like. This is essentially the distinction between examining sources of variation between individuals, and examining mean values in the population. The methods best suited to the former are not necessarily also appropriate for the latter.

The distinction between causes of mean or average values, with causes of variation around mean values can be confusing, to both psychologists and parents. For some characteristics, there is very little individual variation around the mean, but, for other characteristics, there is a broad distribution of results, for which a mean and a variance can be described. For example, there are some human characteristics for which there is no normal variation at the chosen level of analysis; such as having bilateral limbs, two eyes, and a cerebral cortex. Every normal member of the species has these characteristics. At another level of analysis, however, all of these species-typical characteristics show variation (e.g. limb length, eye shape, brain size). The structural genes that cause the development of species-typical characteristics may have no normal variants; but there may be regulatory genes that influence the developmental patterns and the eventual amount of each characteristic a given individual has. There is no necessary association between the structural causes of species-typical character-istics and the regulatory causes of variation. Research on variation has no necessary implications for the causes of the average value of the population (but see Turkheimer, 1990).

This distinction is particularly important to remember when considering analyses of heritability, as pointed out by Arthur Jensen (1989):

Hence, the results of any heritability analysis are necessarily limited to statements concerning variation around the overall *mean* of the group in which the analysis is performed, and it affords no information whatsoever about the factors responsible for the particular value of the group mean (p. 241).

Similarly, as McGuffin & Gottesman (1985) emphasize, heritability estimates have no meaning for a given individual. Such estimates simply tell us the proportion of variance of some trait that is due to genetic variation in that particular population. They cannot tell us what percentage of individual A's limb length is due to genetic influences.

To see the effects of no parents (or parent-surrogates), one would have to return to the orphanages of long ago (or study those in use today in the Soviet Union), or see children trapped in crack houses of inner cities in the United States, locked in basements and attics by vengeful, crazy relatives (see Clarke & Clarke, 1976). Really deprived, abusive, and neglectful environments do not support normal development for any child. Having no parental figures, or being reared in terribly deprived circumstances, have clear detrimental effects on child development, regardless of the child's genetic background (Dumaret & Stewart, 1985). The important point here is that variations among environ-ments that support normal human development are not very important as determinants of variations in children's outcomes.

COMMON AND UNCOMMON ASSUMPTIONS

The prevailing belief among both psychologists and parents is that variations in normal environments, particularly those provided by their families (1) shape children's development and (2) determine their adult futures. Fig. 2.1 shows the commonly accepted model, in which parental characteristics (phenotypes, Pp) determine the child's environment (Ec), which, in turn, determines the child's behavioural outcomes (Pc).

A more complete version of this model is shown in Fig. 2.2. Here the transmission of genes from parents to child is recognized, and the role of genes

$$P_{\overline{p}} \longrightarrow E_{\overline{c}} \longrightarrow P_{\overline{c}}$$

Fig. 2.1. A common model of parent–child effects.

in determining (in part) phenotypes is included in the model. In this model, the parents still determine the child's environment, which affects the child's behavioural development.

It is also commonly assumed that parental characteristics and home environments are arbitrarily or even randomly associated with individual children's characteristics (Bandura, 1982). Parents are, in this sense 'the luck of the draw'. The structure of experience is assumed to be given in the environment, which acts as stimuli that impinge and shape children, regardless of who they are. The uncorrelated nature of people and environments is challenged by constructivist views of how people determine their own experiences and by the hypothesis that experiences are largely correlated with people's own characteristics.

In fact, several lines of research in cognitive, clinical, and social psychology have been based on theories about individual differences in experience and on the idea that, not only do individual's responses to environments differ, but that people construct their own experiences. Some brief examples follow:

1 In cognitive psychology, Bower has pursued the idea that people construct their own experiences and personal histories (Bower, 1987). Faced with the same brief story, different individuals remembered and recalled different versions of the story.

2 Clinical psychology has found that people differ in their emotional responses to situations (e.g. Eysenck (1982, 1983) on psychopaths versus normals in their emotional reactivity to punishment and reward; Wexler et al. (1986) on stress reactions) that shape their behaviours in those situations.

3 Social psychology has presented evidence that personal characteristics affect how others respond to the stimulus person (Langlois & Roggman, 1990). Physical attractiveness may be in the eye of the beholder, but there is a great deal of cultural consensus in judgments about what constitutes physical attractiveness. People judged to be physically attractive by others are more likely to be asked for dates, more likely to be hired for jobs, and once hired more likely to be promoted than others judged to be less physically attractive (Bersheid & Walster, 1974).

4 In personality psychology, Henry Murray (Kluckhohn, Murray & Schneider, 1953) pursued for many years the idea that each person constructs a personal myth, which gives coherence to his life, just as larger cultural myths give coherence to a society. Personality characteristics that are moderately heritable (30 to 50%) have been shown to influence how people react across time and situations. Sociable and

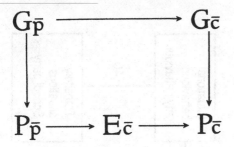

Fig. 2.2. A model of parent–child genetic and environmental effects.

outgoing people experience social interactions with strangers differently than shy, fearful people (Kagan Reznick & Gibbons, 1989; Eysenck, 1983). Optimistic, internally directed older adults cope much better with aging than others who are less optimistic and feel less in control of their lives. A twin study of older adults shows these life-outlook characteristics, like all personality variables, to be moderately heritable (Pedersen et al., 1989).

5 The new field of cultural psychology is actually predicated on the assumption that no sociocultural environment exists apart from the meaning that human participants give it (Shweder, 1990). Nothing real 'just is'; realities are the product of the way things get represented, embedded, implemented, and reacted to.

Although cultural psychology uses non-Platonic, philosophical constructivism to explore ethnic differences in personality, intelligence, and social behaviour, the same ontological and epistemological principles apply to individual differences within cultures (Scarr, 1985). Different people, at different developmental stages, interpret and act upon their environments in different ways that create different experiences for each person. In this view, human experience is the construction of reality, not a property of a physical world that imparts the same experience to everyone who encounters it.

Thus, there are contradictory theories in psychology about how people are influenced by their environments and how they construct their own experiences from those environments. One source of confusion is the nature of the phenotype (observable characteristics) that is the outcome to be predicted. Some behaviours are indices of enduring personality and intellectual characteristics of the person, traits that show considerable stability across many years. Other behaviours are temporally less stable but are consistent responses to contemporary contexts in which development is occurring. Still more transitory behaviours are situation specific. Fig. 2.3 shows a model of how development can be construed at different levels of behavioural analysis from enduring traits to situational behaviours.

In this model or peer relations and peer behaviours, species-normal genes and species-normal social rearing environments are correlated, because normal

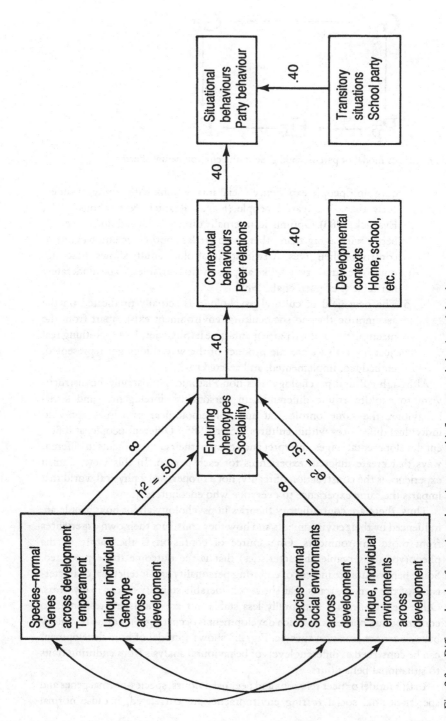

Fig. 2.3.   Different levels of genetic and environmental influences on behavioural development.

organisms evoke different rearing than abnormal ones. They combine with unique individual environments, which are caused by individual genetic characteristics, to produce enduring phenotypes (measurable traits, such as sociability). Enduring traits are hypothesized to combine with developmental contexts (long-range contexts, such as home and school) to produce contextual behaviours, such as relationships with peers. Finally, relationships with peers are predicted to combine with situations to produce specific, situational behaviours. Genes may predict contextual and situational behaviours directly through paths other than the measured personality trait (here, sociability), such as impulsiveness, emotionality, and so forth.

Trying to predict one or another of these kinds of personal traits or behaviours will have great influence on the level of genetic and environmental characteristics one should choose to include in the prediction. Much of the 20-year debate about situation-specific behaviours versus enduring personal traits was mired in the confusion between relatively stable traits and situationally determined behaviours. Discussions of genetic and environmental variability in 'behaviour' risk the same misunderstandings unless the level of behaviour is defined.

THE AVERAGE EXPECTABLE ENVIRONMENT

A resolution of the seeming contradictions in theories about how families affect their children can be found in the concept of the 'average expectable environment' (Hartmann, 1958). Based on evolutionary theory, there are three components that describe normal organisms in normal environments (LeVine, 1987).

Pre-adaptation Infants and children are preadapted by their human species genetic inheritance to respond to a specific range of environmental opportunities for stimulation and knowledge acquisition.

Variation Within the genetically specified range of normal environments, a variety of environmental patterns of stimulation can all act to promote normal human developmental patterns. A wide variety of variations in environments within this normal range are 'functionally equivalent' opportunities for people to construct their own experiences (Scarr & Weinberg, 1983).

Limits Environments that fall outside of the species-normal range will not promote normal developmental patterns.

Thus, normal development does occur in a wide variety of human environments, but not in those which are abusive or neglectful or in those without 'average expectable' conditions, in which the species has evolved. For infants, species-normal environments include parenting adults and a surrounding social group to which the child will be socialized. The exact details and specifications

Table 2.1. *Risk of schizophrenia for offspring of discordant MZ and DZ twins*

	Co-twins	
	Schizophrenic twin	Normal twin
MZ	16.8%	17.4%
DZ	17.4%	2.1%

Source: From Gottesman and Bertelsen (1989).

of the socialization patterns are not crucial to normal development (although they are crucial to understanding the meaning people give to their experiences), but having a rearing environment that falls within the limits of normal environments is crucial to normal development.

Although I argue that genotype–environment correlations are more pervasive and important than gene–environment interactions, there are, in the human literature, a few examples of how different genotypes respond to the 'same' rearing environment. A striking example of genotype–environment interaction has been reported by Gottesman and Bertelsen (1989) in their follow-up study of offspring of identical and fraternal twins discordant for schizophrenia. As shown in Table 2.1, they found that the risk for schizophrenia in the offspring of schizophrenic fraternal twins was 17.4%, and those of their normal co-twins was 2.1%. However, the risk for the offspring of schizophrenic identical twins was 16.8%, and for those of their normal co-twins was 17.4%.

Gottesman & Bertelsen concluded that 'discordance in identical twins may primarily be explained by the capacity of a schizophrenic genotype or diathesis to be unexpressed unless it is released by some kinds of environmental, including non-familial, stressors' (p. 867).

Thus, it is clear from research in many areas of psychology, most notably cultural psychology, and from the investigation of organism–environment interaction, that the 'environment' does not necessarily have the same meaning for all individuals, regardless of who they are.

A TRIARCHIC THEORY OF EXPERIENCE

How might individuals create their own experiences? In earlier publications (McCartney, in press; Scarr, 1985; Scarr & McCartney, 1983; Scarr & Weinberg, 1983), we have proposed that people make their own environments in three ways. First, children's genes are necessarily correlated with their environments because parents provide both, so that their experiences are constructed from opportunities that are positively correlated with their personal characteristics; secondly, people evoke from others responses that are correlated with the

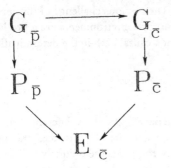

Fig. 2.4. A model of parent–child transmission in which genes determine experience.

person's own characteristics; and thirdly, people actively select environments that are correlated with their interests, talents, and personality characteristics.

Although the proposed theory is based on the idea that, given the same 'objective' environment, individuals will react differently, Scarr (1989) has argued that genotype–environment correlations, rather than gene–environment interactions, predominate in the construction of experiences. Many environmental opportunities are taken in by some individuals and not by others, depending on the individuals' characteristics. This selective use of environmental opportunities is better thought of as genotype–environment correlation than as genotype–environment interaction.

The theory of genotype→environment effect has three propositions:

1 There are three kinds of genotype→environment effects, as described above:
   (a) passive
   (b) evocative
   (c) active

2 The balance of genotype→environment effects changes from passive to active with development, as children move out from the family to make their own choices of interests and activities.

3 Genetic differences become more important across development, as people actively make their own environments.

The theory of genotype→environment effects holds that genotypes drive experiences. Following Hayes (1962), we proposed that the state of development and the individual characteristics of people share the experiences they gather from exposures to their environments. Fig. 2.4 shows a radical model of how genes determine experience.

In this model, parental genes determine their phenotypes; the child's genes determine his/her phenotype; and the child's environment is merely a reflection of the characteristics of both parents and child. Here, differences among children's environments, within the normal species range, have no effect on differences among children's outcomes. The obvious challenge of this model is to demonstrate that differences among normal environments are a product of parental and child characteristics and not a causal path in the determination of children's behavioural phenotypes.

GENERAL THEORY

People are both individually different and developmentally different in the ways they encode and experience their environments. Experiences the person constructs from exposures to various environments are uniquely correlated to that person's perceptions, cognition, emotions, and more enduring characteristics of intelligence and personality.

Following Plomin, DeFries and Loehlin's (1977) analysis of variances in behaviour genetic studies, we proposed that the same concepts could be used in our developmental theory of the determinants of development and individual differences (Scarr & McCartney, 1983). In this theory, there are three ways by which genotypes and environments become correlated.

Firstly, one must take into account the fact that most biological parents provide their children with both genes and home environments. The fact that parents provide both genes and environments means that the child's genes and environments will necessarily be positively correlated. For example, parents who read well, who like to read will be likely to subscribe to magazines and papers, buy and borrow books, take books from the local library, and read to the child. Parents who have reading problems are less likely to expose themselves to this world of literacy, so that their children are likely to be reared in a less literate environment. Those same children are also more likely to have reading problems themselves and to prefer non-reading activities. Thus, the reading abilities of parents are likely to be correlated with the reading abilities of their children and with the environments parents provide for their children – a positive genotype–environments effect.

Secondly, each person at each developmental stage evokes, from others, responses that reinforce positively or negatively that person's behaviours. Evocative effects have profound effects on a person's self-image and self-esteem throughout the life-span. Smiling, cheerful infants who evoke positive social interactions from parents and other adults (Wachs & Gruen, 1982) seem likely to form positive impressions of the social world and its attractions. Infants who are fussy, irritable, and who receive negative or neutral interactions with their caregivers and others would seem less likely to form the impression that social interactions are a wonderful source of reinforcement. School-age children from disadvantaged families who are more intelligent and more 'spunky' (Garmezy, Masten & Tellegen, 1984) are more likely to be given positive attention and encouragement by teachers than less intelligent or less 'spunky' children. Adults who are considered physically attractive by others are more likely to be chosen as dates and mates than others considered less attractive. Attractive adults are also more likely to be hired for jobs and more likely to be promoted on those jobs than their less physically attractive peers. Thus, people's own characteristics evoke from others responses that are correlated with that person's developmental status and individual differences.

Thirdly, each person makes choices about what environments to experience. Past infancy, people who are in a varied environment[1] choose what to attend to and what to ignore. Depending on their personal interests, talents, and personality, people choose pursuits, whether educational, occupational or leisure activities.

The idea that people assort themselves into environments according to their interests, talents, and personality has a long history in industrial/organizational psychology. People choose occupational environments that correlate with their personal preferences for social interaction or solitary work, for independent or supervised work, salesmanship or social service. Preferences for one kind of work environment or another are correlated with other aspects of personality (Grotevant, Scarr & Weinberg, 1977; Holland, 1973).

Differences in preferences for work environment turn out to be just as heritable as other aspects of personality (Bouchard, Scarr & Weinberg, in preparation). Thus, differences in choices among various kinds of environments have been shown to be, in part, functions of the personal characteristics of the individual.

A test of the notion of gene–environment correlation can be seen in a study of reading (Hayes et al., 1989). Pervasive differences in reading choices and amount of reading were found by age, gender, and ability levels – all of which are consistent with the theory that people choose and make their own environments.

These measurements on popular children's books showed: (a) the most able British children read approximately 50% more than their less able peers (within that four-week period), and (b) the average text grows more demanding (lexically) and longer in the older age cohorts. . . . The most able children not only read more books than their peers, those books were slightly more difficult. When this one month language experience is multiplied across years, the highest ability students must have accumulated a huge advantage over their less able peers. They encountered many more uncommon terms and non-mundane topics from their reading. Even if these most able children were no more efficent in extracting, integrating and retrieving information from what they read than their less able peers, they would still have the much richer language experience from their book reading. If it can be shown that they are also more efficient, their advantage over their peers would be still greater (p. 13).

The g→e effects theory predicts that developmental differences are very important, pervasive, and large, based on the same principles as individual differences. For many behaviours, developmental changes, based on genotype and environmental changes (genes are turned on; environments are perceived and experienced differently) will be much larger than individual variations at any one age. All of this is in accord with the theory of developmental and individual differences in the selection and construction of experience.

FAMILIES AS ENVIRONMENTS

The idea of correlated personal and environmental characteristics has been ignored, and even opposed in developmental psychology (e.g. Rheingold & Cook, 1975). Most attention has been focused on differences among families in the opportunities they provide for their children. Beginning with family differences in social class, however measured, it has been assumed that observations of ubiquitous correlations between family education, occupational status, and income and children's intellectual and other outcomes were caused by differences among families' environments (Scarr, 1985). Clearly, there are family differences; it is not clear that most of those differences are environmental. In fact, among families in the mainstream of Western European and North American societies, differences in family environments seem to have little effect on intellectual and personality outcomes of their children.

This point is worth pondering. How can it be that parents have few long-term effects on the intellectual or personality development of their children? As parents who care, it seems impossible that this could be the case. This is not to say that parents may not have effects on children's self-esteem, motivation, ambitiousness, and other important characteristics. It is to say that parental differences in rearing styles, social class, and income have small effects on the measurable differences in intelligence, interests, and personality among their children. And parents' influences wane across development, as older children and adolescents become more influenced by peers and the larger community than they were as pre-schoolers. Only longitudinal behavioural genetic research can show these effects persuasively.

THE DATA

Family resemblances have been reported for intelligence and personality measures for relatives who vary in genetic and environmental resemblances. Table 2.2 summarizes much of the data on IQ test score similarities of late adolescent and adult relatives who are genetically identical, of those related by half of their genes, and of those genetically unrelated individuals.

Let us focus on genetically identical pairs reared together and apart, and on adopted pairs of siblings reared together since infancy. These are the most startling findings. Identical (MZ) twins reared together score as much alike (.86) on IQ tests as the same person tested twice (.87). MZ twins reared in different families are slightly less similar (.76). The remarkable studies of MZ twins reared in different families challenge many cherished beliefs in developmental

Table 2.2. *IQ and degrees of relatedness: similarities of genetically related and unrelated persons who live together and apart*

Relationship	Correlation	Number of pairs
Genetically identical		
Identical twins together	.86	1300
Identical twins apart	.76	137
Same person tested twice	.87	456
Genetically related by half of the genes		
Fraternal twins together	.55	8600
Biological sisters and brothers	.47	35 000
Parents and children together	.40	4400
Parents and children apart	.31	345
Genetically unrelated		
Adopted children together	.00	200
Unrelated persons apart	.00	15 000

Note:
Based on data from Scarr and Weinberg (1978) on older adolescents who are comparable in age to other samples in this table. Younger adopted children resemble each other to a greater degree, with correlations around .24, according to samples of 800 pairs.
Source: Adapted from Plomin (1980).

psychology (but fit very nicely in the genotype→environment theory). That these twins, in four studies, are nearly as similar intellectually as identicals reared together, and are just as similar in personality, raises critical questions about what observed family differences really mean for development. Table 2.3 shows the IQ correlations for MZ twins reared apart in four studies.

By contrast, genetically unrelated siblings, reared from infancy to adulthood in the same family, do not resemble each other at all in IQ. This result based on two studies has been exactly replicated in two additional studies of late adolescents and young adults (Horn, Loehlin & Willerman, 1982; Kent, 1985). Studies of younger adopted siblings show that they do have some intellectual· resemblance (.24), about half that of biological siblings (.47). A major reason for the greater resemblance of younger adoptees is that families have greater effects on their younger than older children, as will be explained in later sections. Another reason for greater resemblance of younger adoptees is selective placement, as shown in Table 2.4.

In this sample (Scarr & Weinberg, 1978, 1983), 75% of the 101 adoptive families also had their own biological offspring. Thus, one can examine the resemblances of biological and adoptive relatives, living together and apart. Correlations of parents and their biological children range from .33 to .43,

Table 2.3. *Sample sizes, and intraclass correlations for all IQ measures and weighted averages for five studies of MZA twins*

Study and test used (primary/secondary/tertiary)	N for each test	Primary test	Secondary test	Tertiary test	Mean of multiple test
Newman *et al.* (1937) (Stanford-Binet/Otis)	19/19	.68	.74	—	.71
Juel-Nielsen (1965) (Wechsler-Bellevue/Raven)	12/12	.64	.73	—	.69
Shields (1962) (Mill-Hill/Dominoes)	38/37	.74	.76	—	.75
Bouchard *et al.* (1990) (WAIS/Raven-Mill-Hill/ First principal component	50/45/44	.69	.78	.78	.75
Weighted average	119/113/112	.70	.76	.78	.74

Table 2.4. *Comparisons of biological and unrelated parent–child IQ correlations in 101 transracial adoptive families*

	N (pairs)	r
Parents–unrelated children		
Adoptive mother–adopted child	174	.21 (.23)[a]
Natural mother–own child of adoptive family[b]	217	.15
Adoptive father–adopted child	170	.27 (.15)[a]
Natural father–own child of adoptive family[b]	86	.19
Parents–biological children		
Adoptive mother–own child	141	.34
Natural mother–adopted child[b]	135	.33
Adoptive father–own child	142	.39
Natural father–adopted child[b]	46	.43

Notes:
[a] Early adopted only ($N = 11$).
[b] Educational level, not IQ scores.
Source: Scarr and Weinberg research.

whether the (natural) parents have never seen the children since birth or whether the parents (adoptive parents, but the biological parents of these children) have reared them to the average age of 7 years.

The intellectual resemblances of adoptive parents and their adopted children are .21 and .27, but this similarity must be modified by the correlation between the natural parents of the adopted child in this family and the biological offspring of the adopted parent (.15 and .19). There is absolutely no environmental or genetic reason why birth parents of adopted children should bear any resemblance to biological children of the families who adopted their children, except for selective placement by adoption agencies.

Social workers are likely to try to match their expectations for children's intellectual development to the adoptive families' educational levels. Thus, by being more likely to place an illegitimate child of two university students with a college-educated family and to place a child of two high school drop-outs with a working class family, adoption agencies create a correlations between the child's probable abilities and the adoptive home environment.

The implication of this unexpected resemblance between birth parents and biological children in the family who adopted their children is that the resemblance of adoptive parents and adopted children must be corrected for selective placement (.21–.15 and .27–.19), which reduces adoptive family correlations to very small effects (.06 and .08), even in early childhood.

A recent 10-year follow-up study (Weinberg, Scarr & Waldman, 1992; Scarr, Weinberg & Waldman, in press) demonstrates the value of longitudinal research in behavioural genetics. Not only could we observe the changes in

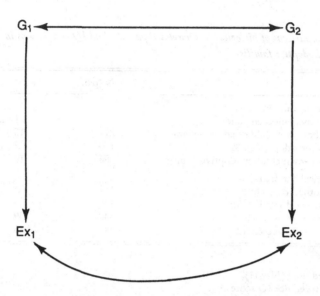

Fig. 2.5.   Genetic similarity determines similarity in experience.

intellectual and personality development from childhood to adolescence, but we could study changes in familial similarities and parental influences across time. Briefly, we found the black/interracial adoptees' IQ scores did not decline from an average age of 7 years to an average age of 17 years, even though adopted parent–child and genetically unrelated siblings' IQ scores were virtually uncorrelated by late adolescence. By contrast, genetically related parents and children and biological siblings remained intellectually similar to the degree predicted by their genetic resemblance. Without longitudinal research on these adoptive families, we could not have known whether or not sampling differences or real changes in parental influences made the difference.

The theory of genotype→environment effects can explain the slight resemblances among adopted relatives and the great resemblances between MZ twins, reared together and apart. If genes drive experience, then the degree to which relatives have similar experiences will depend upon their degree of genetic resemblance. Fig. 2.5 shows the model.

Identical twins, whose genetic correlations is 1.00, evoke similar responses from others, and they make similar choices in their environments. They respond cognitively and emotionally in similar ways, and they construe their experiences in similar ways. By contrast, adopted children, who are genetically unrelated, have uncorrelated experiences even within the same household, school, and neighbourhood environments. This part of the theory explains the family data from behaviour genetic studies more satisfactorily than any other model.

DEVELOPMENTAL PATTERNS

Longitudinal studies of twins, most notably the Louisville, Kentucky study headed for many years by the late Ronald S. Wilson, have contributed to understanding the role of genetic variability in regulating developmental patterns. Wilson (1983) reported on mental development tests administered on nine occasions to infants and young children from 3 months to 6 years. Overall results were that MZ twins scored very similarly (correlations in the mid-80s throughout early childhood) and DZ twins less similarly (correlations declining from the mid-70s in infancy to the low 60s over the pre-school years). But the longitudinal pattern of mental development was also strikingly similar for MZ co-twins, as shown in Fig. 2.6.

Although each pair had a different pattern of spurts and lags in mental growth, the similarity between co-twins was very high within each pair. The four pairs presented by Wilson in Fig. 2.6 were representative of the several hundreds of twin pairs studied over 20 years. Fig. 2.6 also shows the typical patterns of mental developmental resemblance for DZ twins. Because they are siblings with about half of their genes in common, their developmental patterns are similar but not as parallel as those of MZ twins.

OPTIMISM AND PESSIMISM

It is fashionable in developmental circles to believe that professionally approved environments can have enormously facilitating effects on children's development, compared to less middle-class settings. This model of development proposes that facilitative environments can promote the optimal development of even vulnerable organisms. In fact, little difference in outcome is attributed to the intactness of the biological organism; rather, there is supposed to be overwhelming interaction between vulnerable organisms and non-facilitative environments that produce minimal development. Invulnerable organisms are little affected by differences between facilitative or non-facilitative environments. Vulnerable organisms are said to develop well in facilitative environments.

I present the more pessimistic, and realistic, view in Fig. 2.7. The major implication of this model is that vulnerable or impaired organisms are not likely to reach high levels of development in even facilitative environments – they develop better in facilitative than in non-facilitative environments but do not reach high level outcomes. Intact or invulnerable organisms are not very susceptible to potentially bad effects of non-facilitative environments. There are main effects of both organisms and environments, and an interaction between them, because vulnerable organisms are posited to be more susceptible to negative environments and more in need of supportive ones than robust organisms, who are better able to make their own environments in positive ways.

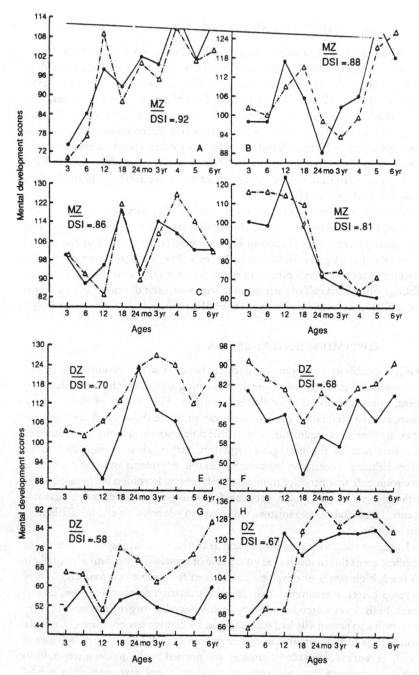

Fig. 2.6.   Trends in mental development during early childhood for four MZ and four DZ Pairs (Wilson, 1983).

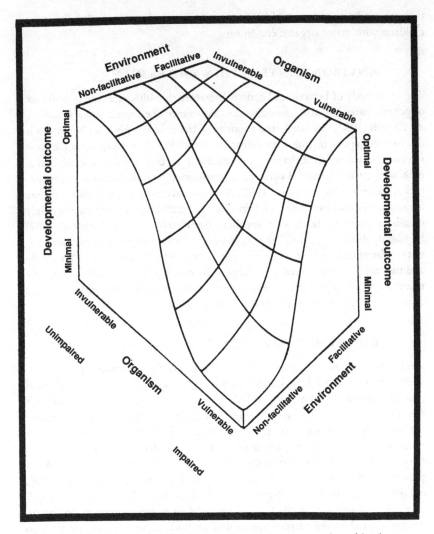

Fig. 2.7.   A developmental model of organism and environmental combinations leading to normal and abnormal development.

The implications of the two models are quite different for parental expectations and for intervention programs. The second, perhaps more pessimistic model recognizes that not every child can become a normally functioning adult, even if parents provide a facilitative environment. Developmental models that ignore biological influences lead to blaming parents of children with developmental problems, because the only way a child could have a poor developmental outcome is to have been reared in a non-facilitative environment. We all know this cannot be true for children with genetic and chromosomal defects, for children with major organic conditions.

ENVIRONMENTS WITHIN THE FAMILY

The same body of behavioural genetic literature that illustrates the importance of genetic variation, also highlights the importance of environmental variation. As Plomin (1990) indicated, 'the majority of the variance for most behaviors is due to non-genetic factors, the environment' (p. 117). However, one of the most striking findings of the behaviour genetic literature is that, for a variety of traits, most of the environmental variance is contributed by non-shared environmental influences (Scarr & Grajek, 1982). Non-shared environmental influences are those that are not shared by members of a family; that is, they act to make family members different from one another. As Plomin and Thompson (1987) highlight, this finding 'implies that the unit of environmental transmission is not the family, but rather micro-environments within families' (p. 20). I would add that micro-environments are largely the construction of individual family members in the ways they evoke responses from others, actively select or ignore opportunities, and construct their own experiences.

GOOD ENOUGH PARENTS

Ordinary differences between families have little effect on children's develop-ment, unless the family is outside of a normal, developmental range. Good enough, ordinary parents probably have the same effects on their children's develoment as culturally defined super-parents (Rowe, in press). This comfort-ing idea gives parents a lot more freedom to care for their children in ways they find comfortable for them, and it gives them more freedom from guilt when they deviate (within the normal range) from culturally prescribed norms about parenting. As Richard Weinberg and I said (Scarr & Weinberg, 1978), children's outcomes do not depend on whether parents take children to the ball game or to a museum as much as they depend on genetic transmission and on having a good enough environment that supports children's development to become themselves.

The idea of good enough parents is a constructive step toward recognizing that parents do not have the power to make their children into whatever they want, or in John Watson's terms, to ruin them in so many ways. Fortunately, evolution has not left development of the human species, nor any other, at the easy mercy of variations in their environments. We are robust and able to adapt to wide-ranging circumstances – a lesson that seems lost on many ethnocentric psychologists. If we were so vulnerable as to be led off the normal developmen-tal track by slight variations in our parenting, we should not long have survived.

The flip side of this message is that it is not easy to intervene deliberately in children's lives to change their development unless their environments are outside the normal species range. We know how to rescue children from extremely bad circumstances and to return them to normal developmental pathways, by providing rearing environments within a normal range. But, for children whose development is on a normal trajectory and whose parents are providing a supportive environment, interventions have only temporary and limited effects (Clarke & Clarke, 1989). Should we be surprised? Feeding a well-nourished but short child more and more will not make him a basketball player. Feeding an average intellect more and more will not make her brilliant. Exposing a shy child to socially demanding events will not make him feel less shy. The average intellect and the shy child may gain some specific skills and helpful knowledge of how to behave in specific situations, but they will not be fundamentally changed.

The associations between a child's characteristics, those of the parents, and the rearing environment they provide are neither accidental nor a likely source of fruitful intervention, unless the child's opportunities for normal development are quite limited. Given a wide range of opportunities, our research and that of the past 25 years in behavioural genetics supports the idea that people make their own environments, based on their own heritable characteristics.

Only longitudinal research can give us a full picture of the role of genetic and environmental factors in development – how they work together to shape both typical human development and individual variations on that modal pattern. In the field of behaviour genetics, we are just beginning to use longitudinal methods to study these issues; in developmental psychology, investigators who use longitudinal methods are just beginning to realize the importance of genetic differences in shaping human development. By combining longitudinal methods with behaviour genetic designs, developmental studies have a powerful approach to the further understanding of both typical human development and individual differences.

NOTE

1. The entire theory depends on people having a varied environment from which to choose and construct experiences. The theory does not apply, therefore, to people with few choices or few opportunities for experiences that match their genotypes. This caveat applies particularly to children reared in very disadvantaged circumstances and to adults with little or no choice about occupations and leisure activities.

REFERENCES

Bandura, A. (1982). The psychology of chance encounters and life paths. *American Psychologist*, **37**, 747–55.

Bell, R. Q. (1968). A reinterpretation of the direction of effects in studies of socialization. *Psychological Review*, **75**, 81–95.

Bell, R. & Harper, L. (1977). *Child effects on adults*. Lincoln, NB: University of Nebraska Press.

Bersheid, E. & Walster, E. (1974). Physical attractiveness. In L. Berkowitz (ed.), *Advances in experimental social psychology*. New York: Academic Press.

Bower, G. H. (1987). Commentary on mood and memory. *Behavior Research and Therapy*, **25**, 443–55.

Breitmayer, B. J. & Ricciuti, H. N. (1988). The effect of neonatal temperament on caregiver behaviour in the newborn nursery. *Infant Mental Health Journal*, **9(2)**, 158–72.

Clarke, A. M. & Clarke, A. D. B. (1976). *Early experience: myth and evidence*. New York: Free Press.

Clarke, A. M. & Clarke, A. D. B. (1989). The later cognitive effects of early intervention. *Intelligence*, **13**, 289–97.

Clarke-Stewart, A. (1989). Infant day care: maligned or malignant? *American Psychologist*, **44**, 266–73.

Dumaret, A. & Stewart J. (1985). IQ, scholastic performance and behaviour of sibs raised in contrasting environments. *Journal of Child Psychology and Psychiatry and Allied Disciplines*, **26**, 553–80.

Dunn, J., Plomin, R. & Nettles, M. (1985). Consistency in mothers' behaviour towards infant siblings. *Developmental Psychology*, **21**, 1188–95.

Eysenck, H. J. (1982). Why do conditional responses show incrementation, while unconditional responses show habituation? *Behavioural Psychotherapy*, **10**, 217–20.

Eysenck, H. J. (1983). Human learning and individual differences: the genetic dimension. *Educational Psychology*, **3**, 169–88.

Garmezy, N., Masten, A. & Tellegen, A. (1984). The study of stress and competence in children: a building block for developmental psychopathology. *Child Development*, **55**, 97–111.

Gottesman, I. I. & Bertelsen, A. (1989). Confirming unexpressed genotypes for schizophrenia. *Archives of General Psychiatry*, **46**, 867–72.

Grotevant, H. D., Scarr, S. & Weinberg, R. A. (1977). Patterns of interest similarity in adoptive and biological families. *Journal of Personality and Social Psychology*, **35**, 667–76.

Hartmann, H. (1958). *Ego psychology and the problem of adaptation*. New York: International Universities Press.

Hayes, D., Whitehead, F., Wellings, A., Thompson, W., Marschlke, C. & Moran, M. (1989). *How strongly do genes drive children's choice of experiences?* Cornell University: Technical Report Series 89–13, November 1989, pp. 16–17.

Hayes, K. J. (1962). Genes, drives, and intellect. *Psychological Reports*, **10**, 299–342.

Holland, J. L. (1973). *Making vocational choices: a theory of careers*. Englewood Cliffs, NJ: Prentice Hall.

Horn, J. M., Loehlin, J. C. & Willerman, L. (1982). Personality resemblances between unwed mothers and their adopted-away offspring. *Journal of Personality and Social Psychology*, **42**, 1089–99.

Jensen, A. R. (1989). Review. Raising IQ without increasing g? *Developmental Review*, **9**, 234–58.

Kagan, J., Reznick, J. S. & Gibbons, J. (1989). Inhibited and uninhibited types of children. *Child Development*, **60**, 838–45.

Kent, J. (1985). *Genetic and environmental contributions to cognitive abilities as assessed by a telephone test battery*. Unpublished doctoral dissertation, University of Colorado, Boulder.

Kluckhohn, C., Murray, H. A. & Schneider, D. M. (eds.). (1953). *Personality in nature, society, and culture.* 2nd edition. New York: Knopf.

Langlois, J. H. & Roggman, L. A. (1990). Attractive faces are only average. *Psychological Science,* 1, 115–21.

LeVine, R. A. (1987). *Beyond the 'average expectable environment' of psychoanalysis: cultural differences in mother–infant interaction.* Paper presented at American Anthropological Association Meeting, Chicago, Illinois.

Lytton, H. (1980). *Parent–child interaction.* New York: Plenum.

Magnusson, D., Stattin, H. & Allen, V. L. (1985). Differential maturation among girls and its relation to social adjustment: a longitudinal perspective. In D. L. Featherman & R. M. Lerner (eds.), *Life-span development and behavior* (vol. 7). New York: Academic Press.

McCartney, K. (in press). Mothers' language with first- and second-born children: A within-family study. In K. Pillemer and K. McCartney (eds.), *Parent–child relations across the life span.*

McGuffin, P. & Gottesman, I. I. (1985). Genetic influences on normal and abnormal development. In M. Rutter & L. Hersov (eds.) *Child and adolescent psychiatry*, pp. 17–35, Oxford: Blackwell Scientific.

Pedersen, N. L., Gatz, M., Plomin, R. & Nesselroade, J. R. (1989). Individual differences in locus of control during the second half of the life span for identical and fraternal twins reared apart and reared together. *Journal of Gerontology,* 44(4), 100–5.

Plomin, R. (1986). *Development, genetics, and psychology.* Hillsdale, NJ: Lawrence Erlbaum Associates.

Plomin, R. (1990). *Nature and nurture.* Pacific Grove, CA: Brooks/Cole.

Plomin, R., DeFries, J. C. & Loehlin, J. C. (1977). Genotype–environment interaction and correlation in the analysis of human behaviour. *Psychological Bulletin,* 84, 309–22.

Plomin, R. & Thompson, R. (1987). Life-span developmental behavioural genetics. In P. B. Baltes, D. L. Featherman and R. M. Lerner (eds.), *Life-span development and behavior,* vol. 8. Hillsdale, NJ: Lawrence Erlbaum Associates.

Rheingold, H. L. & Cook, K. V. (1975). The contents of boys' and girls' rooms as an index of parents' behaviour. *Child Development,* 46, 459–63.

Rowe, D. C. (in press). As the twig is bent?: the myth of child rearing influences on personality development. *Journal of Counseling and Development.*

Scarr, S. (1985). Constructing psychology: making facts and fables for our times. *American Psychologist,* 40, 499–512.

Scarr, S. (1989). How genotypes and environments combine: development and individual differences. In G. Downey, A. Caspi, & N. Bolger (eds.), *Interacting systems in human development.* New York: Cambridge Press, pp. 217–244.

Scarr, S. & Grajek, S. (1982). Similarities and differences among siblings. In M. Lamb and B. Sutton-Smith (eds.), *Sibling relationships.* Hillsdale, NJ: Lawrence Erlbaum Associates, pp. 357–381.

Scarr, S. & McCartney, K. (1983). How people make their own environments: a theory of genotype→environment effects. *Child Development,* 54, 424–35.

Scarr, S. & Weinberg, R. A. (1978). The influence of 'family background' on intellectual attainment. *American Sociological Review,* 43, 674–92.

Scarr, S. & Weinberg, R. A. (1983). The Minnesota adoption studies: genetic differences and malleability. *Child Development,* 54, 260–7.

Scarr, S. Weinberg, R. A. & Waldman, I. D. (in press). IQ correlations in transracial adoptive families. *Intelligence.*

50   S. SCARR

Shepard, R. N. (1987). Toward a universal law of generalization for psychological science. *Science*, **237**, 1317–23.

Shweder, R. A. (1990). Cultural psychology – what is it? In J. W. Stigler, R. A. Shweder & G. Herdt (eds.), *Cultural psychology*. New York: Cambridge University Press.

Silbereisen, R. K. & Noack, P. (1988). On the constructive role of problem behaviour in adolescence. In G. Downey, A. Caspi & N. Bolger (eds.), *Interacting systems in human development*. New York: Cambridge Press, pp. 152–180.

Turkheimer, E. (1990). Individual and group differences in adoption studies of IQ: One (and only one) realm of development. Paper submitted for publication.

Wachs, T. D. & Gruen, G. (1982). *Early experience and human development*. New York: Plenum Press.

Weinberg, R. A., Scarr, S. & Waldman, I. D. (1992). The Minnesota Transracial Adoption Study: a follow-up of IQ test performance at adolescence. *Intelligence*, **16**, 117–35.

Wexler, B. E., Schwartz, G., Warrenburg, S., Servis, M. & Tarlatzis, I. (1986). Effects of emotion on perceptual asymmetry: interactions with personality. *Neuropsychologia*, **24**, 699–710.

Wilson, R. S. (1983). The Louisville Twin Study: developmental synchronies in behaviour. *Child Development*, **54**, 298–316.

3 The human brain and longitudinal research in human development

PAUL CASAER

INTRODUCTION

Knowledge in the field of human developmental neurobiology has grown considerably during recent years. This chapter will selectively review only data and concepts which I consider to be helpful in designing longitudinal research in human development.

Human brain growth can be described as the increase in weight and volume of the brain in pre-natal and post-natal life. A first idea about the magnitude and speed of human brain growth can be obtained by looking at the changes in the shape of the human brain and the complexity of the gyri on its surface during the latter part of gestation (Cowan, 1979). The fetus in the womb shows a growth spurt of the brain, but this can also happen post-natally when a child is born prematurely. Pre-natal growth can be studied by ultrasound measurement of the biparietal diameter of the head. Post-natal growth can be assessed by measuring head circumference. The values obtained should be placed on growth charts and should be compared with the changes in body weight and height over the same period.

A longitudinal study on biological risk factors, and its relation with later psychosocial development is of little value without anthropometric data. One could even argue that each longitudinal study should include a minimum of biological growth variables to explain some of the age-related variations in the non-biological variables.

Longitudinal studies to elucidate the link between peri-natal risk factors and later outcome should not only assess the intensity of the peri-natal care required for the support of adequate breathing and adequate circulation (Casaer & Eggermont, 1985), but should also pay careful attention to the quality of nutritional support (Lucas et al., 1992) and to the efficiency of feeding behaviour (Casaer, 1982). The quality of nutritional support and the efficiency of feeding behaviour enable the brain to follow genetically determined growth capacities (Casaer, DeVries & Marlow, 1991).

HISTOGENESIS: THE INCREASE IN CELL NUMBERS

Maximum acceleration in the increase of the numbers of glial cells and neurons takes place between the gestational ages of 25 to 40 weeks, and during the first months after birth. These facts are derived from a series of post-mortem analyses of DNA concentration in brain tissue as a marker of cell numbers (Dobbing & Sands, 1973).

For longitudinal research in human development, the most interesting findings are the regional differences in the human brain growth spurt. The growth spurt of the spinal column, the brain stem and also of large parts of the forebrain, is almost finished at 40 weeks gestation. In contrast, the cerebellum and, more specifically, the neo-cerebellum has its maximum growth spurt, at birth and during the first year of life (Dobbing & Sands, 1973; Jacobson, 1991).

The vulnerability of the brain during periods of fast growth, and the regional differences in brain growth, indicate when particular parts are damaged most easily. Major catastrophies at any age can result in overt cerebral palsy and mental retardation. Cerebral palsy syndromes should be more expected from ante-natal injuries in mid-gestation or in early last trimester. (Lyon & Gadisseux, 1991).

Hazards during the peri-natal period will result in disturbances in the determination of temporal and spatial sequencing of movements, and especially of fine movements (finger movements, speech); since these are neo-cerebellar functions. The determination of these movements, and especially of the fine movements are prerequisites for expression of the higher cortical capacities such as intelligence and social behaviour. We suggest that damage of, or interference with, development of cerebral–cerebellar circuits are a possible explanation for some of the recent findings of neo-cerebellar underdevelopment or atrophy visible on magnetic resonance imaging in children with mental retardation.

Different neurological outcome variables should thus be used in longitudinal research, based on the age, or the stage of development, in which expression of a genetic or an environmental factor is supposed to interfere with brain development.

MIGRATION

All glial cells, and all neurons of the cerebrum, are born in a small zone close to the inner side of the neural tube or, later, close to the lateral ventricular system. In the early phases, rapid and almost synchronous migration of adjacent neurons leads to the cells spanning the full thickness of the cortical plate in a simple radial alignment (Jacobson, 1991). In the later stages of cortex histogenesis, the itinary of migrating neurons would be very difficult without a fine network of radially organized glial cells to guide them. These glial cells are attached both at the inner side of the germinal zone and at the outer side of the cortical zone. The newly formed neurons glide along those glial fibres from the germinal layer to the cortex (Rakic, 1972).

The formation of the cortical layers results from an inward–outward migration. The first migration forms the deepest cortical layer, the next population of neurons moves through the deepest cortical layer to form the second zone, the third population moves through the two previous zones and this continues until the six cortical layers are formed. In the cerebellum, migration results from two germinal zones. One is close to the fourth ventricle and a second one, appearing somewhat later during development and located externally, lies immediately under the pia mater. Cells in the cerebellum thus move both outwards and inwards. In the human, the external granular layer remains active until 600 days after birth (Jacobson, 1991).

During development, neurons come into very close contact with each other. During migration, surface molecules interact, and this forms a base for later synaptic connections and cytoarchitectural organization. The neural cell adhesion molecule (N-CAM), the glycoproteins laminin and the surface receptor integrin are probably only the first of a series of molecules regulating neurite extension and adhesion (Dodd & Jessel, 1988; Smith, 1988).

From a pathophysiological viewpoint, it is no longer justifiable to sub-divide disorders of brain development into so-called structural and metabolic disorders; both are the expression of an underlying disorder in programming, or they are the result of an external interference with the ongoing genetic programme. A good example is the disorders of migration seen in Zellweger syndrome – a disturbance of peroxisomal assembly.

In recent years, detailed neuropathological studies have demonstrated that genetic disturbances interfere with migration both in animals (Jacobson, 1991) and in humans (Evrard et al., 1988; Lyon & Gadisseux, 1991), but disorders of migration can also be acquired. Viral infections and disturbances in circulation of the brain during specific periods can interfere with migration, or can destroy an already migrated zone of cortical layers. Neuropathological findings of these migration disorders can be very specific (Lyon & Gadisseux, 1991).

At present, brain imaging techniques, can hardly differentiate between genetic and acquired disorders of migration. Only together with a detailed clinical history and a systematic clinical assessment can brain imaging help to define specific aetiological categories. In designing such studies, it should not be overlooked that imaging will never replace post-mortem neuropathology, and vice versa.

The importance of these detailed analyses is obvious for both individual genetic counselling and for longitudinal research attempting to differentiate 'nature' and 'nurture'.

Correlating neurological and behavioural observations with imaging during human development opens fascinating areas for developmental neurobiology. The combined use of structural and functional imaging during specific behavioural paradigms allows direct analysis of the morphological–physiological state of the brain for the first time. Longitudinal study, which emphasizes comparisons within the same individual over time, substantially minimizes the dilemma posed by individual structural variation in the brain. (see Caviness et al., in this volume, Chapter 4).

CELL DIFFERENTIATION

Neurons that reach their destination will start to grow and to differentiate. They will form their dendritic arborization, each cell developing into a very specific 'tree'. The pyramidal cell will take its optimal spatial structure to become the basic cell for the cortical functional unit, the columnar organization. The Purkinje cell will become the basic cytoarchitectural unit for the complex circuits which enable the cerebellum to distinguish a very specific input from a wide range of aspecific inputs; from these comparisons the programmes for well-organized motor behaviour in time and space will later be initiated.

An exact timetable for these cell differentiations is not yet available. In the cerebral cortex, more specifically in the primary visual cortex, Golgi staining techniques have shown that some of these changes occur between the 25th and the 32nd week of gestation, or, in the premature, with a post-menstrual age of 25 to 32 weeks (Purpura, 1975). In the cerebellum, differentiation of Purkinje cells and of the other cerebellar local circuits come much later and last until the end of the second year of life. Arborization of the cells is the mandatory cell surface enlargement which enables the multiple synaptic contacts to take place at the precise sites and in the correct sequence.

From experimental pathology in animals and from some data in human developmental neuropathology there is strong evidence that, during initial stages of development, synaptic density is very high. A redundancy in synaptic connections would be the rule during early brain development, securing the many complex short and long distance connections. However, once the final connections are made, the redundant synaptic connections disappear.

The hypothesis of early synaptic redundancy, and later elimination of synapses, is supported by recent positron emission tomography (PET) studies, using local cerebral glucose metabolism, as an estimate of overall cellular activity and thus also of synaptic metabolic activity. As expected, there is an enormous increase in glucose metabolism during the first years of life. Surprisingly, however, the value of glucose uptake is significantly higher from the second year of life and to a lesser degree until puberty than in young adults. A plausible explanation is the redundancy in synapses and the elimination of redundant synapses towards adult life (Chugani, Phelps, Mazziotta, 1987).

In vivo positron emission tomography (PET) studies confirm previous hypotheses, derived from neuropathological studies, that the subtle structural changes in the brain last much longer than the peri-natal period or the first two years of life. Longitudinal studies in puberty, and even in adult life, can thus not consider the brain as invariable in its interaction with environmental and social factors; furthermore, genetic processes can demonstrate their effect on individual brain development in neurobehavioural differences which only become visible in adult life.

CELL DEATH

Not only redundant synaptic connections but also a large number of cells providing these synaptic connections are eliminated during development. A series of detailed experimental studies demonstrates that, in animals, there is a 10 to 50% reduction in neurons of the lateral motor column in the lumbar spinal system. These phenomena have also been demonstrated in suprasinal and visual pathway localizations. They are genetically determined but may be influenced by functional changes such as motor activity or inactivity (curarization) (Oppenheim, 1981). The retrograde axonal transport of nerve growth factor (NFG) from the target back to the cell body is probably one of the factors determining the survival or death of cells that have, or have not, been successful in reaching their target areas (Purves & Lichtman, 1984). The available data on cell death in human development are still limited (Okado & Kojima, 1984).

In human disease, the spinal muscular atrophies, resulting in the loss of motor strength at different ages, can be considered as a genetic determined imbalance between programmes sustaining cells and programmes causing cell death.

The increased availability of cells and cell connections during early human life are possible indicators for a higher degree of plasticity and adaptation in the young brain. If, and how, these phenomena can be influenced by external factors and by training is at present still speculative.

MYELINIZATION

Nerve conduction velocity, the speed available for electronic information transport over an axon, increases from about 2 metres per second to 50 metres per second when an axon becomes myelinated. The process of myelinization is based on the wrapping of glial cell membranes around naked axons. Recent studies show that the chemical composition of the myelin sheet is not identical to a series of superimposed oligodendric glial cell membranes but that significant changes in the lipid and protein structure occur during the development (Van der Knaap, 1990).

Myelinization is the explanation why normal values for nerve conduction velocities in the peripheral nerves are lower in young children than in older children and in adults. Myelinization also explains part of the physiological decrease in latency times for acoustical, visual and somatosensory evoked responses during human development.

Myelinization of central nervous system pathways has been studied in a superb series of neuropathological studies by Yakovlev and Lecours (1967).

From these studies, a myelinization timetable became available, which is found in many articles on developmental biology and psychology. In those articles myelinization is frequently overestimated.

Myelinization as such is not important but the important factor is which centres in the brain, at what age, are interacting so intensively that they are provided with fast signal-conducting pathways. The exciting developmental approach, is to liken myelinization to highways connecting growing cities.

Vestibular and spinal tracts, related to the basic postural control, are myelinated at 40 weeks. Midbrain–cortical visual pathways are myelinated when the visual smile emerges in infants at 2 to 3 months of age. Descending lateral cortical spinal tracts are available at the end of the first year of life when fine motor control appears (Casaer & Lagae, 1991).

Cerebellar–cerebral connections are myelinated only in the second year of life after the cerebellar cell growth spurt of the first year has come to an end. Reticular tracts are still maturing at school age and the tracts connecting specific and associative cortical areas continue to mature during adult life (Yakovlev & Lecours, 1967).

A renewed interest in myelinization came about with the advent of nuclear magnetic resonance imaging and spectroscopy. These methods enable a non-invasive and longitudinal approach to the study of myelinization during normal and abnormal human development (Boesch et al., 1989; Van der Knaap, 1990). For the systematic study of neurobehavioural–structural correlates, the only limitation is that young children need sedation during the study in contrast to adults and older children.

NEUROTRANSMISSION

Chemical neuroanatomy describing brain networks on the basis of the presence or absence of specific neurotransmitters: acetylcholine, amines, aminoacids and peptides, is gradually emerging (Nieuwenhuys, 1985). These neurochemical data are an attractive frame of reference for new positron emission tomographic studies enabling us to learn some aspects of neurotransmission in vivo. A strong limitation is the necessity to use a radioactive tracer.

For the study of brain development there are still other major problems. Small concentrations of almost every known neurotransmitter are detectable in the first weeks of gestation. This early presence does not imply that neurotransmission takes place. Several neurotransmitters act as trophic factors during early ontogenesis. Receptor sites are sometimes present before their neurotransmitters can be detected. The binding site muscinol for γ-aminobutyric acid (GABA) rises in the cerebellum much more rapidly than the activity of the glutamate decarboxylase. The susceptibility for external benzodiazepines or medication interacting with the receptor is thus greater in those early stages of development than interaction with internally produced GABA (Brooksbank, Atkinson, Balazs, 1981).

The fact that external influences are operational so early, when neurotransmitters are still trophic messengers, may explain some of the long-lasting and devastating effects on later neurological and psychosocial development (Swaab, 1991), of medication and toxic substances reaching the human embryo, fetus or child.

MICROCIRCULATION AND NEURONAL ACTIVITY

The interaction between endothelium cells and neurons, frequently with a glial cell in between, is the basic structure for the blood–brain barrier and the specific structures at the choroid plexuses and the outer arachnoid membrane are also part of the blood–brain barrier system.

Restraining of movements of molecules and ions at this physical barrier is largely governed by lipid solubility. In addition to the passive barrier system, these interfaces contain a variety of transport proteins, which can move electrolytes, sugars, amino acids and other non-electrolytes between the blood and brain and CSF, often against the existing concentration gradient. Enzymes in blood and those bound to the cerebral endothelium can degrade molecules. Other intact macromolecules can be transported through the system (Segal & Zlokovic, 1990). Endothelium cells have a subtle interaction with the platelets. Many of the chemical processes involved in these interactions are still under intense experimental investigations. Differences in the barrier and in the interaction between endothelial cell, glial cell and neurons were demonstrated in experimental work on brain oedema in young animals as compared to adults (Ikuta, 1990).

Longitudinal research on the effect of drugs and toxins on the developing brain should consider the differences in transport characteristics of the blood–brain barrier in pre-natal and during early post-natal life, as compared to the situation in older children and adults.

CONCLUDING REMARKS

After this brief review on aspects of brain development, a first conclusion is that the distinction between structural and metabolic normal or abnormal development becomes less and less tenable. Neuro-messengers are early trophic factors; cytoarchitectural development depends on adhesive, guiding, attracting and repulsing molecules. The development of the blood–brain barrier is the result of a fine structural development between blood vessels, glial cells and neurons. Longitudinal studies on human development should take structural and metabolic factors as interacting and not as independent variables.

Optimization of circulation and respiration, adequate nutritional support and feeding efficiency were key factors in a previous review on peri-natal risk factors for psychosocial development (Casaer, de Vries & Marlow, 1991). The importance of nutritional quality, and of an optimal micro-circulation, becomes obvious from the present review on structural and chemical aspects of brain development.

Neuro-imaging has revived interest in developmental neuropathology. Their mutual interaction will pose new fascinating questions. The differences between imaging and morbid anatomy should never be overlooked. Spatial resolution of our best imaging is still a long way from neuronal connectivity.

Studies clearly stating their hypotheses, sometimes derived from studies in primates, and carefully testing them in longitudinal correlative studies between imaging and neurobehavioural development will further age appropriate assessment and understanding of the human brain (Casaer & Lagae, 1991).

ACKNOWLEDGEMENTS

This study is part of the Developmental Neurology Research Project, KULeuven, Belgium. This research project is mainly supported by a grant of the Medical Research Council Belgium (FGWO) and by a grant from Janssen Research Foundation, Beerse, Belgium.

REFERENCES

Boesch, C., Gucetter, R., Martin, E., Duc, G. & Wülthrib, K. (1989). Variations in the in vivo P-31 MR Spectroscopy of the developing brain during postnatal life. Work in progress. *Radiology*, **172**, 197–9.

Brooksbank, B. W. L., Atkinson, D. J. & Balazs, R. (1981). Biochemical development of the human brain. *Development in Neuroscience*, **4**, 188–200.

Casaer, P. & Eggermont, E. (1985). Neonatal clinical neurological assessment. In Harel, S. (ed.). *The at-risk infant*. pp. 197–220, New York: Paul Brooks.

Casaer, P. & Lagae, L. (1991). Age specific approach to neurological assessment in the first year of life. *Acta Paediatrica Japonica*, **33**, 125–38.

Casaer, P., de Vries, L. & Marlow, N. (1991). Pre- and peri-natal risk factors for psychosocial development. In Rutter, M. & Casaer, P. (eds.), *Biological risk factors for psychosocial disorders*. pp. 139–74, Cambridge University Press.

Casaer, P., Daniëls, H., Devlieger H., De Cock, P. & Eggermont, E. (1982). Feeding behaviour in pre-term neonates. *Early Human Development*, **7**, 331–466.

Chugani, H. T., Phelps, M. E. & Mazziotta, J. C. (1987). Positron emission tomography study of human brain functional development. *Annals of Neurology*, **22**, 487–97.

Cowan, W. M. (1979). The development of the brain. *Scientific American*, **241**, 113–33.

Dobbing, J. & Sands, J. (1973). The quantitative growth and development of the human brain. *Archives of Disease in Childhood*, **48**, 757–67.

Dodd, J. & Jessel, J. M. (1988). Axon guidance and the patterning of neuronal projections in vertebrates. *Science*, **242**, 692–9.

Evrard, P., de Saint-Georges, P., Kadhim, H. J. & Gadisseux, J. F. (1988). Pathology of prenatal encephalopathies. In French, J. H., Harel, S. & Casaer, P. (eds.), *Child neurology and developmental disabilities*. Paul Brooks, pp. 298.

Goodman, R. (1991). Developmental disorders and structural brain development. In Rutter, M. & Casaer, P. (eds.), *Biological risk factors for psychosocial disorders*. pp. 20–49, Cambridge University Press.

Ikuta, F. (1990). Fetal Neuropathology. *Brain and Development*, **12**, 587.

Jacobson, M. (1991). *Developmental neurobiology* (3rd edn.) New York: Plenum Press, pp. 753.

Lucas, A., Morley, R., Cole, T. J., Lister, G. & Leeson-Payne (1992). Breast milk and subsequent intelligence quotient in children born preterm. *Lancet*, **339**, 261–5.

Lyon, G. and Gadisseux, J. F. (1991). Structural abnormalities of the brain in developmental disorders. In Rutter, M. & Casaer, P. (eds.), *Biological risk factors for psychosocial disorders*. pp. 1–19, Cambridge University Press.

Nieuwenhuys, R. (1985). *Chemoarchitecture of the brain*. Berlin Springer-Verlag, pp. 246.

Okado, N. & Kojima, T. (1984). Ontogeny of the central nervous system; neurogenesis, fibre connection, synaptogenesis and myelinisation of the spinal cord. In Prechtl, H. F. R. (ed.), *Continuity of neural functions from prenatal to postnatal life. Clinics in Developmental Medicine*, **94**, 31–45.

Oppenheim, R. W. (1981). Ontogenetic adaptations and retrogressive processes in the development of the nervous system and behaviour: a neuroembryological perspective. In: Connolly K. J., Prechtl, H. F. R. (eds.) *Maturation and development: biological perspectives. Clinics in developmental medicine* Nrs 77/78. pp. 73–109, London SIMP with Heinemann Medical Philadelphia, Lippincott.

Purpura, D. P. (1975). Dendritic differentiation in human cebral cortex. In Kreutzberg, G. W. (ed.) *Advances in neurology*. pp. 91–98, New York, Raven Press.

Purves, D. & Lichtman, J. W. (1984). *Principles of neural development*. Sinauer Ass. Inc. Publishers, Sunderland Massachusetts, pp. 433.

Rakic, P. (1972). Mode of cell migration to the superficial layers of fetal monkey neocortex. *Journal of Comparative Neurology*, **145**, 61–84.

Segal, M. B. & Zlokovic; B. V. (1990). *The blood–brain barrier, amino acids and peptides*. Dordrecht, Boston Kluwer Academic Publishers, pp. 201.

Smart, J. L. (1991). Critical periods in brain development. In Bock, G. R. & Whelan, J. (eds.), *The childhood environment and adult disease*. (Ciba Foundation Symposium 156) pp. 109–24, John Wiley and Sons.

Smith, S. J. (1988). Neuronal cytomechanics: the actin-based motility of growth cones. *Science*, **242**, 708–15.

Swaab, D. F. (1991). Relation between maturation of neurotransmitter systems in the human brain and psychosocial disorders. In Rutter, M. & Casaer, P. (eds.), *Biological risk factors for psychosocial disorders*. pp. 50–66, Cambridge University Press.

Van der Knaap, M. S. (1990). MR imaging of the various stages of normal myelinization during the first year of life. *Neuroradiology*, **31**, 459–70.

Yakovlev, P. I. & Lecours, A. R. (1967). The myelogenetic cycles of regional maturation of the brain. In Minkowski, A. (ed.), *Regional development of the brain in early life*. pp. 3–70. Oxford Blackwell.

4 Longitudinal research and a biology of human brain development and behaviour

VERNE S. CAVINESS, JR, MD, D PHIL
PAULINE A. FILIPEK, MD
DAVID N. KENNEDY, MS, PHD

Maladaptive behaviour reflecting impaired socialization, school performance, language and motor skills are broadly pervasive disabilities among children. Such disabilities in childhood may become transformed in young adulthood into varied forms and levels of societal incompetence and anti-social behaviour. Underlying these disabilities is the abnormal operation of the human central nervous system. Our task is to understand the maladaptive workings of this remarkable organ system as it evolves normally and abnormally in the course of a child's development. We consider this challenge here in the general framework of human brain science with emphasis upon cognitive neuroscience and developmental neurobiology. We propose a set of programmatic expectations and strategies that draw upon the critical advantages of longitudinal study of subjects through a substantial portion of the developmental epoch.

We envision a developmental brain science of child behaviour that is built upon models of brain operation which have arisen in cognitive neuroscience. A developmental brain science of child behaviour must also proceed within the analytic limits of the set of tools with which we may study the living human brain. These guiding constraints shape the perspective of the present discussion.

We will accept, as our working cognitive science model, the view that the brain is a computational map (Churchland & Sejnowski, 1988; Kosslyn, 1987; Changeux & Dehaene, 1990). By this we mean that behaviour reflects the operation of information processing algorithms, and that these algorithms depend upon the workings of discrete and definable processing components organized into sub-systems. The individual components and their sub-systems serving each algorithm are mapped in distributed fashion upon the brain. That is, each has an assigned discrete localization within the central nervous system (Mountcastle, 1978; Damasio, 1990). The various interdependent sub-systems are interconnected by local and long distance axonal connections. It is assumed that the normal adult brain has a constant set of such operators and that these are distributed in specified patterns with respect to the cytoarchitectonic subdivisions of the normal adult brain (Mesulam, 1985).

Those algorithms sub-serving the complex behaviours of principal interest here, that is, those sub-serving perception, language, memory, cognition, skilled motor behaviour and socialization, are viewed to be mapped predominantly, though not exclusively, in the forebrain. By illustration, the processing components serving an algorithm of visual information processing is proposed to be hierarchical and organized in parallel with elementary processing components located in the lateral geniculate nucleus of the thalamus and primary visual and unimodal visual association cortex of the occipital lobe of the cerebral hemisphere (Fig. 4.1; Kosslyn, et al., 1990). Intermediary processors are viewed as located in the parietal and temporal lobes and the highest order associative processors in the frontal lobes. Acoustic and more specialized linguistic processors are distributed principally through the region of the sylvian opercula (Caplan, 1991) while systems concerned with affective state and socialization may have additional strong representation in the limbic lobe (Mesulam, 1985). The entire cerebrum, but the polymodal cortical regions in particular, will contribute to attentional mechanisms and cognitive processes (Mesulam, 1981, 1990).

PATHOLOGICAL PROCESSES AND MODES OF NERVOUS SYSTEM INJURY

The various disease processes to which the central nervous system is subject can be viewed schematically to degrade neural tissue in two principal ways. For the purposes of this discussion, we will consider this to be the case whether the disorder acts during the developmental epoch or later in adult life. At the two extremes are focally acting destructive disorders, on the one hand, and diffusely acting processes leading to functional disability and death of large numbers of neurons, on the other. The focally destructive processes include ischaemia, tumour, certain infections, and trauma; a host of acquired and heritable systemic or neuropathological processes represent the model of diffusely acting neuronal disease. Hepatic encephalopathy or the encephalopathy of phenylketonuria are but two recognized examples of what is certainly an extended set of classified and unclassified conditions belonging to the latter class of pathological process.

How will these different classes of pathological process affect the operation of the central nervous system, and will the effects be different in the adult and developing child? We emphasize here that the approach to these questions is not simply to determine whether behaviour is abnormally modified by a neuropathological process. It is rather to understand in what ways the resulting abnormal behaviour represents specifically the disordered operation of information processing algorithms of the central nervous system.

The adult brain as a reference

The relationships between abnormal behaviour and abnormalities of the supporting processing systems is more predictable for the adult than the

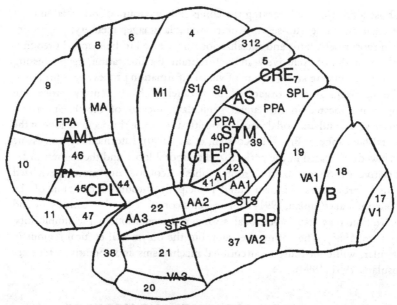

Fig. 4.1.   Three different neocortical maps are represented in a lateral view of the cerebral hemisphere. Map 1: The numbered architectonic subdivisions according to the system of Brodmann. Map 2: Functional hierarchies based upon the primary sensory modalities (vision, hearing, somatic sensation) and motor function. Thus, for each sensory and motor function modalities there is a primary cortical region corresponding to a Brodmann architectonic field. A region adjacent to the primary region of the cortex, involving multiple architectonic fields, is principally concerned with processing information relayed through the primary field and is referred to as a unimodal association area. Thus, for the visual system, the primary region (VI) corresponds to architectonic field 17 and the unimodel association areas (VA 1–3) correspond to multiple architectonic fields involved in visual information processing and distributed through the occipital and temporal lobes. Finally, polymodal association areas concerned with the highest order, or multimodal processing, are distributed through architectonic fields located adjacent to the unimodal association areas. Thus the parietal polymodal association region (PPA) lies in the posterior parietal lobe at the interface of occipital and temporal lobes and the frontal polymodal association region (FPA) lies in the frontal polar region. Map 3: A selected set of subsystems involved in visual information processing and indicated by abbreviations in capital letters are distributed through the primary and unimodal visual association areas and also in the polymodal association areas. The visual buffer (VB) is found in the VA1 region. Visual information is fed forward through the VB in two general streams. One stream, directed temporally through a preprocessing subsystem (PRP), is concerned with object recognition in terms of shape, color and other object features. Another stream is directed parietally where it is processed by spatiotopic mapping (STM), coordinate relations encoding (CRE), and categorical relations encoding (CTE) subsystems. The fed forward information is compared to, and further processed in relation to, experientially acquired and stored visual information coming from associative memory (AM) and the coordinate and categorical property lookup (CPL) subsystems which are distributed in the frontal polymodal association region (see Kosslyn, 1987; Kosslyn et al., 1990).

developing brain. When a frankly destructive process strikes the elementary processing components or unique sets of connections in the fully developed brain, there is typically an associated elementary perceptual or behavioural deficit. For example, destruction of a component of cytoarchitectonic area 17, the lateral geniculate nucleus of the thalamus or the intervening geniculocalcarine radiation will be followed by a visual field defect corresponding to that portion of the retinotopic representation which has been destroyed. Destruction of the pre-central cortex or its descending corticospinal projections will be attended by contralateral hemiparesis.

Focal destruction of unimodal or polymodal association areas, or their interconnections, will have consequences for the operation of neural systems which, though admittedly little understood, may be expected to be substantially more complex. Thus, elementary perceptual or motor functions may be expected to survive such injury but higher order functions may be substantially degraded. For example, pre-frontal injury may result in slowness and impoverishment in the quality of skilled and swift movement.

The consequences of disruption of the operation of the algorithm of visual information processing is illustrated by findings from an analysis in a subject with infarction in the left (dominant) centrosylvian region (Kosslyn et al., in preparation). In this brain, there was no direct impingement of the lesion on the putative subcomponents of the visual processing system. However, the subcortical extent of the lesion was such that the axonal systems interconnecting the lower level visual processors, located post-centrally, and the higher levels banks of associative visual memory, located in the frontal region of the brain, were interrupted. The subject had impairment in performance on sub-sets but not all test paradigms sensitive to visual pattern recognition. Thus, the lesion affected differentially the sub-systems involved in visual information processing. The impairment was one of degraded efficiency or speed of test performance and not one of accuracy. This last aspect of the impaired performance is consistent with the view that the processing system is parallel and distributed.

Widespread neuronal degenerations acting in the adult brain may have differential effects upon selected processors, but this is typically encountered in relatively early stages of disease. For example, differential impairment of a hierarchic array of semantic processes has been encountered in early stages of Alzheimer's Disease (Huff et al., 1986).

The developing brain

The interrelationship between neuropathological process and disruption of neural systems supporting algorithms of information processing may be expected to be less determinant for the developmental period of life. The straightforward elimination of primary perceptual or motor functions by focal lesions, though certainly encountered, may be only incidental to the pervasive and generally disabling disorders of perception, cognition, language, complex motor function and socialization which are of central interest here. Typically for the behavioural disabilities arising from these realms of brain dysfunction, neither the nature of the underlying pathological process nor its time course of action are confidently known.

The uncertainty relating to the neural processing deficits underlying complex behavioural disability in childhood has its most substantial basis in developmental plasticity. The varied phenomena gathered under the rubric of 'plasticity' direct our attention to the full set of cellular processes in development through which neural systems are assembled. Experimental study in animals informs us as to the principal sequences of cellular events and interactions through which the structure of the nervous system develops under normal circumstances. Much is known of the modulating effect of neural circuit function upon the development of the brain. Function of neural systems is, in turn, driven by the experiences of post-natal life. This entire array of cellular processes, variably modulated by experience and neural circuit operation, may be expected to participate variably in the plastic revisions of neural circuitry associated with pathological process.

The principal cellular events of brain development include both progressive and regressive processes (Purves, 1988). Among the former are cell generation and migration, the elaboration of dendritic and axonal neuronal processes, the formation of synaptic junctions, and subsequent growth and differentiation of networks of neural systems. There are, in addition, a series of regressive processes which overlap the regressive processes in time. These appear to be indispensable to the fine tuning of systems organization and interaction. These regressive processes include programmed cell death, which leads to reduction in neuronal number, trimming back of 'exuberant' axonal and dendritic arbors and reduction in synaptic number and density. Both the progressive and regressive processes, particularly those late processes which are critical to fine tuning of neural systems wiring diagrams, appear to be strongly modulated by primary perceptual and perhaps even by more complex experiences and behaviours.

The timetables for these events in brain structures critical to behaviour in man have been estimated to a rough approximation. Thus, cytogenesis and neuronal migration in the human forebrain are largely completed by the sixth month of gestation (Sidman & Rakic, 1973, 1982; Gadisseux & Evrard, 1985). In the cerebellum, these most elementary developmental processes continue well into the first post-natal year of life. The collective set of processes contributing to growth and differentiation of the forebrain accelerate in tempo late in the second trimester as cytogenesis and cell migrations come to completion. Thus, the human brain weighs only about 100 g at 20 weeks gestation, approximately one-fifteenth its adult weight (Gilles, Leviton & Dooling, 1983; Lemire et al., 1975). The weight rises sharply to 400 g by the time of birth at 40 weeks. Rapid growth continues to age 2–3 years by which time brain weight is 1200 g. A period of decelerating growth extends to age 12–14 by which time the adult weight of 1200 to 1500 g is achieved.

The terminal regressive processes may be largely delayed until post-natal life at which time experience driven, systems operation may become a dominant determinant of circuitry revision and design. By illustration, reduction in the number and density of synaptic junctions in the human visual cortex proceeds rapidly through the second two years of post-natal life and then more slowly until about the sixth year (Huttenlocher & de Courten, 1987; Huttenlocher et al., 1982, 1982–83). It is especially during this earliest segment of post-natal life that the development of normal binocular vision is critically dependent upon perfect ocular alignment. It is plausible that all aspects of the child's experiences during this early critical period similarly shape the hardwiring of his or her nervous system itself and thus set the character and limits of future adaption in life (Huttenlocher, 1984).

We will review here three separate classes of plastic phenomena. Although these illustrations of plasticity have been extrapolated from experimentation in animals, they are reasonably expected to operate also in the developing human nervous system. We emphasize, in this selection, the processes impinging principally upon terminal events of neural systems assembly where the progressive cellular events of terminal axon sprouting and synaptogenesis are proceeding concurrently with the regressive processes of pruning of exuberant connections and elimination of redundant synapses (Innocenti, 1981; Koppel & Innocenti, 1983). The first two classes of plasticity are drawn from experiments where there has been either restriction of peripheral information access to, or destruction of, central processing centres and pathways. These disruptions are associated with substantial rewiring of major neuronal circuits. The process of rewiring resulting from these manipulations may lead to circuits which may, or may not, support adaptive behaviours. Our general quest is an elaboration of principles which govern the modification of processing circuitry and its consequences for behaviour (Purves, 1988).

Disruption of the normal flow of sensory input   The most completely explored and informative paradigms here have been monocular visual deprivation in monkeys or cats (Hubel, 1978; Hubel, Wiesel & LeVay, 1977) and destruction of the mystacial vibrissal pad in rodents. These experimental manipulations reformat the patterns of axonal arborization and synaptology in target nuclear and neocortical structures. These systems become 'rewired' so as to achieve a match with the experimentally modified receptotopia. With regard to the visual projection developing under conditions of monocular deprivation, the entirety of neocortical architectonic area 17 in each hemisphere is taken over by the projection arising from the sighted eye and at the expense of the zone normally innervated by the non-sighted eye (Hubel et al., 1977; LeVay Wiesel & Hubel, 1980). With regard to the consequences of elimination of mystacial vibrissae in the rodent, again the wiring diagram of the CNS is modified in that the nuclear and cortical targets of the eliminated vibrissae are themselves eliminated (Simons, Durham & Woolsey, 1984; Van der Loos, Dorfl & Welker,

1984; Durham & Woolsey, 1984). These paradigms illustrate plastic revisions of internal receptotopic mappings within cytoarchitectonic units. The phenomena are, in principle, strongly adaptive in that they optimize the connectional–functional match between receptotopia and central target. As far as is known, this occurs without modification of signal processing itself, neither that in the revised primary cortical target nor that of derivative processing at more elaborated levels of the information processing algorithm.

Focal brain destruction Remarkable degrees of recovery or acquisition of function are characteristic where there has been focal injury to the developing brain. Amputation of the pre-frontal cerebral regions of macaque fetuses just after neuronal migration to the neocortex is completed (Goldman-Rakic, 1978; Goldman & Galkin, 1978; Rakic, 1974) has little or no behavioural sequelae in post-natal life. Central nuclear structures normally connected to the ablated cortex retain their normal volumes. In contrast, this same pattern of pre-frontal ablation undertaken in post-natal life in this species is followed by profound impairment in spatial mnemonic functions and also by atrophy of central nuclear masses bereft of their connections as result of the cortical ablations. It is an implication of these observations that the brain damaged early in its development is able to establish effective information processing systems different from, and effectively alternative to, those that normally support behaviours in the normal brain.

Whereas early ablation of the pre-frontal neocortex may be followed by rewiring of the cerebral circuitry and the revised circuitry may support adaptive behaviour indistinguishable from normal, quite anomalous and maladaptive behaviour may attend other plastic circuitry reconstructions. Thus, the retinal projection may be routed into the somatosensory thalamus if its principal thalamic and tectal targets, and the ascending somatosensory lemniscal axons are experimentally destroyed at earliest stages of development of the retinofugal axonal system (Frost, 1990; Metin & Frost, 1989; Bhide & Frost, 1991). This rewired retinothalamic projection supports a retinotopic physiologic representation in the somatosensory thalamus which is projected upon the somatosensory neocortex. In some animals, the regenerating fibres of the damaged sensory lemnisci may also re-establish a somatotopic representation which becomes stabilized with the visuotopic representation within the somatosensory cortex. Although the behavioural consequences of this anomalous circuitry reconstruction are not yet defined, one may assume that the functional properties of the rewired system are in no sense adaptive. Here the primary visual field representation has been transformed in a way that may be assumed not to support useful vision; further, there is probably no liaison achieved between the retinal projection and the cerebral sub-systems that support visual information processing.

In the developing brain, in contrast to that of the adult, more diffusely acting encephalopathic processes may be expected to impair generally the growth and differentiation of neurons and supporting glial populations (Huttenlocher, 1991). Here, circuitry functions will become downgraded in broadly pervasive ways, not obviously reflected in defective information processing within specific systems. General impairments in cerebral processing functions with impoverishment of all higher functions including socialization has been suggested to be the most characteristic direct consequence. In other circumstances, perhaps when there has been a net impairment of inhibitory systems or impaired capacitance properties of excitatory neurons, systems hyperexcitability may result. Seizures would be among the behavioural correlates.

THE LONGITUDINAL STUDY DESIGN

We envision the following as the essence of a programme of longitudinal study of the biological basis of child behaviour. Analysis structured from principles of cognitive science will be mounted correlatively with an integrated, direct analysis of the morphology and physiological state of the brain. Such analyses will be executed serially in the same subjects throughout critical stages of systems maturation. The most elementary objective will be to define and map within the brain, at each stage of analysis, the sub-components of neural systems which support complex behaviours in the developing child. The behavioural analyses must be constructed in such a way that broad sets of behavioural paradigms depend selectively upon and 'activate' specific information processing circuits, for example, those supporting the operation of algorithms involved in visual or linguistic processing, or skilled motor performance. Within each set of systems selective paradigms, individual paradigms must activate in selective, or at least biased, fashion the individual sub-components that contribute to the overall processing system. For example, behavioural paradigms within the visual processing domain might differentially be dependent upon processing sub-components concerned with spatiotopic mapping or pattern activation at intermediate levels of processing or visual associative memory at higher levels of processing (Kosslyn et al., in preparation). In the linguistic domain, the separate paradigms might be differentially selective for varied semantic or syntactic operators (Caplan, 1991).

A developmental neurobiology concerned with circuit organization and operation in the developing human brain in relation to human brain function is beset by formidable methodological obstacles. These derive from the dilemma that the primary structure and cellular physiology of the human nervous system are directly accessible to neurobiological study only after death. Yet, the very questions of interest relating to cellular organization and operation of the nervous centre are rendered inaccessible by the death process. There is a compounding dilemma that animal experimentation provides relatively unsatisfactory models for the study of the neurobiology of specific maladaptive human behaviours.

With regard to direct study of the morphology and functional states of the brain itself, advancing technology promises both the sensitivity and selectivity to be required for correlational analysis with the behavioural paradigms. Magnetic resonance imaging will provide the basis for morphological analysis (Caviness, Filipek & Kennedy, 1989; Filipek et al., 1989; Filipek, Kennedy & Caviness, 1992). The procedure is non-invasive and without risk and thus suitable for repeated application in the child. Rapid sequencing schedules now provide, with imaging times on the order of 10 minutes, imaging data sets for the complete brain with high grey matter–white matter contrast at spatial resolutions approaching 1 mm. Computer-assisted algorithms, now at advanced stages of development and application, allow efficient segmentation of grey-white subdivisions or of focal lesions with separate computations of volumes and shapes of segmented structures (Fig. 4.2).

Behavioural paradigm induced activation of information processing subsystems within the brain may be detected by an array of technological means, each with its characteristic sensitivity and spatiotemporal resolution (Churchland & Sejnowski, 1988). Magnetoencephalography (MEG) (Papanicolaou et al., 1990; Cohen et al., 1990) and electroencepholographic (EEG) detection of event related potentials (ERP) (Lovrich et al., 1986; Lovrich, Novick & Vaughn, 1988; Wood et al., 1988) offer temporal resolutions in the range of milliseconds. The recording methods mark the cranial surface locations overlying activated cerebral regions with spatial resolutions in centimetres. Experience to date indicates that these methods are sufficiently sensitive to detect behavioural paradigm driven activation of sub-systems concerned with visual, acoustic and linguistic processing. Positron emission tomography (PET) (Lueck et al., 1989; Mintun, Fox & Raichle, 1989; Petersen et al., 1988, 1990; Posner et al., 1988) offers a spatial resolution approximating to that of MEG and ERP but temporal resolution in minutes. This technology has the advantage that it provides an imaged reconstruction of the full volumes of cerebral regions where increase in blood flow or glucose uptake has been activated by paradigms delineating the operation of visual system or linguistic processors. Echo planar magnetic resonance imaging, now in only initial stages of application, holds promise for imaged reconstructions similar to, but at higher spatial resolution than, those obtained with PET and temporal resolutions approaching those obtained with MEG and ERP. Thus far, it is clear that this potentially revolutionary technology is virtually as sensitive as PET to pattern shift activation of the primary visual cortex (Belliveau et al., 1991). The full range of its sensitivity and potential applications remains to be determined.

The mapping process, that is the process by which the location of physiologically detected activations is registered with the MRI defined anatomic substrate, is achieved by embedding both morphological and physiological data sets in a common set of stereotactic coordinates. It must be emphasized that this stratagem does not reliably map to underlying systems based architectonic subdivisions of the cerebrum, in particularly the cerebral cortex. This is because inter-individual variation, indeed the inter-hemispheric variation in the same

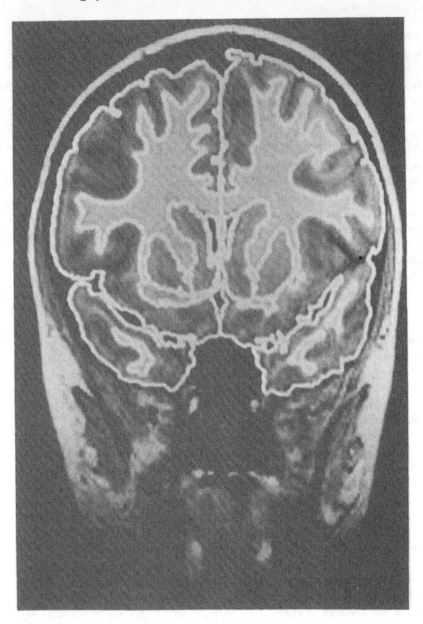

Fig. 4.2. A coronal view through the frontal region of a normal adult human brain as represented in a magnetic resonance imaging data set. The cortical and nuclear grey matter structures have a lower signal intensity than that of white matter structures. Grey and white matter structures have been delineated from each other (or segmented) by a computer-assisted program. The segmentation operation is the initial step in a series of computations that provide the basis for measures of volume, shape and mapping position (cf. Fig. 4.1) within the hemisphere.

subject with respect to the coordinate designation of architectonic fields, is substantial. Thus the cordinate values for a given cytoarchitectonic field for a standard or 'atlas brain', may be expected to correspond to quite different cytoarchitectonic localizations in other brains. We propose that this inconvenience will be largely overcome by an individual systems-based parcellation of the cerebrum of each subject brain according to a method that is based on 'limiting fissures' and/or constant topographic landmarks which may be confidently identified in magnetic resonance images (Jouandet et al., 1989; Rademacher et al., 1992, 1993). The longitudinal study design which emphasizes comparisons within the same individual over time, substantially minimizes the dilemma posed by individual variation.

We assemble here a set of expectations as to the classes of observations that may be the earliest harvest of this study programme. These expectations focus upon processing sub-component identification and their systems-based mapped locations within the brain. It should be understood here that the precedents that allow these expectations have been realized only in the adult, and generally in the normal adult brain. Thus, it is not simply that one must reconstruct the computational map supporting complex behaviours in childhood; one must construct the normal ontogeny of this map. This may be expected to require the investigator to extend the developmental window of observation into the first post-natal years to define the critical ontogenetic events and their sequences. At a purely morphological level, one may expect that the parcellated different systems components will acquire their mature volumes and configurations at differential rates. Patterns of processing sub-component activation, nested within these morphological sub-divisions, may also be expected to develop differentially with time.

The following phenomena might be encountered. Certain sub-components, activatable at some stage of normal maturation might not be so at earliest stages of analysis or, obviously, their level of activation might yield signals below the threshold for detection with the available technology. Multiple sub-components initially activatable, might at first not be spatially resolvable. The topographic extent of a sub-systems-related activation, as well as the amplitude, duration and latency of activation, might be additional variable parameters which are typical and unique for the separate sub-systems.

A prospectus for such a programme of study of the abnormal brain carries us even further beyond guiding precedent. It is to be expected that the design of behavioural paradigms will be greatly challenging and a principal constraint upon the conduct of study. It is to be expected that manifestly different disabilities will be associated with detectably different systems pathology. The more restricted disorders grouped together as dyslexias may be expected to be associated with sub-component anomalies in the sylvian opercular region, an expectation to some extent already anticipated by correlative behavioural–morphological (Filipek et al., 1989, 1992; Jernigan & Tallal, 1990) and behavioural–physiological (Lou, Henriksen & Bruhn, 1990) analyses. Also under scrutiny are the general regional localizations posited earlier for disabled sub-systems underlying autism or general cognitive impairment, and those associated with more selective limitations in visual, acoustic processing or skilled motility.

Within the appropriate regions of the brain such disorders might be associated with frank absence of certain processors with anomalous routing of the information processing vector. Delayed emergence or anomalies of the parameters of sub-component activation are additional readily imaginable correlates of maladaptive behaviours.

Finally, it is to be considered, both for the normal and for the handicapped child, that the methods available will be sufficiently sensitive to allow us to detect the workings of manipulable determinants of the rate and degree of sub-systems development. At the simplest level there is the possibility that there may be 'education' or pharmacologically induced modulations of development which are favourable and within the power of resolution of the methods brought to bear upon the analysis. Such an eventuality would provide a powerful and much desired rational basis for education and longitudinal management of the child with developmental disabilities in the domain of complex behaviour.

ACKNOWLEDGEMENTS

This work is supported in part by NIH grants NINDS PO1 20489 and NINDS PO1 24279. The authors thank Ms. Virginia Tosney for her expert assistance with the manuscript preparation.

REFERENCES

Belliveau, J. W., Kennedy, D. N., McKinstry, R. C., Buchbinder, B. R., Weisskopf, R. M., Cohen, M. S., Vevea, J. M., Brady, T. J. & Rosen, B. R. (1991). Functional mapping of the human visual cortex by magnetic resonance imaging. *Science*, **254**, 716–19.

Bhide, P. G. & Frost, D. O. (1991). Stages of growth of hamster retinofugal axons: implications for developing axonal pathways with multiple targets. *Journal of Neuroscience*, **11**, 485–504.

Brodmann, K. (1909). *Vergleichende Lokalisationslehre der Grosshirnrinde.* Leipzig: Barth.

Caplan, D. (1991). *Language: structure, processing, and disorders.* MIT Press, Cambridge, MA.

Caviness, V. S. Jr., Filipek, P. A. & Kennedy, D. N. (1989). Magnetic resonance technology in human brain science; blueprint for a programme based upon morphometry. *Brain and Development*, **1**, 1–13.

Changeux, J. P. & Dehaene, S. (1990). Neuronal models of cognitive functions. In *Neurobiology of Cognition*, pp. 64–109. A. M. Galaburda and P. D. Eimas (eds.). MIT Press, Cambridge, MA.

Churchland, P. S. & Sejnowski, T. J. (1988). Perspectives on cognitive neuroscience. *Science*, **242**, 741–5.

Cohen, D., Cuffin, B. N., Yunokuchi, K., Maniewski, R., Purcell, C., Cosgrove, G. R., Ives, J., Kennedy, J. G. & Schomer, D. L. (1990). MEG versus EEG localization test using implanted sources in the human brain. *Annals of Neurology*, **28**, 811–17.

Damasio, A. R. (1990). Time-locked multiregional retroactivation: a systems-level proposal for the neural substrates of recall and recognition. In A. M. Galaburda & P. D. Eimas (eds.), *Neurobiology of Cognition*, pp. 25–62. MIT Press, Cambridge, MA.

Durham, D. & Woolsey, T. A. (1984). Effects of neonatal whisker lesions of mouse central trigeminal pathways. *Journal of Comparative Neurology*, **223**, 424–47.

Filipek, P. A., Kennedy, D. N., Caviness, V. S. Jr., Rossnick, S. L., Spraggins, T. A. & Starewicz, P. M. (1989). Magnetic resonance imaging-based brain morphometry: development and application to normal subjects. *Annals of Neurology*, **25**, 61–7.

Filipek, P. A., Kennedy, D. N. & Caviness, V. S. Jr. (1992). Neuroimaging in child neuropsychology. In Boller, F. and Grafman, J. (eds.), *Handbook of Neuropsychology*, vol. 6 *Child neuropsychology*. Rapin, I. & Segalowitz, S. (topic eds.), Amsterdam: Elsevier, in press.

Frost, D. O. (1990). Sensory processing by novel, experimentally induced cross-modal circuits. *Annals of the New York Academy of Science*, **608**, 92–109; discussion 109–112.

Gadisseux, J.-F. & Evrard, P. (1985). Glial–neuronal relationship in the developing central nervous system. *Developmental Neuroscience*, **7**, 12–32.

Gilles, F. H., Leviton, A. & Dooling, E. C. (1983). *The developing human brain*. John Wright PSG, Inc, Boston.

Goldman, P. S. & Galkin, T. W. (1978). Prenatal removal of frontal association cortex in the fetal rhesus monkey: anatomical and functional consequences in postnatal life. *Brain Research*, **152**, 451–85.

Goldman-Rakic, P. S. (1978). Neuronal plasticity in primate telencephalon: anomalous projections induced by prenatal removal of frontal cortex. *Science*, **202**, 768–76.

Hubel, D. H. (1978). Effects of deprivation on the visual cortex of cat and monkey. *Harvey Lecture*, **72**, 1–51.

Hubel, D. H., Wiesel, T. N. & LeVay, S. (1977). Plasticity of ocular dominance columns in monkey striate cortex. *Philosophical Transactions of the Royal Society of London (Biol.)*, **278**, 377–409.

Huff, F. J., Corkin, S. and Growdon, J. H. (1986). Semantic impairment and anomia in Alzheimer's disease. *Brain and Language*, **28**, 235–49.

Huttenlocher, P. R. (1984). Synapse elimination and plasticity in developing human cerebral cortex. *American Journal of Mental Deficiency*, **88**, 488–96.

Huttenlocher, P. R. (1991). Dendritic and synaptic pathology in mental retardation. *Pediatric Neurology*, **7**, 79–85.

Huttenlocher, P. R. & de Courten, C. (1987). The develoment of synapses in striate cortex of man. *Human Neurobiology*, **6**, 1–9.

Huttenlocher, P. R., de Courten, C., Garey, L. J. & Van der Loos, H. (1982). Synaptogenesis in human visual cortex – evidence for synapse elimination during normal development. *Neuroscience Letters*, **33**, 247–52.

Huttenlocher, P. R., De Courten, C., Garey, L. J. & Van der, Loos, H. (1982–83). Synaptic development in human cerebral cortex. *International Journal of Neurology*, **16–17**, 144–54.

Innocenti, G. M. (1981). Growth and reshaping of axons in the establishment of visual callosal connections. *Science*, **212**, 824–7.

Jernigan, T. L. & Tallal, P. A. (1990). Late childhood changes in brain morphology observable with MRI. *Developmental Medicine and Child Neurology*, **32**, 379–85.

Jouandet, M. L., Tramo, M. J., Herron, D. M., Hermann, A., Loftus, W. C., Bazell, J. & Gazzaniga, M. S. (1989). Brainprints: computer-generated two-dimensional maps of the human cerebral cortex in vivo. *Journal of Cognitive Neuroscience*, **1**, 88–117.

Koppel, H. & Innocenti, G. M. (1983). Is there a genuine exuberancy of callosal projections in development? A quantitative electron microscopic study in the cat. *Neuroscience Letters*, **41**, 33–40.

Kosslyn, S. M. (1987). Seeing and imagining in the cerebral hemispheres: a computational approach. *Psychology Reviews*, **94**, 148–75.

Kosslyn, S. M., Flynn, R. A., Amsterdam, J. B. & Wang, G. (1990). Components of high-level vision: a cognitive neuroscience analysis and accounts of neurological syndromes. *Cognition*, **34**, 203–77.

Lemire, R. J., Loeser, J. D., Leech, R. W. & Alvord, E. C., Jr (1975). *Normal and abnormal development of the human nervous system*. Harper and Row, New York.

LeVay, S., Wiesel, T. N. & Hubel, D. H. (1980). The development of ocular dominance columns in normal and visually deprived monkeys. *Journal of Comparative Neurology*, **191**, 1–51.

Lou, H. C., Henriksen, L. & Bruhn, P. (1990). Focal cerebral dysfunction in developmental learning disabilities. *Lancet*, **335**, 8–11.

Lovrich, D., Novick, B. & Vaughn, H. G., jr (1988). Topographic analysis of auditory event-related potentials associated with acoustic and semantic processing. *Electroencephalography and Clinical Neurophysiology*, **71**, 40–54.

Lovrich, D., Simson, R., Vaughn, H. G., jr & Ritter, W. (1986). Topography of visual event-related potentials during geometric and phonetic discriminations. *Electroencephalography and Clinical Neurophysiology*, **65**, 1–12.

Lueck, C. J., Zeki, S., Friston, K. J., Deiber, M. P., Cope, P., Cunningham, V. J., Lammertsma, A. A., Kennard, C. & Frackowiak, R. S. (1989). The colour centre in the cerebral cortex of man. *Nature*, **340**, 386–9.

Mesulam, M. M. (1981). A cortical network for directed attention and unilateral neglect. *Annals of Neurology*, **10**, 309–25.

Mesulam, M. M. (1985). Patterns in behavioural neuroanatomy: association areas, the limbic system, and hemispheric specialization. In M.-M. Mesulam (ed.), *Principles of Behavioral Neurology*, pp. 1–70. F. A. Davis Company, Philadelphia.

Mesulam, M. M. (1990). Large-scale neurocognitive networks and distributed processing for attention, language, and memory. *Annals of Neurology*, **28**, 597–613.

Metin, C. & Frost, D. O. (1989). Visual responses of neurons in somatosensory cortex of hamsters with experimentally induced retinal projections to somatosensory thalamus. *Proceedings of the National Academy of Science (USA)*, **86**, 357–61.

Mintun, M. A., Fox, P. T. & Raichle, M. E. (1989). A highly accurate method of localizing regions of neuronal activation in the human brain with positron emission tomography. *Journal of Cerebral Blood Flow and Metabolism*, **9**, 96–103.

Mountcastle, V. (1978). An organizing principle for cerebral function: the unit module and the distributed system. In Edelman & V. Mountcastle (eds.), *The mindful brain: cortical organization and the group-selective theory of higher brain function*, pp. 7–50. MIT Press, Cambridge, MA.

Papanicolaou, A. C., Bauman, S., Rogers, R. L., Saydjari, C., Amparo, E. G. &

Eisenberg, H. M. (1990). Localization of auditory response sources using magnetoen-cephalography and magnetic resonance imaging. *Archives of Neurology*, **47**, 33–7.

Petersen, S. E., Fox, P. T., Posner, M. I., Mintun, M. & Raichle, M. E. (1988). Positron emission tomographic studies of the cortical anatomy of single-word processing. *Nature*, **331**, 585–9.

Petersen, S. E., Fox, P. T., Snyder, A. Z. & Raichle, M. E. (1990). Activation of extrastriate and frontal cortical areas by visual words and word-like stimuli. *Science*, **249**, 1041–4.

Posner, M. I., Petersen, S. E., Fox, P. T. & Raichle, M. E. (1988). Localization of cognitive operations in the human brain. *Science*, **240**, 1627–31.

Purves, D. (1988). *Body and brain*. Harvard University Press, Cambridge, M.A.

Rademacher, J., Caviness, V. S. Jr., Steinmetz, H. & Garaburda, A. M. (1993). Topographical variation of the human primary cortices: implications for neuroimaging brain mapping and neurobiology. *Cerebral Cortex*, in press.

Rademacher, J., Garaburda, A. M., Kennedy, D. N., Filipek, P. A. & Caviness, V. S. Jr. (1992). Human cerebral cortex: localization, parcellation, and morphometry with magnetic resonance imaging. *Journal of Cognitive Neuroscience*, **4**, 352–74.

Rakic, P. (1974). Neurons in rhesus visual cortex: systematic relation between time of origin and eventual disposition. *Science*, **183**, 425–7.

Sidman, R. L. & Rakic, P. (1973). Neuronal migration, with special reference to developing human brain: a review. *Brain Research*, **62**, 1–35.

Sidman, R. L. & Rakic, P. (1982). Development of the human nervous system. In W. Haymaker & R. D. Adams (eds.), *Histology and histopathology of the nervous system*, pp. 3–145. Charles C. Thomas, Springfield.

Simons, D. J., Durham, D. & Woolsey, T. A. (1984). Functional organization of mouse and rat SmI barrel cortex following vibrissal damage on different postnatal days. *Somatosensory Research*, **1**, 207–45.

Van der Loos, H., Dorfl, J. & Welker, E. (1984). Variation in pattern of mystacial vibrissae in mice. A quantitative study of ICR stock and several inbred strains. *Journal of Heredity*, **75**, 326–36.

Wood, C. C., Spencer, D. D., Truett, A., McCarthy, G., Williamson, P. D. & Goff, W. R. (1988). Localization of human sensorimotor cortex during surgery by cortical surface recording of somatosensory evoked potentials. *Journal of Neurosurgery*, **68**, 99–111.

5 Cognitive, social and emotional development

F. E. WEINERT AND W. SCHNEIDER

Every developmental psychologist knows it, many developmental psychologists have explicitly said it over the years, but only a few researchers have paid attention to this fact in their own work: most of our theories of developmental change are not based on empirical study of these changes, but rather on inferences derived from studies of developmental differences between groups of subjects of different ages. It is well known that more than 90% of published data arise from cross-sectional studies; in contrast, the results from longitudinal studies play only a secondary role.

Why is developmental research so strongly dominated by cross-sectional designs? Three advantages of these designs come first to mind.

The first advantage is a pragmatic one. Modern science is in some ways like a factory for the fast and efficient production of the most data possible. Cross-sectional studies offer a very effective medium for fulfilling this requirement. All one needs for a fair chance of getting successful results is a good idea about possible developmental changes or age differences, two, three or four samples from different age groups and a relatively uncomplicated and reliable measurement that avoids floor and ceiling effects. It is only reasonable to expect that some of the many variables measured in childhood will increase with age, that no interesting age differences will be apparent in early and middle adulthood, and that mean decreases in cognitive competence, and increases in behavioural problems, occur in old age. Of course, the characterization of cross-sectional designs as just a vehicle for allowing more and more developmental psychologists to publish more and more articles is too simplistic and biased an evaluation.

The second advantage of cross-sectional designs is that they can characterize and describe typical characteristics across different ages very well. Behavioural and mental changes that are otherwise difficult to describe, and often only moderately correlated with age become, through age-group comparisons, very concise and clear contrastive developmental differences. However, the validity of taking mean age differences as an indicator of individual change is generally an untested presumption that is reasonable only when it applies to universal developmental phenomena that apply to (nearly) all members of our species.

This brings us to the third advantage of cross-sectional designs: they fit into a methodological framework arising from a theoretical perspective in which development is conceived as species-specific, universal, and unavoidable. Many developmental phenomena, at least in early childhood and old age, obey such biological rules and constraints or follow a (psycho-)logical sequence.

A characterization of the advantages of cross-sectional designs also implicitly refers to their limits and disadvantages. Assuming that research has the goal of providing scientifically appropriate descriptions, explanations and predictions of cognitive, social and emotional development, there are five problem areas where no satisfactory solution is possible without longitudinal data.

(a) Current developmental laws are not based on data aggregated over changes within individuals, but rather on inferences from mean, variance, and covariance data from two or more age groups. As a consequence, those phenomena for which the detection of developmental change on the basis of mean age differences is not possible or not reliable will be overlooked or misinterpreted. One typical example for this is that underlying the linear increase of average memory performances there are enormous intra- and inter-individual differences in the development of memory skills that were ignored for over a century (Weinert, 1991).

(b) Both the overemphasis on universal development and the resulting cross-sectional methodology reinforce the tendency to reduce the definition and analysis of interindividual differences to acceleration or retardation in the pace of development within a universal, age-related developmental sequence. This means that qualitative differences in developmental change are generally not taken into account, and, more importantly, it is not even possible to test whether there are qualitative differences in patterns of change at all. This is well illustrated by the many studies and debates about possible qualitative developmental differences among normal, disabled and gifted children (Weisz & Yeates, 1981; Weiss, Weisz & Bromfield, 1986; Weinert & Waldmann, 1986).

(c) The third problem area is that cross-sectional designs tend to promote psychological theories of development that are variable- rather than person-centred, because changes in the intra-individual structure or pattern of variables cannot be assessed. Any person-centred claims made on the basis of cross-sectional data are usually empirically untested inferences from the patterns of correlations between independent samples. To illustrate: a focus on variable-centred theories has, no doubt, contributed to the fact that personality development is described either in terms of cognitive models that assume a universal developmental course, or as the sum of changes in single characteristics, such as anxiety, shyness and the like.

(d) We lack theoretical models and empirical studies that address themselves to predicting individual developmental sequences. This is not just a problem directed to academic research: it also severely hinders the application of results from developmental research (Kohlberg, LaCrosse & Ricks, 1972).

(e) A lack of models concerning change at the individual level applies not just to predictions but also to explanations of developmental change. For example, socialization research has been separate from mainstream developmental research for some time, because of its focus on socialization conditions as the explanatory basis for inter- and intra-individual variance in the development of psychological characteristics. Of course, the extent of this variance is largely unknown, because there is a lack of empirically grounded models for the description of intra- and inter-individual developmental variance (Weinert, 1990).

Enough of the familiar complaints about the limitations of cross-sectional designs. Longitudinal researchers are inclined to think that their methodological approach can make a great contribution to developmental psychology. Longitudinal studies, however, at least with the current methodology, can not quickly and satisfactorily solve all of the obvious theoretical problems either. To achieve this, we still need to do a great deal of work. We will argue, though, that this work will pay off. We will address this claim in the rest of the chapter, addressing four points.

TYPES OF LONGITUDINAL ASSESSMENTS OF PSYCHOLOGICAL DEVELOPMENT

A general problem with evaluating the relevance of longitudinal studies for the description and explanation of human development concerns the definition of what is considered as 'longitudinal'. This term does not describe a single method but a large variety of methods. The spectrum of methods ranges from single-case studies in time-series arrangements to broad-band panel designs including many measurement points and thousands of subjects. The only common denominator of longitudinal research is variation of time and repeated observation of a given entity (cf. Baltes & Nesselroade, 1979).

Given the lack of definitional clarity, it makes sense to distinguish among different types of longitudinal approaches that seem to follow different goals. There is a general agreement in the developmental literature that two basic types of longitudinal inquiry can be differentiated. One type concerns what Wohlwill (1973) called the 'developmental function', that is, changes in the average and/or individual value of a dependent variable over time. The second type of longitudinal inquiry concerns the issue of individual differences. Here, the major issue is how stable or unstable individual differences remain over time.

It is important to note that the issue of stability or instability of individual differences over time is conceptually independent from the issue of continuity or discontinuity in the developing psychological entity. A continuous developmental function for an entire sample might still occur despite significant instability in individual differences. Whether the two are related or not is always an empirical question (cf. Appelbaum & McCall, 1983). Longitudinal researchers have often overlooked the fact that the continuity of a developmental function and the stability of individual differences over time represent two separate aspects of the same problem (see for a more systematic treatment of this topic Asendorpf 1992a; Schneider, 1989).

How can we relate the existing types of longitudinal studies to these two aspects of inquiry? A review of longitudinal studies (Schneider & Edelstein, 1990; Verdonik & Sherrod, 1984) reveals that the majority of studies focus on the stability issue. That is, these studies concentrate on the question of whether individual subjects maintain approximately the same relative rank ordering within their group over time. Differences among studies of this type concern how the stability concept is treated: whereas some researchers differentiate between the stability of a variable and the stability of an individual (Wohlwill, 1973), others define stability of the individual as ipsative stability, that is, the persistence of a pattern of variables for an individual subject over time (cf. Asendorpf & Weinert, 1990; Asendorpf & van Aken, 1991; Rutter, 1987).

In a few longitudinal studies the second aspect of longitudinal inquiry, that is, the issue of continuity/discontinuity of development has been investigated. Here, the major difficulty is that the same instruments must be used on each testing occasion, and one must be able to prove that the instruments do not change their meaning over time (cf. Kagan, 1980; Magnusson, 1981). Asendorpf (1992a) has recently suggested a methodology for studying this problem empirically. Other approaches include (nomothetical) single-case studies, investigating the growth of a specific psychological function over an extended period in time; and so-called 'micro-genetic' longitudinal studies, based on a few subjects and focusing on quantitative as well as qualitative changes in a specific developmental area (for a more systematic characterization of this treatment and for some illustrative examples, see Siegler & Jenkins, 1989; Siegler & Crowley, 1991).

WHAT KIND OF PSYCHOLOGICAL KNOWLEDGE DOES LONGITUDINAL RESEARCH GENERATE?

What is the 'new' knowledge that longitudinal studies can add to that already acquired through cross-sectional research? As emphasized by Baltes and Nesselroade (1979), longitudinal research can improve our understanding of developmental processes because it is particularly suited to describe and explain individual development in several aspects: (a) intraindividual change can be directly identified; (b) causes of intra-individual change can be analysed; (c) inter-individual differences in intra-individual change can be directly identified; (d) possible causes of inter-individual differences in intra-individual change can be analysed, and (e) interrelationships among classes of behaviour and their common patterns of change can be assessed. Another advantage of longitudinal studies over cross-sectional designs is that individual differences in one domain can be predicted from individual differences in another domain. For example, with longitudinal designs one can explore the impact of early risk factors like delay in language acquisition (domain 1) on later reading and writing skills (domain 2).

In our view, it is questionable whether large-scale, broad-band longitudinal analyses can provide new information on general or universal developmental trends. The same results could probably be obtained via cross-sectional studies (for specific problems see Schaie, 1989). Accordingly, the costs of longitudinal research may appear too great for researchers predominantly interested in the exploration of universal developmental trends (cf. De Ribaupierre, 1989).

However, there is no doubt that the longitudinal approach is the only suitable method for investigating individual differences and their stability over time. That is, longitudinal research must be used to assess whether development takes the same form for all individuals. As already mentioned above, the issue of the continuity/discontinuity of development is conceptually unrelated to the issue of stability/instability of individual differences. The relationship between these two aspects of development can only be tested empirically: although it could be that a continuous developmental function (e.g. a linear increase in competence over time) is accompanied by stable inter-individual differences over time, this need not be the case. The exact nature of this relationship can only be assessed via longitudinal designs.

Another advantage of the longitudinal studies is that the single-case and microgenetic studies mentioned above provide tools for investigating the issue of identification of intra-individual change in specific psychological functions. When planned carefully, such studies give important information on the typical developmental course of a psychological function that is based on growth curve patterns aggregated across several individuals. Statistical models (growth curve models) that suggest the type of the developmental function in question (e.g. linear versus nonlinear), and that are helpful in identifying underlying causes of individual differences in intra-individual change can be used with these data (see Bryck & Raudenbush, 1987). Information of this kind cannot be obtained through cross-sectional analyses.

Fine-grained longitudinal analyses of this type are generally restricted to small-scale, short time-span investigations. Microgenetic studies are not feasible over a long time period or with many subjects.

A final important advantage of longitudinal designs is that they allow the estimation and testing of developmental models. Usually, predictions/hypotheses concerning stability and change in patterns of variables are derived from cross-sectional research and tested through longitudinal assessments. The importance of this approach for the acquisition of new knowledge about long-term developmental trends has been demonstrated in many cognitive and social domains (cf. Magnusson, 1988).

EXAMPLES OF LONGITUDINAL RESEARCH ON COGNITIVE AND SOCIAL DEVELOPMENT BASED ON LONGITUDINAL DATA

In the following, we will discuss a few selected examples that we think show how longitudinal research has enriched our knowledge of developmental processes.

Consistency and stability of memory development in early childhood

The first example concerns the development of cognitive processes and is taken from the longitudinal study on the genesis of individual competencies (LOGIC) which has been conducted at our institute (cf. Weinert & Schneider, 1989). The study started in 1984 with about 200 4-year-old children who have been followed annually. From the very beginning, children were tested with a broad range of measures assessing cognitive skills like intelligence, memory, and problem solving, motivational tendencies, and social–emotional constructs like social inhibition or social competence in various settings.

One question concerned the development of memory in children. At the first measurement point, memory span, performance in a sort–recall task and memory for scripted texts (e.g. a birthday party, playing with friends) were assessed. When inter-correlations among these memory measures were computed for this first measurement point (see Table 5.1), it was found that, with the exception of the inter-relationship between recall for the two stories, intertask consistency in pre-schooler's memory performance was remarkably low (cf. Weinert, Schneider & Knopf, 1988).

Table 5.1. *Intercorrelations among various memory performance measures obtained for four-year-old children (N = 185)*

Variables	(2)	(3)	(4)
1. Memory span	.21	.20	.25
2. Recall in a sort-recall task		.23	.36
3. Text recall 1 (birthday party)			.64
4. Text recall 2 (playing with friends)			—

Source: Data from Weinert *et al.* 1988, p.59.

Over the subsequent pre-school and kindergarten years, the same measures were repeated at least twice. An inspection of the means and standard deviations suggested an approximately linear increase in performance for most memory measures. However, the analysis of synchronic (cross-sectional) and diachronic

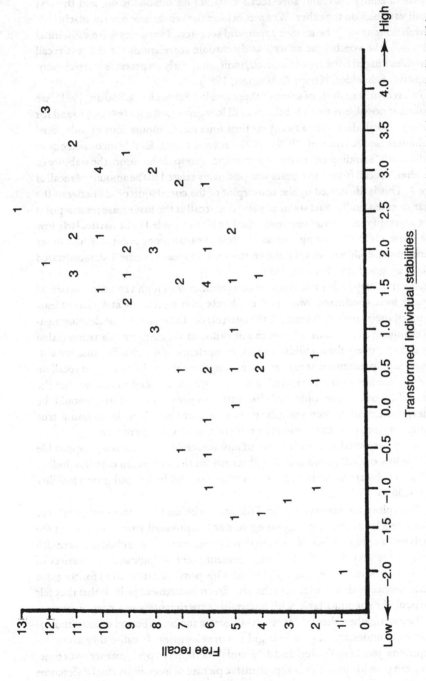

Fig. 5.1. Scatterplot of the bivariate distribution of children's individual stabilities in free recall and their initial scores in this variable. (Data from Schneider & Sodian, 1991, p.23.) *Note* Numbers displayed on scatterplot indicate number of observations at each position.

(across-measurement points) correlations revealed different patterns of stability for the memory span and sort–recall variables on the one hand, and the text recall variables on the other. Whereas neither the synchronic nor the diachronic correlations among the memory span and sort–recall variables were substantial ($rs < .40$), the synchronic as well as diachronic correlations for the text recall variables ranged between .40 and .60, indicating fairly respectable interrelationships (cf. Schneider, Knopf & Weinert, 1989).

In a recent reanalysis of some of these results (Schneider & Sodian, 1991), we looked at possible reasons for the overall low group stability ($r = .38$) found for the sort–recall data over a two-year time interval. Computations of individual stabilities (see Asendorpf, 1989a, 1990c) revealed considerable inconsistency in individuals' standing relative to the reference group. In addition, the stability of children's recall from 4 to 6 years was positively related to the amount of recall at age 4. This is illustrated by the scatterplot of the correlation of .24 between the (transformed) individual stabilities and free recall at the first measurement point at 4 years. Fig. 5.1 shows that individual stabilities tended to be particularly low for those children scoring low at the first measurement point. On the other hand, most children scoring above the sample mean at time 1 demonstrated relatively good stability over time.

As a next step, sub-group analyses on children with high versus low scores at 4 years were conducted. Most of the subjects who scored low at 4 years at least doubled their recall by 6 years. Although this could be due to true developmental change in these children's mnemonic skills, an alternative explanation is that we did not assess these children's true competence at 4 years. Because we also found highly inconsistent results when comparing these children's text recall on the two similar stories presented at 4 years, we are inclined to believe that the instability over time observed for this sub-group of children should be interpreted more as stemming from measurement problems in assessing true competence than as fluctuations in rates of true developmental change.

As we suspected, the small group of unstable children was mainly responsible for the low overall group stability observed for the sort–recall data. Excluding these 24 subjects from the sample of almost 200 children raised group stability from .36 to .65.

To explore the reasons for the difficulties with assessing these subjects' true competencies at the very beginning of our longitudinal study, we carried the analyses one step further. We found that the majority of these children were also classified as very shy at the first measurement point, as indicated by a variety of shyness assessments (Asendorpf, 1990a). One possible explanation for the poor performance of these children at the very first measurement point is that they felt particularly uncomfortable with unfamiliar experimenters in a new situation.

Taken together, then, these results illustrate the contribution of longitudinal studies in understanding early cognitive development. Because they allow in-depth analyses of individual and differential stabilities of performance over time, they can provide us with a comprehensive picture of inter-individual differences in developmental change, thereby going beyond the information obtained from cross-sectional studies.

STABILITIES, OPPORTUNITIES AND LIMITATIONS OF COGNITIVE DEVELOPMENT IN ADULTHOOD AND OLD AGE

It is well known that the results from cross-sectional studies in the first decades of this century helped support a generally accepted deficit model of cognitive aging. More recent research in this area can be described as a successful effort to overcome this stereotype. In this effort, different sorts of longitudinal studies have played an important role.

Convincing evidence for a 'new look' in research on adult intelligence within the psychometric paradigm comes from two conclusions from the results of the Seattle Longitudinal Study (Schaie, 1983). In this study, subjects between 25 and 81 years of age were tested regularly every seven years on intelligence tests that were constructed according to the construct of primary mental abilities. The two conclusions were:

- A considerable portion of age-typical decreases in intellectual achievement found in cross-sectional studies is not an effect of aging, but of cohort group. What this means is that differences in the acquisition of cognitive competence result from differences in the culture, school, and work-related learning opportunities available to people in different generations. Indeed, on the basis of changes in these opportunities, Schaie expected that in the future 'the large ability differences between young and old adults that are observed currently will be much reduced' (1990, p. 299).

- Changes in performance competence in adulthood may be due to individual differences in experience even more than to cohort differences. For example, among the 60 year-olds in the Seattle Longitudinal Study, 75% of the participants maintained their performance level for at least four out of five of the primary abilities tested 7 years later, as did more than half of the 80 year-olds. From this result Schaie concluded 'that rates of change in cognitive behavior is a highly individuated phenomenon' (1989, p. 84).

The data from studies using an information processing paradigm support and strengthen the role of individual differences in cognitive aging suggested by psychometrically oriented longitudinal studies. This approach assumes that the solution of demanding tasks and problems depends less on general intellectual abilities than on the quantity and quality of content-specific declarative and procedural knowledge. Indeed, in their modification of a conclusion made famous by Flavell, Hatano and Inagaki wrote: 'What develops? It is domain specific knowledge that develops" (1986, p. 267).

It is often assumed that the exclusive importance of domain specific knowledge is confirmed by studies comparing novices and experts. Many cognitive psychologists interpret novice–expert performance differences (where subjects are equated for IQ, memory span and education) exclusively as a consequence of the experts' increased and different content-specific knowledge within a particular domain (e.g. chess, physics, radiology). This explanation, however, is not accurate, because interpreting results from such contrastive studies runs into the same problems as interpreting results from cross-sectional studies. Specifically, it is not clear whether differences between novices and experts are valid indices for individual processes of change. In fact, it is quite likely that group differences between novices and experts arise because some proportion of novices drop out during the long process of acquiring expertise, perhaps because the cognitive demands are too hard, or because the long term motivation is missing. Thus, novices and experts may differ in more than just the possession of rich domain specific knowledge. Thus, to explain the influence of knowledge acquisition on changes in cognitive performance at an individual level, longitudinal studies are necessary. Different sorts of longitudinal methodologies can be useful in this context.

First of all, there are quasi-longitudinal designs, in which pre-experimental knowledge is carefully analysed. In this case, both the intra-individual knowledge profile and inter-individual differences in knowledge are predicted to play an important role. Not only will meaningful individual differences in the solution of cognitive tasks depend on how comprehensive domain specific expertise is but an individual's performance level will remain more stable with increasing age when an elaborated knowledge base can be used. This hypothesis has generally been confirmed in empirical studies (Knopf, Kolodziej & Preussler, 1990). It is both theoretically and pragmatically interesting that such expert skills can help compensate for age-related deficits in basic cognitive functions in the production of more complex outcomes (Salthouse, 1984).

A second longitudinal procedure is to provide systematic and controlled training in a specific expertise. Because of the enormous amount of effort required, this is usually realized in a single subjects design. A good example of such a design is a study by Staszewski (1990), who turned a single subject into a digit span memory expert by systematically training him for more than five years. Beginning with an average span of 8 digits, the subject finally achieved a span of 104 numbers, correctly repeated after a single presentation. Even more interesting than this incredible achievement, is the theoretically oriented study of the memory skills that the subject acquired from a mixture of practice, knowledge and strategies.

An example of a third variation of longitudinal designs shows how the results of such single case studies can be generalized to all age-groups. This example is of testing-the-limits experiments with unselected samples of different ages (Kliegl, Smith & Baltes, 1989). The experiments were concerned with extending word span through combining and automatizing different mnemonic techniques.

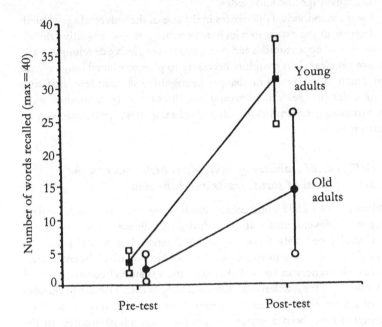

Fig. 5.2. Age × time of assessment interaction for serial recall of words in Experiment 1 (combining performance at 10 s and 4 s rates), showing the magnification of age and individual differences at post-test. (Bar lines indicate range of scores.) (Data from Kliegl et al., 1989, p.250.)

Fig. 5.2 shows that young and old adults showed equivalently large training effects and both achieved a criterion of outstanding performance. None the less, clear age differences in the extent to which maximum performance could be achieved were apparent, so that improvements in memory performance at the end of training by young and old subjects equated for IQ no longer overlapped. This pattern of results provides good evidence both for the possibility of age-independent improvement in memory performance as a consequence of acquiring expertise, and also for age-dependent limitations in the learning skills necessary for acquiring expertise. As Fig. 5.2 also makes clear, individual differences in these age-related limitations were also quite large.

If one summarizes the findings from the longitudinal studies on cognitive aging mentioned here as well as many others, some general conclusions about the meaning of individual differences for cognitive development in adulthood are possible.

- There are age-invariant individual differences in the cognitive potential to acquire new cognitive competencies.
- There are individual differences in domain specific zones of proximal

change that seem to depend on general intellectual resources as well as on domain specific knowledge.

- There are individual differences in the size of the universal age-related decrease in the extent to which one can acquire new cognitive skills.

How the individual opportunities and constraints on cognitive development are related is not yet clear. It is therefore necessary to plan combined longitudinal studies in which investigation of changes in cognitive skills in representative samples of different ages under natural conditions can be combined with specialized training programmes for selected subsamples with particular cognitive characteristics.

Differential stability of individual differences in the development of social traits and behaviour

The development of social competence is closely related to, when not dependent upon, cognitive development, at least during childhood. However, social behaviour results not only from 'social intelligence' but also depends on motivational and emotional processes and on social experience. The emergence of individual differences in social behaviour, the situational consistency and temporal stability of these differences, the continuity or discontinuity of changes in social behaviour, and the internal or external conditions governing developmental patterns have been a preferred area for longitudinal studies. In the following description of some basic questions and results, we will rely heavily on the work of Jens Asendorpf. This work stems from the Munich Longitudinal Study on the Genesis of Individual Competencies (LOGIC) mentioned above.

The following constructs were assessed in the LOGIC study of social development:

Social competence   This is a set of skills for interacting adequately and effectively with other people in the environment and an ability to influence the behaviour of another person so that it matches one's own interests. This construct was measured in the kindergarten group as well as in dyadic play with familiar and unfamiliar peers.

Social inhibition   This is an individual disposition to react by inhibiting interactive behaviour in certain social situations. This construct was measured in the kindergarten group, in the school class, and in a standardized laboratory situation. In addition, children's aggression in peer groups was both directly observed and was rated by the parents.

Personality profile   This is as measured by the California Child Q Sort. It was measured each year on the basis of ratings by the preschool/kindergarten teacher. In the discussion that follows, we will focus on some data concerning the development of social inhibition.

A central concern of most longitudinal studies, including those concerned with social inhibition, is the question of the temporal stability of individual differences. Many believe that a relatively high stability of individual differences despite age-related developmental changes means that long-term prediction of behaviour in the individual case is possible.

Even when one overlooks this misconception, the scientific yield of the many studies on stability is disappointing. What Wohlwill wrote continues to be valid: 'With only very few exceptions, work on stability . . . has consisted in the endless proliferation of correlation coefficients, to indicate the degree of relationship between measures of behavior obtained over some given time interval . . . The result has been that we have learned a little about the "behavior" of *variables* over age, but nothing concerning the behavior of individuals' (1973, pp. 358–359).

A step-by-step description of Asendorpf's research programme on social inhibition will illustrate how such pitfalls can be avoided.

The first prerequisite for a developmental analysis is to clarify the theoretical constructs one wants to investigate and to specify their behavioural indices. For example, if social inhibition is defined as 'an emotional state that is characterized by inhibited approach motivation', it must be possible to differentiate this behavioural pattern from others such as unsociability or social avoidance. The emotional state indicating social inhibition is primarily manifested as inhibition toward strangers and as inhibition in social-evaluative situations (Asendorpf, 1989*c*, in press).

The second pre-requisite for developmental analysis is an empirical test of whether the chosen behavioural indices tap the same construct at different ages. Asendorpf (1992) showed that there is a relatively perfect continuity across age in how shyness and social inhibition are expressed and are perceived.

The third step is the investigation of the general developmental sequence of the trait. In the case of social inhibition, it is possible to discern three stages: 'In the first stage, inhibition towards adult strangers is aroused by rather simple physical characteristics of the situation . . . and social evaluative inhibition is restricted to conditioned cues for punishment of frustrative non-reward. . . . In the second stage, beginning around the age of 20 months, the emerging new ability of spontaneous perspective taking arouses inhibitions towards peer and adult strangers due to a perceived uncertainty of the strangers' intentions, and social–evaluative inhibition due to the anticipation of negative or insufficiently positive social evaluations. Later on, in the third stage of the development of inhibition, the reflections about one's own self-presentation reaches awareness and becomes particularly intense during adolescence' (Asendorpf, in press).

Inter-individual differences in inhibition toward strangers are very stable over time. This is based not only on a systematic review of the literature (Asendorpf, 1989*b*, p. 79), but also on the results of the LOGIC study (Asendorpf, 1990*a*, 1993). The average, that is aggregated stability increases with increasing age from the second year of life on, and decreases only temporarily in adolescence.

Inhibition toward strangers is a personality trait that shows considerable situational and, as noted above, temporal consistency. This trait, however, loses its behavioural effect when situations and persons become more familiar, for example, in a kindergarten or school class. Table 5.2 shows the relevant results for this point from the LOGIC study (Asendorpf, 1990*b*, p. 11; Asendorpf, 1993).

Whereas the stability of individual differences in inhibition toward strangers remained stable across five measurement points, social inhibition in kindergarten and school classes was less stable, and decreased continuously between measurement points. As the correlation pattern shows, the consistency between behaviour with strangers and behaviour with familiar classmates also changed. In the first year of kindergarten and in the first year of grade school (when classmates were unfamiliar) there was a clear positive relation between inhibition toward strangers and inhibition toward classmates. However, in the third year of kindergarten and at the end of the second grade (when classmates were familiar), these correlations were no longer significant.

The temporal stability of individual differences in a sample should be assessed not only at the aggregate level, but individual social inhibition scores should also be used to assess differential stability, that is individual differences in stability (Asendorpf, 1989*a*). From a developmental perspective, data concerning the stability of inter-individual differences in intra-individual change are especially interesting because they would make the identification of differential developmental patterns possible. Asendorpf (1992*b*) showed that the stability of children's peer network was positively related to the one-year stabilities of their inhibition toward peers (as judged by their parents) for three successive one-year intervals. This finding demonstrates that the stability of individual characteristics can be profitably related to an individual's environmental stability.

The steps of the research programme described thus far have all been variable-centred, that is, they have been focused on the variable 'social inhibition', not on the organization of the personality within which social inhibition is but one trait among many. To tap the important person-centred level, Asendorpf used a Q-sort profile procedure. The Q-sort profiles showed large inter-individual differences in temporal stability, producing individual stability coefficients that, in studies from Asendorpf and van Aken (1991), varied from − .09 to .83.

How can one explain the large interindividual differences in the stability of personality patterns? A first answer to this question comes from the surprisingly strong correlations between a measure of two-year stability of the personality profile and a profile of the 'ideal child' provided by kindergarten teachers. In general, the more a child's profile approached that of the 'ideal child', the more stable was that child's profile over time (Asendorpf, 1990*b*).

In a further analysis of data from the LOGIC project, it was possible to show that children with socially inhibited behaviour increasingly tended to prefer

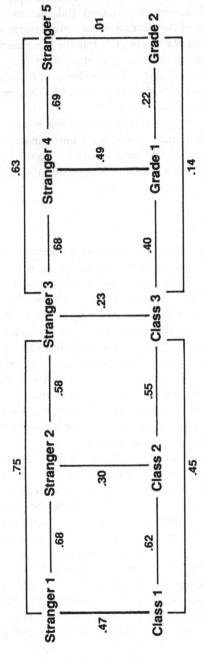

Table 5.2.　Stabilities and consistencies of social inhibition towards strangers and classmates. (Data from Asendorpf, 1990a, p.11.)

passive solo activities to social involvement. This finding suggests that an initially independent tendency to be socially inhibited becomes increasingly associated with unsociability on the overt behavioural level (Asendorpf, 1991).

One should not interpret such patterns of relations and changes in the features of social behaviour in terms of a simple causal chain. For example, social inhibition is not the only determinant of social behaviour in the peer group. The social skills and the social status of an individual also play an important role. Asendorpf (1990a), for example, found that the social inhibition of children in a classroom became more pronounced when they were ignored by their peers or when their attempts at contact initiation were rejected.

Future longitudinal studies will have to decide whether one is justified in speaking of children who are at risk for future social development in such cases. To be sure, Hymel et al. (1990) recently reported data that supported earlier findings (Kohlberg et al., 1972; Parker & Asher, 1987) that peer difficulties in early childhood are predictive of later maladjustment.

CONCLUDING REMARKS

It would be completely inappropriate to try to undermine the current preference for cross-sectional designs with a new myth of longitudinal designs. The three examples we presented should have made it very clear that a better understanding of development and individual differences in cognitive, social and emotional areas does not arise simply from testing subjects longitudinally. Rather, longitudinal studies must fulfill certain theoretical criteria and methodological standards to avoid being simply a series of cross-sectional studies with repeated measures spread out over time. In saying that good longitudinal studies must meet certain criteria, we do not refer to the usual and obvious features of good empirical research, but rather to some particular specific requirements of longitudinal designs, that are best described here as statements about the necessity of combining different research perspectives, not in a single study of course, but within a comprehensive research programme.

Variable- and person-centred approaches should be combined. This allows two things: first, on the variable-centred level, independent of the person as a structural entity, one can test psychological laws longitudinally; second, on the person-centred level, one can test hypotheses about the development of the person as an organized pattern of variables or as an intentional actor and self-reflective subject. The Swedish research project 'Individual development and adjustment' is a convincing and noteworthy example of the productivity of this research approach (Magnusson, 1988; Magnusson & Bergman, 1990).

Single-subject and large-scale designs should be combined. Using longitudinal data to fully analyse quantitative and qualitative changes in developmental functions, and to study the stability of inter-individual differences in intra-individual change is possible only when one combines the micro- and macro-genetic levels.

The potential of longitudinal research for explaining change and stability has not been sufficiently exploited. Whereas longitudinal designs are preferred for *describing* continuity and discontinuity in developmental functions, changes in individual characteristics, the stability of individual differences, and variations of inter-individual differences in intra-individual changes, the few examples of research possibilities outlined in the discussion of social development should serve as a stimulant for exploring the potential of longitudinal designs to further *explain* inter-individual differences in intra-individual change.

Longitudinal studies should generally be theoretically grounded and should allow specific hypotheses to be tested. However, longitudinal data also provide a source of hard-won data that may be used to uncover new or overlooked developmental phenomena and that may lead to the formulation of new theoretical ideas. Therefore, a combination of confirmatory and exploratory procedures in longitudinal studies should not only be an important criterion when planning single projects, but should become a dominant goal for all longitudinal research.

REFERENCES

Appelbaum, M. I. & McCall, R. B. (1983). Design and analysis in developmental psychology. In P. H. Mussen (ed.), *Handbook of child psychology: history, theory, and methods* (3rd ed.), vol. 1, pp. 415–476. New York: Wiley.

Asendorpf, J. B. (1989*a*). Individual, differential, and aggregate stability of social competence. In B. H. Schneider, G. Attili, J. Nadel & R. Weissberg (eds.), *Social competence in developmental perspective*, pp. 71–86. Dordrecht, NL: Kluwer.

Asendorpf, J. (1989*b*). *Soziale Gehemmtheit und ihre Entwicklung*. Berlin, Heidelberg, New York: Springer-Verlag.

Asendorpf, J. B. (1989*c*). Shyness as a final common pathway for two different kinds of inhibition. *Journal of Personality and Social Psychology*, **57**, 481–92.

Asendorpf, J. B. (1990*a*). Development of inhibition during childhood: Evidence for situational specificity and a two-factor model. *Developmental Psychology*, **26**, 721–30.

Asendorpf, J. B. (1990*b*). Soziale Kompetenzentwicklung zwischen dem 4. und 8. Lebensjahr. In F. E. Weinert (ed.), *Die Entwicklung kognitiver, motivationaler und sozialer Kompetenzen zwischen dem 4. und 8. Lebensjahr*. Paper Nr. 16/1990. München: Max-Planck-Institut für psychologische Forschung.

Asendorpf, J. B. (1990*c*). The measurement of individual consistency. *Methodika*, **4**, 1–23.

Asendorpf, J. B. (1991). Development of inhibited children's coping with unfamiliarity. *Child Development*, **62**, 1460–72.

Asendorpf, J. B. (1992*a*). A Brunswikean approach to trait continuity: application to shyness. *Journal of Personality*, **60**, 53–77.

Asendorpf, J. B. (1992*b*). Beyond stability: predicting interindividual differences in intraindividual change. *European Journal of Personality*, **6**, 103–17.

Asendorpf, J. B. (1993). Beyond temperament: a two-factorial coping model of the development of inhibition during childhood, pp. 265–89. In K. H. Rubin & J. B. Asendorpf (eds.), *Social withdrawal, inhibition, and shyness in childhood*. Hillsdale, EJ: Erlbaum.

Asendorpf, J. B. (in press). Social inhibition: A general-developmental perspective. In J. Pennebaker & H. C. Traue (eds.), *Emotional expression and inhibition in health and illness*. Toronto, Canada and Lewiston, NY: Hogrefe and Huber.

Asendorpf, J. B. & van Aken, M. A. G. (1991). Correlates of the temporal consistency of personality patterns in childhood. *Journal of Personality*, 59, 689–703.

Asendorpf, J. & Weinert, F. E. (1990). Stability of patterns and patterns of stability in personality development. In D. Magnusson & L. R. Bergman (eds.), *Data quality in longitudinal research*, pp. 181–197. Cambridge: Cambridge University Press.

Baltes, P. B. & Nesselroade, J. R. (1979). History and rationale of longitudinal research. In J. R. Nesselroade & P. B. Baltes (eds.), *Longitudinal research in the study of behavior and development*, pp. 1–39. New York: Academic Press.

Bryk, A. S. & Raudenbush, S. W. (1987). Application of hierarchical linear models of assessing change. *Psychological Bulletin*, 101, 147–58.

De Ribaupierre, A. (1989). Epilogue: on the use of longitudinal research in developmental psychology. In A. De Ribaupierre (ed.), *Transition mechanisms in child development*, pp. 297–317. Cambridge: Cambridge University Press.

Hatano, G. & Inagaki, K. (1986). Two courses of expertise. In H. Stevenson, H. Azuma & K. Hakuta (eds.), *Child development and education in Japan*, pp. 262–272. New York: Freeman.

Hymel, S., Rubin, K.H., Rowden, L. & LeMare, L. (1990). Children's peer relationships: longitudinal prediction of internalizing and externalizing problems from middle to late childhood. *Child Development*, 61, 2004–21.

Kagan, J. (1980). Perspectives on continuity. In O. G. Brim, Jr. & J. Kagan (eds.), *Constancy and change in human development*, pp. 26–74. Cambridge, MA: Harvard University Press.

Kliegl, R., Smith, J. & Baltes, P. B. (1989). Testing-the-limits and the study of adult age differences in cognitive plasticity and of mnemonic skill. *Developmental Psychology*, 25, 247–56.

Knopf, M., Kolodziej, P. & Preussler, W. (1990). Der ältere Mensch als Experte – Literaturübersicht über die Rolle von Expertenwissen für die kognitive Leistungsfähigkeit im höheren Alter. *Zeitschrift für Gerontopsychologie und-psychiatrie*, 4, 233–48.

Kohlberg, L., LaCrosse, I. & Ricks, D. (1972). The predictability of adult mental health from childhood behavior. In B. B. Wolman (ed.), *Manual of child psychopathology*, pp. 1217–1284. New York: McGraw-Hill.

Magnusson, D. (1981). Some methodology and strategy problems in longitudinal research. In F. Schulsinger, S. A. Mednick & J. Knop (eds.), *Longitudinal research – methods and uses in behavioral science*, pp. 192–215. Boston: Martinus Nijhoff Publishing.

Magnusson, D. (1988). *Individual development from an interactional perspective: a longitudinal study*. Hillsdale, NJ: Erlbaum.

Magnusson, D. & Bergman, L. R. (1990). A pattern approach to the study of pathways from childhood to adulthood. In L. N. Robins & M. Rutter (eds.), *Straight and devious pathways from childhood to adulthood*, pp. 101–115. Cambridge: Cambridge University Press.

Parker, J. G. & Asher, S. R. (1987). Peer relations and later personal adjustment: are low-accepted children at risk? *Psychological Bulletin*, 102, 357–89.

Rutter, M. (1987). Continuities and discontinuities from infancy. In J. D. Osofsky (ed.), *Handbook of infant development*, vol. 2, pp. 1256–1296. New York: Wiley.

Salthouse, T. A. (1984). Effects of age and skill in typing. *Journal of Experimental*

Psychology: General, **113**, 345–71.

Schaie, K. W. (1983). The Seattle Longitudinal Study. In K. W. Schaie (ed.), *Longitudinal studies of adult psychological development,* pp. 64–135. New York: Guilford.

Schaie, K. W. (1989). Individual differences in rate of cognitive change in adulthood. In V. L. Bengtson and K. W. Schaie (eds.), *The course of later life. Research and reflections,* pp. 65–85. New York: Springer.

Schaie, K. W. (1990). Intellectual development in adulthood. In J. E. Birren & K. W. Schaie (eds.), *Handbook of the psychology of aging,* (3rd ed.), pp. 291–309. San Diego: Academic Press.

Schneider, W. (1989). Problems of longitudinal studies with children: Practical, conceptual, and methodological issues. In M. Brambring, F. Lösel and H. Skowronek (eds.), *Children at risk: assessment, longitudinal research, and intervention,* pp. 313–335. New York: De Gruyter.

Schneider, W. & Edelstein, W. (1990). *Inventory of European longitudinal studies on the behavioral and medical sciences.* Berlin: Max-Planck-Institut für Bildungsforschung.

Schneider, W. & Sodian, B. (1991). A longitudinal study of young children's memory behaviour and performance in a sort–recall task. *Journal of Experimental Child Psychology,* **51**, 14–29.

Schneider, W., Knopf, M. & Weinert, F. E. (1989). Interrelationships among measures of memory and measures of intellectual development. In F. E. Weinert & W. Schneider (eds.), *The Munich Longitudinal Study on the Genesis of Individual Competencies (LOGIC). Report No. 6: psychological development in the preschool years: longitudinal results of wave one to three,* pp. 108–113. Munchen: Max Planck Institute for Psychological Research.

Siegler, R. S. & Crowley, K. (1991). The microgenetic method: a direct means for studying cognitive development. *American Psychologist,* **46**, 606–20.

Siegler, R. S. & Jenkins, E. (1989). *How children discover strategies.* Hillsdale, NJ: Erlbaum.

Staszewski, J. J. (1990). Exceptional memory: the influence of practice and knowledge on the development of elaborative encoding strategies. In W. Schneider & F. E. Weinert (eds.), *Interactions among aptitudes, strategies, and knowledge in cognitive performance,* pp. 252–285. New York: Springer-Verlag.

Verdonik, F. & Sherrod, L. R. (1984). *An inventory of longitudinal research on childhood and adolescence.* New York: Social Science Research Council.

Weinert, F. E. (1990). Entwicklungsgenetik und Sozialisationsforschung: Widersprüche, Probleme und Perspektiven. *In Entwicklung und Lernen – Beiträge zum Symposium anläßlich des 60. Geburtstages von Wolfgang Edelstein,* pp. 13–36. Berlin: MPI für Bildungsforschung.

Weinert, F. E. (1991). *Stability and variability in change of memory functions in childhood.* Paper presented at the International Conference on Memory, Lancaster, July 1991.

Weinert, F. E. & Schneider, W. (eds.) (1989*a*). *The Munich Longitudinal Study on the Genesis of Individual Competencies (LOGIC), Report No. 6: Psychological development in the preschool years: Longitudinal results of wave one to three.* München: Max Planck Institute for Psychological Research.

Weinert, F. E. & Schneider, W. (eds.) (1989*b*). *The Munich Longitudinal Study on the Genesis of Individual Competencies (LOGIC), Report Nr. 5: Results of wave three* (Technical Report). München: Max Planck Institute for Psychological Research.

Weinert, F. E. & Waldmann, M. R. (1986). How do the gifted think: intellectual abilities and cognitive processes. In A. J. Cropley, K. K. Urban, H. Wagner & W.

Wieczerkowski (eds.), *Giftedness: A continuing worldwide challenge*, pp. 49–64. New York: Trillium Press.

Weinert, F. E., Schneider, W. & Knopf, M. (1988). Individual differences in memory development across the life span. In P. B. Baltes, D. L. Featherman & R. M. Lerner (eds.), *Life-span development and behavior*, vol. 9, pp. 39–85. Hillsdale, NJ: Erlbaum.

Weiss, B., Weisz, J. R. & Bromfield, R. (1986). Performance of retarded and nonretarded persons on information processing tasks: tests of the similar structure hypotheses. *Psychological Bulletin*, **100**, 157–75.

Weisz, J. R. & Yeates, K. O. (1981). Cognitive development in retarded and non-retarded persons: Piagetian tests of the similar structure hypothesis. *Psychological Bulletin*, **90**, 153–78.

Wohlwill, J. F. (1973). *The study of behavioral development*. New York: Academic Press.

6 Developmental psychopathology: some historical and current perspectives

NORMAN GARMEZY, PHD

INTRODUCTION

Developmental psychopathology has been described as an 'emergent discipline' (Cicchetti, 1984) one 'truly . . . born over the past five years' (Zigler, 1989). What characterizes this newcomer that seeks an integration of the developmental and clinical sciences? Many characterizations have been offered, (Lewis & Miller, 1990) and these vary in complexity and coverage. On the side of simplification are the offerings of Achenbach (1990) ('. . . a general approach to understanding relations between development and its maladaptive deviations') and Lewis (1990) ('. . . the study of the prediction of maladaptive behavior and processes.')

Two definitions provide a better offering given the complexity of this growing arena of research. One has been provided by Sroufe & Rutter (1984) in a seminal article on *The domain of developmental psychopathology* in which they present both a definition and the boundaries of the field from their perspective as developmental researchers/theorists:

The very name of the discipline provides a starting point for defining the scope and particular quality of this field. First, it is concerned with development and is therefore closely wedded to the whole of developmental psychology. The methods, theories, and perspectives of developmental psychology are important tools of inquiry. Second, the focus is on pathology, that is developmental deviations. Developmental psychopathology may be defined as *the study of the origins and course of individual patterns of behavioral maladaptation*, whatever the age of onset, whatever the causes, whatever the transformations in behavioral manifestation, and however complex the course of the developmental pattern may be.   (p. 18)

The distinction Sroufe and Rutter noted between developmental psychopathology as opposed to abnormal psychology or clinical psychiatry lies in the greater outreach of its contents to include areas that go beyond the description of the symptomatology of disorders, its differentiation from other behaviours, or its emphasis on treatment all of which are central to traditional psychiatry and clinical psychology.

The focus of developmental psychopathology is on the research enterprise.

From the standpoint of this goal, the origins and time course of mental disorders are of critical importance to the developmental psychopathologist as well as are the behavioural transformations that occur at different transition points in development. (Attie, Brooks-Gunn & Petersen, 1990). Comparisons with normative behaviour at these crucial points in development constitutes a heartland of research from a developmental/psychopathological viewpoint. Both typicality and atypicality are of particular interest in this research orientation. Who are the at-risk persons? What are their behavioural and biological patterns over time? What are the potentiating events in disorder? Who among those presumed to be at-risk individuals fail to manifest a disorder in contrast to those who do? What are the continuities and discontinuities reflected in normal and aberrant development? Who, seemingly not at all viewed as at-risk candidates develop psychopathology somewhere along the developmental trail? What are the sources of competence and vulnerabilities in development? And, above all, what factors, processes, and mechanisms operate to produce seemingly unanticipated outcomes as well as those that are more predictable? This last issue reflects quite a different focus from the traditional one of clinical psychiatry and clinical psychology wherein the emphasis is primarily on those who become disordered. The vision of an invariant future trajectory over time of those who have shown incipient signs of disorder or are considered to be at-risk is not an inevitable one as numerous follow-up studies indicate. (Anthony & Cohler, 1987; Elder, 1974; Festinger, 1983; Watt et al., 1984).

Two consequences follow for developmental psychopathologists from their joint focus on adaptive *and* maladaptive outcomes for at-risk populations. First, there is the need to consider multiple comparison groups that go beyond the traditional control group. Secondly, longitudinal investigations, both short-term and long-term, assume their rightful place as a research method of choice in seeking to pinpoint behavioural transitions at age periods typically marked by more stable vs. more unstable behaviours.

In considering the range of environmental variables that influence development Eisenberg (1977) includes: disorganized homes, lack of environmental stimulation, failure of mother–child bonding, malnourishment, nutritional neglect, poor housing, overcrowdedness in the home, lack of intellectual stimulation, poor schooling, etc.

To cite an example of antecedent and consequent, Eisenberg chose the world-wide problem of nutrition with its multiple effects over time on early neurobiological development, on developmental retardation and the incapacity of the infant to attend to the environment and to engage in information-processing, on the modification of the child's relationships with caretakers and later with peers, on school failure, and the child's restriction of subsequent opportunity.

Malnutrition is inevitably linked to poverty, which in turn brings in its wake a circular pattern of stressors marked by short-term and long-term effects. Fig.

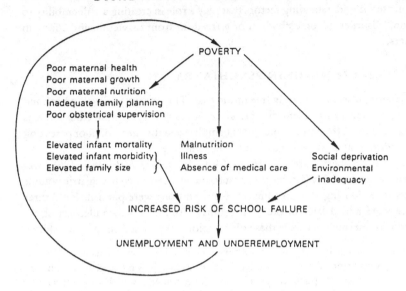

Fig. 6.1.   A model of the negative consequences of poverty. (Birch & Gussow, 1970)

6.1 (Birch & Gussow, 1970) illustrates the life-span developmental consequences of poverty. Long-term poverty initiates an inter-generational cycle in
which poor maternal health, absent or poor obstetrical care during pregnancy,
and inadequate maternal nutrition, all conduce to heighten the probability of
greater infant mortality and morbidity, and the poor health status of the infant
and child. School failure which often characterizes the behavioural patterns of
many impoverished children in the pre-school years (e.g. attention deficits,
inappropriate behaviours, failure to learn to read, poor peer relations) that
insures later inadequate school performance and early dropout. There follow
life-time patterns of unemployment and under-employment and the maintenance of poverty in the adult with its reiteration of the same despairing cycle of
events on the generation to follow.

    The seminal writings on developmental psychopathology of three dis-
tinguished child psychiatrists, Rutter (1979, 1980*b*, 1985, 1988*a*, 1990), Bowlby
(1973, 1980, 1982, 1988), & Eisenberg (1977), provide a picture of current and
projected research activities that reveals the potential contributions that can
stem from the union of the developmental and the clinical sciences. Such a
future inter-disciplinary collaboration, the ultimate scope of developmental
psychopathology, may in time begin to incorporate under its family tree the
contributions of a large body of significant biological, behavioural, and social
sciences and their integration with relevant medical specialties.

    It is difficult at this point to conceive that this infant field in science can be
assisted in its growth by older distinguished forebears but it is important to

recognize that these disciplines do provide a breadth of knowledge that is a requisite for understanding factors that play a role in creating a vulnerability to mental disorder in some children or a freedom from its victimizing effects in others.

BEGINNINGS IN PSYCHIATRY

An emergent science is rarely free of the past. The linkage of development and psychopathology has a lengthy if unsystematic history. One famed example is drawn from a 17th century volume that emphasized the effects of poor parenting in childhood as a precursor to adult 'melancholia'.

In 1621, Robert Burton's (1577–1640) *Anatomy of Melancholy* (1961) was published and quickly became the most frequently reprinted psychiatric volume of its time. During Burton's life-time, five editions were published and three more were added later in the 17th century. Among his formulations of the origins of melancholia were these observations of parental effects on children:

Parents and such as have the tuition and oversight of children, offered many times in that they are too sterne, always threatning, chiding, brawling, whipping, or striking; by meanes of which their poore children are so disheartned & cowed that they never after have any courage, or a merry houre in their lives, or take pleasure in any thing . . .

Others againe in that other extreame does as much harme . . . Too much indulgence causeth the like, many fond mothers especially, dote so much upon their children like Aesops ape, till in the end they crush them to death.

(Cited in Hunter & Macalpine, 1963, p. 97)

This passage initiated accounts of parental blame for mental disorder in the later lives of children – a developmental proposition that has had a centuries' old psychiatric history.

There is a closer and more contributory relative on the family tree of developmental psychopathology, one deeply rooted in 20th century psychiatry and far more relevant to the developmental tradition. It resides in the contributions of Adolf Meyer whose 'commonsense psychiatry' (Lief, 1948) was rooted in psychobiology and the search for the relevant life-history factors that could help to determine those risk factors that might be operative in mental disorder.

The origins of this then uncommon view provides an interesting story that is relevant to contemporary developmental psychopathology. Meyer initially received his medical training in Switzerland, where he came under the tutelage of Professor August Forel at the University of Zurich. Forel's interest lay in brain anatomy and these interests for Meyer were furthered by other faculty members trained in neurology. But despite this primary orientation, Meyer's biographers have noted his concurrent preoccupation with other mentors who provided him with an expanded view of a 'dynamic human organism making adjustments to life.' (Lief, 1948). In one sense, this duality captures part of the essence of developmental psychopathology.

Meyer came to America to pursue his neuropsychiatric goals. He accepted a position as a pathologist in a mid-western state mental hospital where he began his study of the brains of deceased schizophrenic patients. He hoped that this work might yield up the mysteries of that intransigent disease – a hope unrealized, and yet a failure that proved productive. Gradually, Meyer began to formulate a 'psychobiology' of mental disorder in which a confluence of contributions incorporated both a biological/organic and a psychological/ socio-cultural perspective in a formulation of aetiological hypotheses of schizophrenia. Pondering the origins of mental disturbances, Meyer began to gather the early histories of his patients, seeking to insure that both psychogenic and constitutional data were included.

Meyer's biographer, (Lief, 1948) in describing the growth of Meyer's formulation writes:

The roots of a person's good qualities as well as evil anomalies could be found in 'the period of plasticity,' with its early surroundings and lasting impressions. Too much was made of heredity; the significant thing was that 'the child of abnormal parents is apt to be exposed from birth to acquire unconsciously habits of morbid character. (p. 51)

Meyer provided a view of symptomatology that serves the goals of contemporary developmental psychopathology. He urged that symptoms not be misinterpreted for in isolation a given symptom might be observed even in a normal person. What Meyer sought was the connection of a given symptom to other symptoms. That constituted the pathology side; on the recovery side, Meyer sought indications of a person's power to overcome a given symptom. It is this recovery function that has become another arena of investigation for contemporary developmental psychopathologists.

Meyer's scholarship and productivity ultimately carried him to one of America's most prestigious posts in academic psychiatry – the chairmanship of the Department of Psychiatry of the Johns Hopkins' Medical School. From that point on his outreach was formidable. In time he formulated his views of the 'psychobiology' of mental disorder and spread the gospel of a discipline that could include a biological/psychological/socio-cultural perspective in formulating etiologic hypotheses of mental disorders.

On July 12, 1919 in a symposium honouring a legendary physician, Sir William Osler, Meyer (1919) presented a paper that can serve as a landmark article for developmental psychopathology. He titled it 'The Life Chart', as a working instrument that reflected an individual's case study in which the contributions of personality study accompanied by a thorough review of case history materials would focus on the patient's 'life situation'. It incorporated stressful life events and their correlated effects in illness or psychiatric disorder.

These elements that included a view of the social forces acting upon the mental patient slowly began to take hold in American psychiatry. Meyer advocated that an investigation of the patient's life history, if obtained carefully and verified, would lead to a tracing of 'the genesis and development of behavior without the extensive probing of the unconscious'. Central to the success of that task was the need for a 'chronological, longitudinal life-history'. With the acquisition of such a data base, the patient could then be studied as 'an experiment in nature'. To foster his investigation of the individual patient, Meyer drew on multiple fields involved in the development of human behaviour with the goal of opening all 'worthy avenues' in the study of mental disorders.

Figs 6.2 and 6.3 are reproductions of the 'Life Charts' of two of Meyer's cases, the first, that of a schizophrenic patient, the second summarizes a portion of the life history of a patient suffering from 'invalidism'. While schizophrenia has retained a diagnostic similarity over decades, 'invalidism' has not. Current psychiatric classification would likely redesignate invalidism as a somatoform disorder with the specific assignment of a formal diagnosis of Hypochondriasis or Hypochondriacal Neurosis (Campbell, 1989). An essential feature of the disorder is 'preoccupation with the fear of having, or the belief that one has, a serious disease, based on the person's interpretation of physical signs of sensations as evidence of physical illness'. (DSM III-R, 1987, p. 259).

Meyer had the insight to perceive that life stressors throughout one's life-time could play an instrumental role in the development of a mental disorder. Hence, there had to be great care in recording the life-history data, a task that was accompanied by a set of rules that he detailed. (This information will help the reader in perusing the two life charts.)

We begin with the entering of date and year of birth so as to be able to read off easily the individual age and the corresponding calendar years . . . ; we next enter the periods of disorders of the various organs, and after this the data concerning the situations and reaction of the patient. The space on either side of the tracing of the organism is used for explanations, but specifically for the data which constitute the principal situations and reactions expressing the 'mental' record, permitting various degrees of completeness. On the right border near the edge we may note the changes of habitat, of school entrance, graduations or changes, or failures; the various jobs; the dates for possible important births and deaths in the family, and other fundamentally important environmental influences. Brackets indicate the duration of some of these features. Any specific trends of special importance in the evolution of the illness had best be underscored with different colored inks.

It is well to put on the left side the entries concerning special diseases, the sex life, etc. In case the details of illness required more space, certain periods can be chartered on a supplementary chart so as to make the space represent months instead of years.

(Meyer, 1919; pp. 419–422)

Meyer's 'Life Chart' bore in miniature his view of psychiatry's mission, one that partially anticipated tasks we now identify with developmental psychopathology:

1 A life-span developmental view of the mentally disordered with an emphasis on longitudinal accounts of their life-histories on the premise that to comprehend behaviour at any given point in time requires knowledge of what has preceded it;

2 The encompassing belief that development is an integrating theme in psychopathology;

3 The significance of temporally stressful events that either precede or accompany the onset of symptoms of psychopathology;

4 A broadened view of the etiology of psychiatric disorders that incorporated biological, psychological, and socio-cultural contributions in the search for an understanding of their origins and course;

5 A recognition that the mentally disordered patient represents more than a disease process; that significant antecedents are derived from sources that reflect the multiple scientific disciplines that contribute to an understanding of mental disorders;

6 An emphasis on vulnerability and risk factors that are implicated in mental disorder, thus placing psychopathology in the context of a deviation from normative patterns the shaping sources of which are located in 'endowment' (i.e. biogenetics), personality, and the social setting;

To quote one of Meyer's biographers:

'Besides behavior situations and life situations, Meyer saw in the problem of adjusting individual and environment the necessity of studying the patient's energy, endowment, capacity for constructive composure, ability to muster assets in emergencies (judgement), extent of the need of consistency (personality), inclusion of others, tendencies of action in vision, thought, fancy, play, work, prospect, retrospect, and the amount of socialization, as opposed to the mere self-concern and almost obsessive individualism so rampant today.' (Lief, 1948, p. 545)

7 Lastly, Mayer perceived a contemporary image, 70 years in advance of his time, of the role of the community as a protective factor against the incursion of psychopathology. Meyer's view was that 'communities have to learn what they produce in the way of mental problems and waste of human opportunities, and with such knowledge they will rise from mere charity and mere mending or hasty propaganda to well-balanced early care, prevention, and the general gain of health, efficiency, and happiness'. (Meyer, 1930 in Lief, p. 456)

These Meyerian contributions, today reconstructed and demonstrably powerful, have not escaped the attention of scholars of developmental psychopathology. Two of the leaders in this field are: 1) Cicchetti (1984, 1989), who has provided the historical heritage of this new interdisciplinary science; and 2) M. Rutter (e.g. 1983, 1984a, 1984b, 1985, 1986, 1988b, 1989 and Rutter & Garmezy (1983), Rutter & Hersov (1985)) whose numerous writings have established the significance and the place of this emergent discipline. These investigators have written of the historical and contemporary underpinnings of psychopathology in recognizing the contributions of an inter-disciplinary core of sciences. The rapid development of the neurosciences has added further power by heighten-

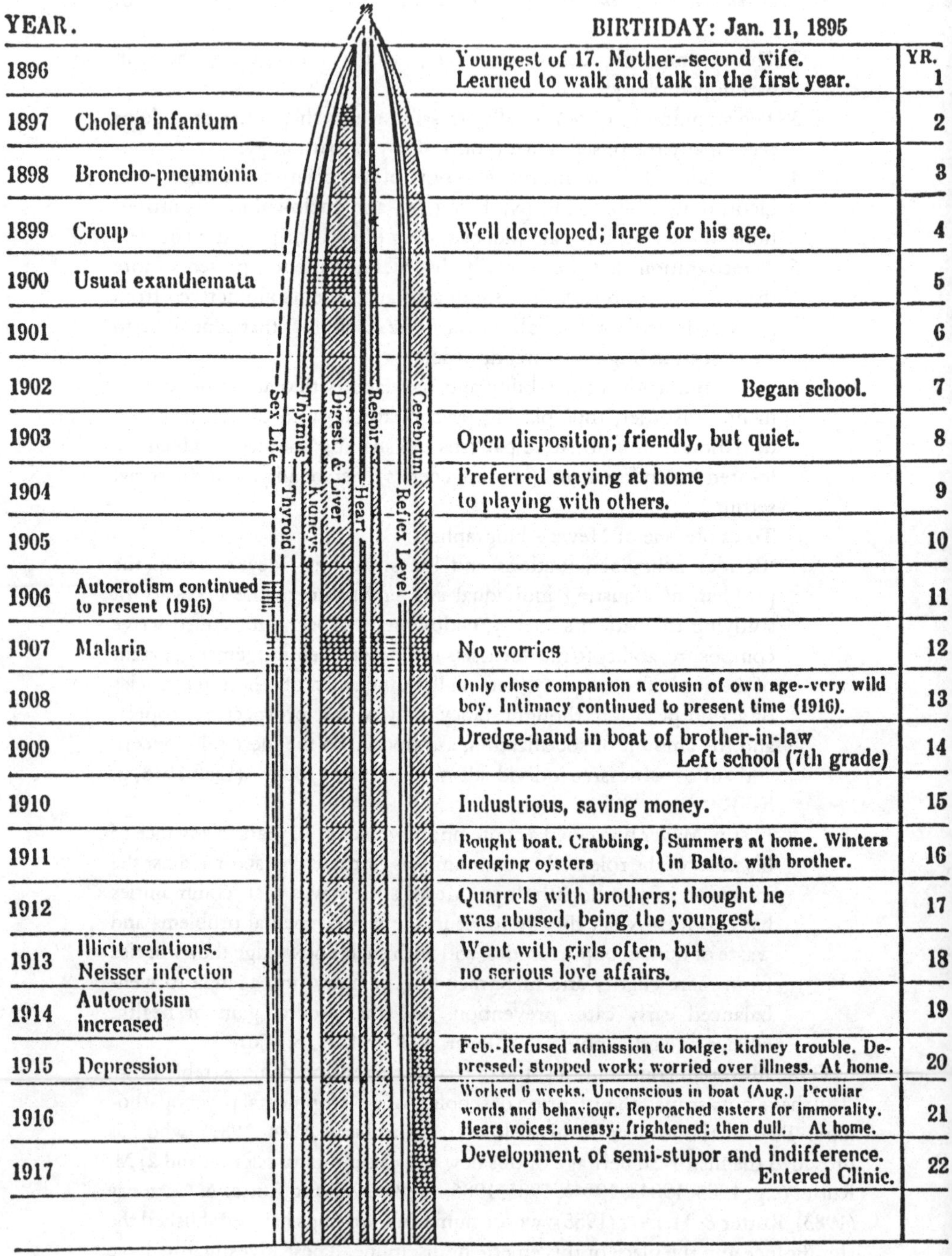

A Case of Schizophrenia

Fig. 6.2.   Meyer's life chart: a case of schizophrenia. (Meyer, 1919)

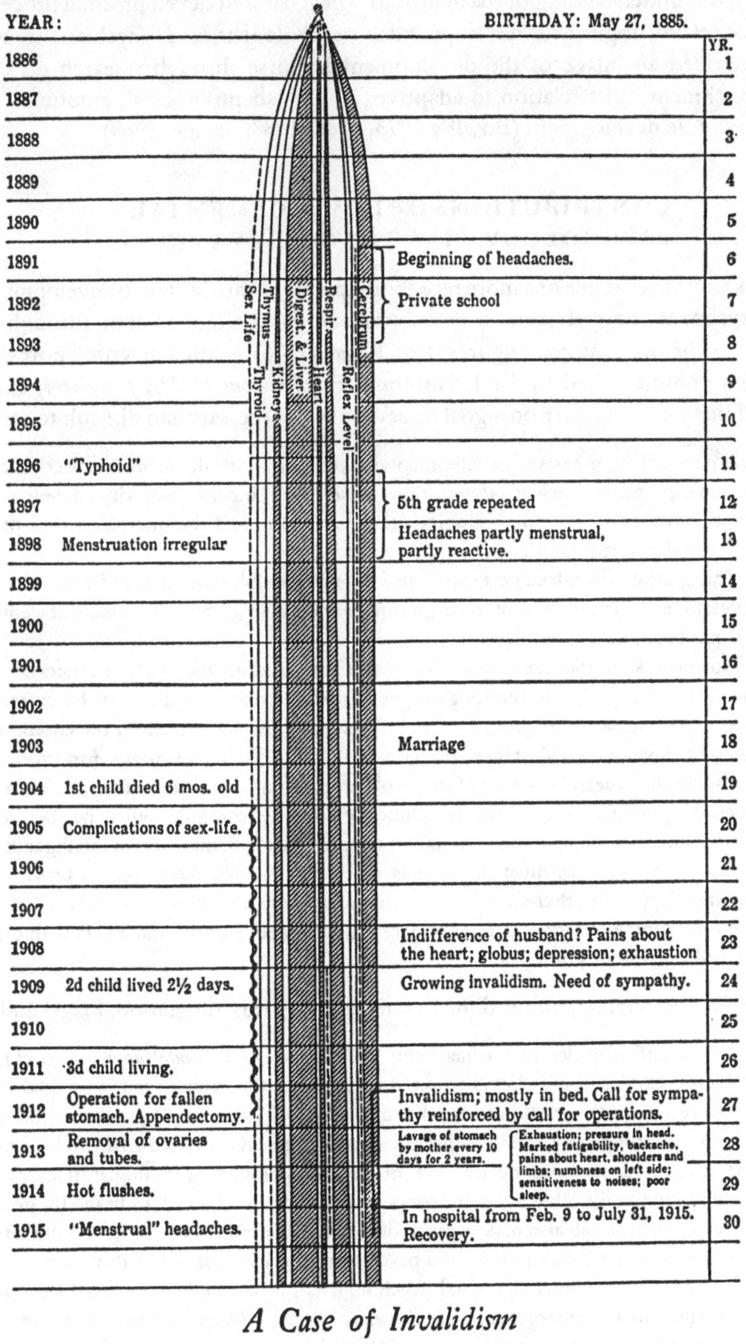
YEAR:
BIRTHDAY: May 27, 1885.
YR.
1886
1
1887
2
1888
3
1889
4
1890
5
1891
Beginning of headaches.
6
1892
Private school
7
1893
8
1894
9
1895
10
1896
"Typhoid"
11
1897
5th grade repeated
12
1898
Menstruation irregular
Headaches partly menstrual, partly reactive.
13
1899
14
1900
15
1901
16
1902
17
1903
Marriage
18
1904
1st child died 6 mos. old
19
1905
Complications of sex-life.
20
1906
21
1907
22
1908
Indifference of husband? Pains about the heart; globus; depression; exhaustion
23
1909
2d child lived 2½ days.
Growing invalidism. Need of sympathy.
24
1910
25
1911
3d child living.
26
1912
Operation for fallen stomach. Appendectomy.
Invalidism; mostly in bed. Call for sympathy reinforced by call for operations.
27
1913
Removal of ovaries and tubes.
Lavage of stomach by mother every 10 days for 2 years.
Exhaustion; pressure in head. Marked fatigability, backache, pains about heart, shoulders and limbs; numbness on left side; sensitiveness to noises; poor sleep.
28
1914
Hot flushes.
29
1915
"Menstrual" headaches.
In hospital from Feb. 9 to July 31, 1915. Recovery.
30
Sex Life
Thymus
Thyroid
Kidneys
Digest. & Liver
Respir
Heart
Reflex Level
Cerebrum
A Case of Invalidism

Fig. 6.3. Meyer's life chart: a case of invalidism. (Meyer, 1919)

ing our understanding of the neurobiological bases of developmental processes just as distinguished developmental psychologists and psychiatrists have provided an image of the developmental course through research on early attachment in its relation to adaptive, and maladaptive social, emotional and cognitive development (Bowlby 1973, 1982, 1988; Sroufe, 1989).

CONTRIBUTIONS OF DEVELOPMENTAL PSYCHOLOGY: PIAGET'S OBSERVATIONS

As another example of a more recent disciplinary contribution to developmental psychopathology I turn to developmental psychology as seen through the vision of one of its great figures, Jean Piaget (1975). Invited to write a Foreword to a volume edited by E. J. Anthony, *Explorations in child psychiatry*, Piaget offered a commentary on a goal he saw as both necessary and difficult to attain:

This goal is the synthesis of developmental psychology with all the other aspects of child psychology into a *science of ontogenetic development* from birth to maturity encompassing three points of view – the biological, the behavioral, and the internalizations of the behavioral into mental life.

This synthesis is indeed necessary since it is not possible to understand a disorder or a developmental arrest without having a sufficient knowledge of the ensemble of elements that has brought it about . . .

However, since there are those who remain normal in situations where others become variously disturbed, the meaning of the disorder to be remedied can be extremely diverse, and in order to grasp it, it is necessary to immerse oneself in the ensemble at different developmental stages, the order of which is by no means fortuitous but resembles the orderly sequence of stages observed in embryogenesis. Thus, for example, when the psychiatrist is confronted clinically with a learning disability, he should not content himself merely with the signs and symptoms or with measures of intelligence and emotionality; what he must discover is the level at which the cognitive process has foundered and must, therefore, examine the patient as to his stage of operational thinking (logical, arithmetical, spatial, temporal, causal, etc.) and integrate these data with others derived from more clinical inquiry.

Then in referring to the difficulty of achieving this integration, Piaget added:

The . . . difficulty lies in the necessity of using an *experimental approach* to clinical problems. Clinicians are always tempted to overstate the value of the individual 'case' and to construct theories on isolated and exceptional instances. If psychopathology is ever to be a completely scientific discipline, it requires an effort and an attitude of mind that approximates more nearly that of the physiologist or biologist than of the practitioner. On the other hand, the cooperation between the 'case' study and the general processes at work can also make a most informative contribution, and we can, therefore, look forward very much to the child psychiatry that develops out of this.

To put it briefly, developmental psychologists . . . are looking forward with great expectation to the emergence of *developmental psychopathology* as a new discipline still struggling to organize its own relevant field of knowledge. They are hoping especially that in spite of all the obstacles in the way and the huge amount of creative effort required for the purpose that this science will constitute itself on an interdisciplinary basis as wide as possible and on a common language that helps to unify what is precise and generalizable. (pp. vii–ix)

Sixteen years later Piaget's hoped-for emergence has begun to be realized.

THE ROLE OF ATTACHMENT IN THE LIFE HISTORY: BOWLBY'S CONTRIBUTIONS

No effort to highlight the contributions of major figures who influenced the early origins of developmental psychopathology would be complete without citing the work of John Bowlby. For half a century Bowlby's concern with the interrelatedness of maternal care and mental health (1951), the impact of pathological processes set in motion by early mother–child separation (1953), separation anxiety (1960*a*), the effects of grief and mourning in infancy and early childhood (1960*b*), the making and breaking of affectional bonds (1979), developmental psychiatry (1988), and three seminal volumes on *Attachment and loss* (Bowlby 1973, 1980, 1982) that were focused in turn on *Attachment* (Vol I), *Separation, anxiety, and anger* (Vol II) and *Loss, sadness and depression* (Vol III) provided the base for an exploration by numerous investigators of short-term and long-range consequences of an effective vs. an inadequate attachment of the infant to the maternal figure. It also served to foster the evolution of a developmental approach to psychopathology.

Bowlby's personal 'attachment' to a life-long developmental psychopathology is contained in the Epilogue to Vol III, and particularly its closing paragraph:

Intimate attachments to other human beings are the hub around which a person's life evolves, not only when he is an infant or a toddler or a school child but throughout his adolescence and his years of maturity as well, and on into old age. From these intimate attachments a person draws his strength and enjoyment of life and, through what he contributes, he gives strength and enjoyment to others. These are matters about which current science and traditional wisdom are at one. (p. 442)

In one of his final articles, presented as the Adolf Meyer Lecture to the American Psychiatric Association, Bowlby (1988), called attention to the reality that 'Developmental Psychiatry' had come of age and that one such manifestation resided in research showing that the degree of a person's vulnerability to life stressors was 'strongly influenced by the development and current state of his or her intimate relationships'. (p. 1) In this article, Bowlby laid stress on testing the hypothesis that a person's resilience or vulnerability to stressful life events is determined to a large extent by patterns of attachment in the early years. But Bowlby's final message took a broader turn. He urged that the contemporary scene was not to be neglected, for the present too provides variable events that can modify the patterns of individual resistance or vulnerability.

To broaden our knowledge of life-span influences on adaptation Bowlby called for an increase in prospective longitudinal studies carried out through 'different phases of the life cycle and in different environments'. (p. 9) He saw the research needs as extending over generations and compared the task ahead as one comparable to past and ongoing studies of immunology. The central task of developmental psychopathology he asserted is analogous to ... 'the degree to which an organism is immune to a wide variety of hazards and the extent to which an existing state of immunity will persist or change over time'. (p. 9)

CONTRIBUTIONS OF PSYCHOANALYSIS: ANNA FREUD AND DEVELOPMENTAL LINES

Having illustrated the vision of major figures in psychiatry and developmental psychology and psychiatry, it is appropriate to turn to another contributor drawn from the field of psychoanalysis. The rise of psychoanalysis followed upon Meyerian psychobiology which gradually moved off centre stage. It was supplanted, in part, by a dynamic psychiatry that placed its emphasis on 1) early development in the form of a topographical model of mind which delineated conscious, pre-conscious and unconscious mental contexts; 2) a structural model of psychological conflict between id, superego, and ego; and 3) a developmental model of stages in the formation of object relations (i.e. oral, anal, phallic, and genital stages).

This 'dynamic' child psychiatry has also made its mark on contemporary developmental psychopathology. In contemplating the role of maturity and mastery so central to the development of resilient behaviour, Anna Freud (1965, 1976) set forth a conception of developmental lines to provide tracings of the growth of the individual's personality from profound early dependency in childhood to ultimate mastery of his or her internal and external worlds.

This concept of developmental lines is wholly consistent with the orientation of contemporary developmental psychopathology. To evaluate a child's performance on a variety of age-appropriate tasks is to accept the significance of inter- and intra-individual variation in multiple behavioural domains. Unlike the earlier psychiatric emphasis on symptomatology, Anna Freud's conception sought to evaluate both deficits and assets in the course of the development of the child. This formulation is consistent with developmental psychopathology's focus both on normative and non-normative development over time. Anna Freud's model emphasizes the multiple contributions to a child's development: motivational factors, ego and superego development, and reactivity to environmental influences.

This important linkage to the current scene, and to Adolf Meyer's views as well, is best realized in the closing sentences of Anna Freud's (1976) Maudsley Lecture:

It has been the object of this paper to pursue some links between mental health and illness, immaturity and maturity. It was its further aim to convince psychiatrists of adults that there is much to be learned from child psychiatry and to convince child psychiatrists that infantile psychopathology should be assessed against the background knowledge of normal development.   (pp. 405–406)

It is this agreed upon context that four major figures, representing very diverse views of the tasks of clinical psychiatry, used to generate a degree of convergence of views within the emergent area of developmental psychopathology.

DEVELOPMENTAL PSYCHOPATHOLOGY: RESEARCH ON CHILDREN AT RISK

In specifying the types of studies that reflect the orientation of developmental psychopathology, Sroufe & Rutter (1984) have cited risk research as 'paradigmatic' of the area.

'Children-at-risk' (now a highly popularized term) defines a status marked by a heightened probability for disorder at some time in the life-span of a child (or an adult) as a consequence of risk factors that may originate in genetic predisposition, personality dispositional attributes, harsh familial circumstances, negative environmental conditions ranging from ghetto life to foster home or institutional placements, physical limitations, disadvantaged socio-cultural backgrounds such as poverty, undesired and unsought for migration to another culture, or severe trauma such as war, sequential dislocations, parental loss, enslavement, holocaust experiences, etc (Robins & Rutter, 1990).

Since these events can occur at various points in the life cycle with unremitting consequences over time, the concept of a life span developmental psychopathology has been recognized as a valid bridging description of retained risk status. To study the range of the temporal antecedents potentially implicated in psychopathology, four research methods have been found useful in studying life-span factors and their effects. (Garmezy & Streitman 1974; Garmezy, 1974)

Type I: the case study

The case study method has been identified as a clinical retrospective method in which single case studies serve as the basis for ascertaining risk status and outcome. More sophisticated methods have supplanted the case study but, as an initial incursion into the area of risk research for purposes of hypothesis formation, the case study remains an instrument of value. (Garmezy, 1982) Examples of contributory case studies are not uncommon. Perhaps the most complete case study ever constructed in psychiatry, and maintained with long-term follow-up was that of the Genain Quadruplets, who were identical quads all of whom at some point exhibited schizophrenia (a highly improbable statistical event) or schizophrenic-like behaviour with varying long-term consequences. Variations in onset, depth of the disorder, and differences in level of functioning and adaptation made evident the complexity of factors that influence the course of psychiatric disorder. (Rosenthal, 1963; Mirsky et al., 1987)

Another page from the literature of schizophrenia is Bleuler's (1984) presentation of a 'paradoxical' case study: Vreni, the daughter of a chronic schizophrenic mother and an alcoholic father, who held her family together, including multiple siblings, despite difficult familial conditions, and did so by dint of her personal characteristics and courage. These cases have pointed the way to explanations based not solely on genetic factors, but also on psychological responses to stress, and socio-cultural elements that can influence mental disorder, but provide evidence of resilience influences as well.

Type II: follow-back studies: the search for childhood origins of risk

These studies are often retrospective reports based on societal records. The beginning point is typically at a later age when manifestations of disordered behaviour that are becoming evident warrant a search of records of the individual's past history such as school records, court assessments, teacher judgments, peer relations data, and significant familial data as an entry point for evaluating early precursor signs of disorder.

A famed quotation by Freud (1955), now well known by repeated citation, raises a basic issue as to the validity of extrapolations from such retrospective methods:

So long as we trace development from its final outcome backwards, the chain of events appears continuous, and we feel we have gained an insight which is completely satisfactory and even exhaustive. But if we proceed the reverse way, if we start from the premises inferred from the analysis and try to follow these up from the final result, then we no longer get the impression of an inevitable sequence of events which could not have been otherwise determined. We notice at once that there might have been another result, and that we might have been just as able to understand and explain the latter . . . Hence the chain of causation can always be recognized with certainty if we follow the line of analysis whereas to predict . . . is impossible.   (pp. 167–168)

Type III: follow-up studies: the child at risk as adult

Follow-up research studies which have a lengthy history, typically provide two time points, the patterns of subject behaviour at an earlier age, usually childhood or adolescence, and then the search to locate those individuals in adulthood to evaluate their contemporary status.

Three decades ago, Stone & Onque (1959) published a *Review of studies of child personality*, which included early follow-up studies, many focused on at-risk children. One such study cited in the early 1920s focused on the outcomes of fostered children. (Theis, 1924) Over a time-span that was variable extending up to 18 years, the author reported successful adjustment in adulthood after release into the community of three-quarters of the children in the study, with the proportion greatest for those placed in better homes prior to age 5. A more recent study by Festinger (1983) of a greater-at-risk group of children (some 70% minority) placed in foster homes and institutional settings is confirmatory of these positive findings derived from earlier research conducted in the 1920s.

The method poses numerous problems. It predisposes to negative outcomes by the selection of the at-risk group, often without adequate and comparable control cases matched to attributes not related to the selection criterion. Secondly, it does not allow a detailed accounting of the many interim events, and the varied patterns of development change that have occurred between selection (Time 1) and follow-up (Time 2). Thirdly, if selection is based on early symptomatology, the processes that might account for the early onset of maladaptive behaviour can no longer be attended to with reliability in follow-up research. The method, however, can provide data on outcomes of at-risk children, but not about the temporal developmental processes implicated in good and poor outcomes.

Type IV: follow-through research

In this fourth type of research, the ascendant method of current investigative choice, the researcher seeks out a cohort of children who exhibit, (often by inferred genetic or environmental factors present in their life-histories), a presumed risk status that may reflect a heightened probability of a negative outcome in adulthood. This is a variant of the 'follow-up' strategy but an important difference is that it typically involves multiple evaluation points concurrent with the age status of the members of the cohort. The longitudinal study best delineates the phenomenon of growth, the role of antecedent and concurrent significant experiences, both stressful and normative, and the impact of such experience on the adaptational efforts of the members of the cohort. It is the most powerful method of the study of lives in which various age-stage characteristics of children or adolescents moving toward adulthood can be studied with special attention given to developmental transitions and transformation, continuities and discontinuities in behaviour, and shifts in status and adaptation over time.

LONGITUDINAL PROSPECTIVE STUDIES OF CHILDREN AT RISK FOR SCHIZOPHRENIA

Most of the studies created by an earlier consortium of research groups focused on developmental studies of children at risk for schizophrenia adopted this research method and thus added significantly to our knowledge of the later consequences for children born to schizophrenic parents. (This was the criterion of presumed risk status used by most of the research programme.) Two sources of information on the results of these diverse research programmes are provided in a lengthy significant volume edited by Watt et al. (1984), with a later follow-up of the findings of these multiple projects reported in an issue of the *Schizophrenia Bulletin* edited by Goldstein & Tuma (1987). Rutter (1966) had earlier anticipated the movement with his monograph on: *Children of sick parents: an environmental and psychiatric study*.

These research programmes (e.g. Mednick, et al., 1984) in their breadth and depth are a clear advance over the tabular genetic studies of an earlier era that provided rates for the occurrence of schizophrenia in offspring born of schizophrenic parentage. They move us closer to the critical issue of the processes and mechanisms that underlie resistance and capitulation factors in high-risk offspring. Developmental studies of adaptation of at-risk children, over time, were these to be joined to future advances in the molecular genetics of schizophrenia there would be the collaborative pairing necessary to provide in time an enhanced understanding of cases in which risk status is actualized into disorder and other cases in which outcomes of disorder for similar risk statuses remain unfulfilled.

To illustrate differences in research approaches to this area of a developmental–psychopathological approach to children at risk for schizophrenia, I present two studies. In one, the genre of developmental psychopathology research is clearly evident, while the other which, although non-developmental in its orientation, is also of significance for inferring some potential barriers to healthy development. Both are contributions to the study of children at risk for schizophrenia, but developmental considerations is the focus of one, while another hints at potential but speculative developmental outcomes.

The illustrative example of a truly developmental study is drawn from an article titled *A process model for the development of schizophrenia* (Marcus et al., 1987; Hans & Marcus, 1987). This study was part of the NIMH–Jerusalem collaborative investigation of children at risk for schizophrenia that was conducted in Israel. This investigation, under the international sponsorship of the National Institutes of Mental Health and an Israeli core of scholars, centred on studying the interactive effects on children at genetic risk for schizophrenia with variations in their rearing conditions. The decision was made at the induction of the study to follow the offspring of two groups of schizophrenic mothers, one group living in the city and the other on kibbutzim, which are rural agricultural collective communities in Israel. In the kibbutzim, children did not live with their parents but in a separate children's house where they were cared for by 'metapelets'. However, the children were in daily contact with their parents. In the comparison condition, the children of schizophrenic mothers were living in their parental homes in town.

David Rosenthal, a distinguished behavioural geneticist was then the Principal Investigator and Head of the Laboratory of Psychology in the NIMH Intramural Research Programme. He believed that the kibbutz environment

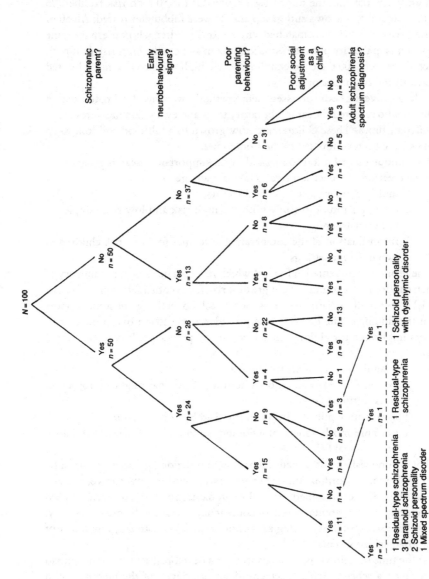

Fig. 6.4. A decision-tree model for the development of schizophrenia: the Israeli high-risk study. (Marcus et al, 1987)

would be a protective factor because negative or uncertainties in behaviour exhibited by the mother would be of a briefer duration (i.e. the result of less contact) and hence would produce a less traumatic effect on the child's development. Further, there would be the positive enhancement and care provided by an adaptable metapelet.

The investigations were systematic and in depth. Fifty families were studied in both the at-risk and the normative groups. Of the 50 high-risk families, 25 were located in an in-town sub-group and 25 were kibbutzim-reared. All 50 of the high-risk children were matched with control children who were in the same school class in the city or in the same kibbutzim as were the high-risk group. In effect, there were 100 matched couplings – two high and two low risk – located in each of the two types of settings.

A large diverse body of assessment methods were used with the paired children who received the same laboratory tasks and evaluation measures albeit at different times. These children are now grown to adulthood and follow-up studies have been conducted of their outcomes.

The unique contribution to method in this important research programme was the creation of a decision tree to take advantage of:

1 multiple potential aetiological factors;
2 the opportunity to study both the high-risk and low-risk samples as individuals; and
3 the evaluation of the comparative outcomes for high-risk children in two different settings.

The results are presented in Fig. 6.4 which reflects a decision tree summary of which children were found to be at greatest risk for eventual schizophrenia. The model is essentially a diathesis–stress theoretical model that gains some support from the findings. The decision tree provides a succession over time of risk factors implicated for children of schizophrenic parentage. In sequence these were:

1 a family history of schizophrenia;
2 evidence of early neurobehavioural deficits that might be rooted in constitutional factors;
3 a stressful family environment marked by poor parenting;
4 poor pre-morbid social functioning as adduced from social withdrawal or antisocial behaviour.

The second risk factor of neurobehavioural functioning was determined by tests of: 1) motor coordination; 2) hyperkinesis (impulsive, overactive, restless, distractible, due to presumed residual brain damage); 3) environmental stress particularly in the parental home (inconsistency, over-involvement, hostility, etc.; 4) the quality of the offspring's pre-morbid social adjustment; 5) presence of diagnosed schizophrenia.

At the time of follow-up, nine offspring had developed schizophrenia or had been given a schizophrenia spectrum diagnosis. Seven of the nine had been exposed to all four risk factors in their childhood history, one person was the victim of three factors (poor social adjustment as a child was absent from the history), one other also had three risk factors present but failed to show early neurobehavioural deficits. The left side of the decision chart shows the sequence eventuating in pathological outcomes; the right side of the diagram where the risk factors were absent failed to produce any cases of a schizophrenic outcome. This research effort suggests the power of a possible linkage test of a genetic/developmental interaction.

Unanswered yet requisite for furthering our understanding of schizophrenia's aetiology are the outcomes of those who were exposed in varying degrees to the risk factors but failed to terminate in a schizophrenic disorder. Here is the other side of the task of developmental psychopathology suggested at the beginning of this chapter – a study of those who escape disorder via a longitudinal analysis of positive life-history factors despite exposure to risk elements that often correlate with disorder.

An interesting contrast with regard to the context of developmental psychopathology is provided by an earlier study conducted by Rodnick and Goldstein (1974). These investigators evaluated the adaptation over time of acute, first-admission schizophrenic women who were treated very briefly in a community mental health centre hospital. The brevity of the period of hospitalization was the result of the state's political decision to close the more traditional long-term mental hospitals and to return patients to the community as rapidly as possible. After discharge and a brief hospital stay, the patients returned home where they were followed for one year after being discharged into the community. These patients varied in their manifest adequacy during the pre-morbid period. One group gave evidence of a good pre-morbid history ($N = 19$), another group had a poor one ($N = 8$). The focus of interest was on the child-care patterns of mothers upon return to their homes. The significance of the earlier pre-morbid history resides in its correlates. Studies of schizophrenic women and men with poor pre-morbid histories (e.g. poor work histories, limited social competence, low level jobs, lack of memberships in community organizations, lower education status) seemingly reflect a possible higher genetic loading in the familial background of such patients. It is also an index that typifies the development of schizophrenia earlier in the patient's life-span. (Phillips, 1968)

Results of the study indicated that the poor pre-morbid mothers on the average were seven years younger than the good pre-morbid patients at the time of hospitalization for their psychotic episode (21:28). Each had at least one infant child who had been left at home. By contrast, the offspring of the good pre-morbid mothers were older (mid-childhood and beyond). For poor pre-morbid mothers that age-range of the children were infancy to four years; for good pre-morbid offspring it was infancy to 13 years. The pattern was clearly one of placing very young children of the poor pre-morbid mothers at greater risk.

Careful attention was given to the mothers' post-hospitalization period through interviews held with the mother and a close relative. The quality of the mother's care-giving, after release from the hospital, was recorded. With mother's return to the family, follow-up visits to the home were made at 30 days, 6 months, and one year. Maternal symptomatology and the adequacy with which the mother met her social and care-giving roles were recorded by raters of maternal adaptation who were blind to the mother's pre-morbid history and the patient's identification. The focus of inquiry and observation was on time for recovery of the mothering function.

Based on interviews and home visits, observers noted that poor pre-morbid mothers tended to be more apathetic to their offspring and more indifferent at the 30-day post-hospital mark than were the goods. At 6 months there was greater recovery in the goods; poors were still indifferent; goods tended to be more anxious and overprotective. At one year post-hospitalization, all mothers were 'conscientious and giving good care', but poors lacked warmth, they were less able to cope with household and child care tasks, and were slower in the recovery of their affective responsivity.

These two studies are both significant for increasing our understanding of children born to schizophrenic mothers. Yet I view the Hans–Marcus study as more adequately meeting the criteria of a developmental psychopathology study because of its longitudinal context and the sequential and cumulative account of risk elements at varying points in the offspring's development.

By contrast, the Rodnick–Goldstein study is not of a developmental nature yet contributory in linking heightened risk status to the younger offspring of a younger mother who was more likely to be at risk for a process-type schizophrenia in contrast to the outcomes of older children of mothers with a more reactive disorder who exhibited greater pre-morbid and post-morbid competencies. The literature (Mednick & Schulsinger, 1968) is supportive that offspring of mothers with a poor pre-morbid history are at greater risk for a schizophrenia-spectrum disorder because of the greater vulnerability that inheres in young children of mothers with a prolonged pattern of maternal incompetence when their children were young.

Systematic longitudinal study of the process of adaptation of such mothers and their children would cast this research effort as one potentially developmental in content and significantly relevant to the field of developmental psychopathology were its focus to be on a continuation of observations of the adaptation of these children at risk over time.

Although many of these consortium studies were exploratory, some were sufficiently longitudinal in scope to take their at-risk children into the period of adulthood when the culmination of risk status could be evaluated. Among these programmes, some 11 in number, were ones led by Mednick and Schulsinger in Denmark (1984), Erlenmeyer-Kimling and Cornblatt and their colleagues in studies conducted in New York City (1984), and Bleuler's (1984) follow-up study of patients and offspring in Switzerland. A number of these and other outcome studies were not truly developmental in their orientation despite their lengthy follow-up qualities. An exception to this general observation is a study at the University of Rochester headed by Sameroff and his colleagues. (Sameroff, Seifer & Zax, 1982; Sameroff, Barocas & Seifer, 1984) This research programme focused on early indicators of schizophrenic outcomes in a group of chronically ill schizophrenic women. A sample of 337 pregnant women with varied degrees of mental illness were studied during the pre-natal period and then invited to participate in a longitudinal study. A substantial sample ($N = 263$) participated, which enabled the investigators to study their offspring at birth, four, 12 and 30 months of age. The children have since been followed into adolescence (Sameroff, Seifer, Baldwin, A., & Baldwin, C., 1993).

Marked attention was paid to diagnosis, severity of symptomatology, and chronicity of intelligence of the mothers. Of interest were the early findings that schizophrenia in the mother did not have the impact on the young child as did the mothers who had been diagnosed as neurotic depressive.

Children of more severely or chronically ill mothers and lower socio-economic status black children performed most poorly. The striking finding was that the newborns of depressed mothers had the worst obstetric status, and, over time, tended to be less adaptive. Seemingly, and unlike the children of schizophrenic mothers, the impact of maternal depression was constant in the early years with negative consequences for the adaptive efforts of their offspring. Severity and chronicity of maternal psychiatric disorders proved to have important effects on children. Sameroff (1989) has followed these children over the years and has recently reported on influencing factors at age 13. These reports indicate that the early characteristics of the child have been 'overpowered' by factors in the subsequent environment. The focus has been on ten environmental risk factors that incorporate maternal elements (a history of mental illness, maternal anxiety, rigidity of mother's beliefs, attitudes, values regarding their child's development, low maternal interaction with the child in infancy, and low educational level of the mother), three socio-economic indicators (unskilled occupation of the head of household, disadvantaged minority status, and reduced family support), large family size, and many stressful life events.

The magnitude of environmental risk relates to children's intelligence at ages 4 and 13 as well as to their social–emotional competence. The correlation of environmental characteristics over that nine year span was $+.76$. The authors conclude that 'whatever the child's ability for achieving high levels of competence, was severely undermined by the continuing paucity of environmental support. The environment limited the opportunities for development.' These findings, that the higher the risk score the lower the IQ, was affirmed by the increase in the number of children in the high-risk group with IQs below 85 from year 4 (22%) to year 13 (46%). Thus high-risk environments would appear to modify the intellectual competence of children over time. The fact that intelligence has been identified as a powerful protective factor for children under stress (Werner, 1989) makes evident that negative environments can heighten risk by reducing the adaptive potential of children. Cultural, familial and environmental variables tend to be correlated and are important elements in the opportunities, or lack thereof, of children in all societies.

The Rochester study speaks to the breadth and complexity of developmental influences on adaptation and growth. Shifting statuses over time whether for children or adults require that a developmental orientation be maintained by risk research investigators. This requires not merely knowledge of experimental techniques but a sophistication about the methods, contents, and processes implicated in development from various disciplinary perspectives.

What has marked the risk-for-schizophrenia studies was the extensive use of experimental methods and techniques that were drawn from the armamentarium of experimental, physiological, cognitive and clinical psychology. That characteristic has not marked the recent surge of research with children at risk for affective disorders.

CHILDREN AT RISK FOR AFFECTIVE DISORDERS

In the 1980s and 1990s, researchers began to direct their attention to the adaptation of children of depressed parents. The result has been an expansion of our knowledge of these offspring at various age points in development. (e.g. Beardslee et al., 1983, Billings & Moos, 1983, 1985; Cohn et al., 1990, Dodge, 1990, Downey & Coyne, 1990; Fendrich, Warner & Weissman, 1990; Goodman & Brumley, 1990; Orvaschel, Walsh-Allis, & Weijai, 1988; Radke-Yarrow et al, 1985; Rutter, 1987*b*, 1990; Weissman et al., 1987.)

The findings of these and related studies make evident that the research orientation of many of these risk investigators has a different cast from those who have studied children of schizophrenic parents. A substantial focus has been on the manifestations of disorder in the offspring of depressed parents. These are some illustrative early findings:

- Children of depressed parents in comparison with offspring of normal parents show increased rates of depression, substance abuse, less adequate social functioning, and a greater frequency of school problems. Further, these children have significantly earlier onsets of depression than do control cases. The more seriously disturbed the parents, the greater the risk for depression in the offspring. Data suggest that an early onset in the pre-puberty period may be related to a greater familial loading for depression. (Weissman et al., 1987)

- Specific family risk factors such as low family cohesion, 'affectionless control', and parental divorce heighten the probability of major depression, conduct disorder, and other psychiatric disturbances in the offspring. (Fendrich et al., 1990)

- Higher rates of insecure attachment in young children of parents with major unipolar or bipolar affective disorder have been reported, but the relationship is not an invariant one, suggesting that insecure attachment may be an early risk factor for depression later in life. (Radke-Yarrow et al., 1985)

- Carefully defined samples of depressed parents suggest that the offspring are at generalized risk for a wide range of adjustment problems, as well as for a specific risk for clinical depression. (Downey & Coyne, 1990)
- Factors operating in these outcomes may be related to other qualities in the depressed mother such as her constricted affect, inadequate control strategies, and patterns of hostile, negative relationships.
- The study of positive characteristics of depressed mothers have been 'totally neglected' with attention given largely to the mothers negative impact upon her child. Yet the ability of many depressed mothers to continue to provide for their children despite their emotional distress, may reflect a protective element for children in some families. (Downey & Coyne, 1990)
- Two protective elements in the children of disordered parents are high social skills and intelligence. The presence of these factors appear to reduce the child's risk for disorder.
- The severity of children's symptomatology appears in some cases to be a joint function of parental disorder and life stress thus reflecting a person × environment interaction in their depressive disorders.

These findings suggest that many researchers of children at risk for depression are currently focused on validating the heightened probability of pathological outcomes. Absent from these reports is the broad set of experimental psychopathology studies that has characterized research with children at risk for schizophrenia. (Garmezy, 1974; Watt et al., 1984) The reasons for this difference may be twofold. Schizophrenia has been associated over decades with a history of experimental studies in the search for psychological, cognitive, social, psychophysiological, and neuropsychological deficits in patients. Further, a strongly supportive psychiatric genetics literature has pointed to a likely genetic transmission of the disorder. Hence, for the researcher of risk for schizophrenia, experimental studies of potentially pre-disposing elements have offered a broad spectrum for developmental study.

This has not been true to the same extent for the affective disorders. Even the issue of whether or not childhood depression exists has evoked pros and cons. Since that question has now been set aside by empirical findings, it is more likely that, in the future, a broader set of studies will be conducted in the search for behavioural and biological characteristics of children of affectively disordered parents. Accompanying such studies, it is hoped, will be several suggestions offered by Rutter (1990): 1) Less heterogeneity in the selection of samples of offspring to be studied; 2) A more adequate recruitment of at-risk families with less reliance on volunteers in order to provide a more appropriate representation of families and offspring at risk for depression.

Finally, there exists a seeming need for a sophisticated awareness among risk researchers of the nature and complexity of human development, of stages of growth, of developmental transitions, and of continuities and discontinuities in behavioural patterns over time.

THE ADAPTIVE FOCUS OF DEVELOPMENTAL PSYCHOPATHOLOGY: THE STUDY OF RESILIENCE UNDER ADVERSITY

Maladaptive and adaptive behaviours are the joint concern of developmental psychopathologists. Sroufe & Rutter (1984) provide the rationale for this broad sweep:

> First, developmental psychopathologists are interested in childhood behavior problems but also in the ties between behavior problems and normal development and socialization especially across time . . . Second, disordered behavior is examined in terms of its deviation from the normal developmental course. Disordered patterns of behavior are illuminated by considering usual patterns of adaptation vis-à-vis the developmental issues of a given period.   (pp. 18–19)

While risk factors and disordered behaviour receive priority it is obvious that normative development must be the baseline against which to evaluate deviations from that standard. Such a view helps to temper premature interpretations of deviance. Thus while life stressors are often evident in the lives of the mentally disordered, similar or identical events frequently typify as well the lives of many adaptable persons. These variations in responsiveness to stressful events have been a factor in initiating studies of protective factors that may serve to temper the effects of risk elements.

It has also given rise to the concept of 'resilience' or 'stress-resistance' to describe the maintenance of adequate behaviour in the presence of major stressful life events. From early beginnings in case descriptions of 'resilient' persons (Goertzel & Goertzel, 1962; Illingworth & Illingworth, 1966), there have followed efforts to study the characteristics and backgrounds of accomplished persons who have been exposed to a variety of markedly stressful experiences such as profound poverty in childhood, racial and ethnic prejudice, affectional deprivation, physical and sexual abuse, a background of familial mental disorder, physical and mental disability, and even criminogenic family backgrounds and neighbourhood settings marked by high rates of delinquency.

In all of these constraining events, there exist accounts of persons who have overcome adversity and demonstrated functional competence over their life-span. While these outcomes reflect the reality of the phenomenon of resilience, they can also serve as a basis for the systematic study of specific trauma shared by groups of individuals with the varied outcomes that follow. The goal is the search for the attributes and underlying processes that are implicated in successful adaptation to disadvantaged and threatening circumstances. (Clark, 1983; Masten, Best & Garmezy, 1990)

Contributing to this new orientation have been the multiple studies of children at risk for mental disorder by virtue of possible familial genetic status (Watt et al., 1984). The findings of a range of adaptability in these presumed-to-be at-risk offspring have accelerated the interest in resilience research. Similarly, the crisis of poverty and its consequences for children, have elicited an international concern for the futures of such children. In this context too, variability in outcomes for children reared in poverty (Long & Vaillant, 1984) has added to efforts to understand factors influencing children's adaptability to dire economic circumstances, single parenting, parental unemployment, poor housing, etc. Parental divorce and family dissolution has been an additional stressor now besetting children. These experiences too, so distressing for children, do not elicit uniform reactions. Children vary in their maintained adaptability under such stressors and the increase in attention to these trying events and their consequences have become the basis for a search for the attributes of resilient and maladaptive responsiveness in children (Hetherington & Furstenberg, 1989).

The meaning given to the term 'resilience' helps to clarify its content. Its dictionary definitions include the following: 'the tendency to rebound or recoil', 'to return to a state', 'to spring back', 'the power of recovery'. None of these suggests a context of 'invulnerability' to stress. Instead, it portrays an underlying process that allows for recovery to a prior level of performance that follows on a stressful imposition. It is assumed that the prior level reflected a higher degree of competence or function – and it is this construct of enhanced competence rather than the more popularized one of 'coping' that is the central element in research into the nature of resilience. (Garmezy & Masten, 1991)

Several years ago (Garmezy, 1985) in an effort to find commonalities descriptive of adaptable children exposed to a variety of stressful situations, I initiated a search of a diverse literature and concluded that four factors recurrent across stressful life situations, helped to insure adaptive behaviour in children under stress. One resided in temperament attributes such as activity level, reflectiveness, responsivity to others, etc. The second was the critical element of intelligence and the utilization of one's cognitive skills, the third was the nature of the family specifically its cohesion, warmth and concern for the child's well-being; and the fourth was the availability of a source of external support such as a teacher, a parental substitute, or an institution such as the school, a social agency, a church etc that fostered ties to a larger community.

At the time I drew these attributes together, they were summary impressions derived from a set of markedly varied stressors and studies. It was gratifying, therefore to read subsequently of Professor Emmy Werner's (1989) recent report on a 30-year follow-up of her longitudinal study of the children of Kuaia. (Werner & Smith, 1982, 1992) The report was of a sub-set of children drawn from her larger sample consisting of those subjects who demonstrated competence, ability and autonomy as young adults. Looking back to data gathered from infancy to adulthood, Werner reported on a triad of characteristics that marked these adaptive young adults who as infants had been born into poverty and endured early peri-natal stress.

In reviewing her findings Werner (1989) reported on the attributes of family and child that she viewed as protective factors that helped to determine the positive adult outcomes:

Three types of protective factors emerge from our analyses of the developmental course of high-risk children from infancy to adulthood: 1) dispositional attributes of the individual, such as activity level and sociability, at least average intelligence, competence in communication skills (language and reading), and an internal locus of control; 2) affectional ties within the family that provide emotional support in times of stress, whether from a parent, sibling, spouse, or mate; and 3) external support systems, whether in school, at work, or church, that reward the individual's competencies and determination, and provide a belief system by which to live.   (p. 80)

Werner's commentary extends to the parents. She reports that good relationships in childhood existed between parent and child. Parents were: a) supportive of their offspring; b) set rules and regulations in the home which were to be obeyed; and c) showed parental respect for their children's individuality, while maintaining the stability and cohesion of the family.

As for the children, theirs was a history of good health, active and social involvement with others, they early exhibited a sense of autonomy, they identified with positive role models, had good peer relationships, engaged in multiple interests and hobbies, early developed reading and reasoning skills, and set goals for themselves.

These accounts are fascinating and they raise a provocative question. In poverty, what makes for a seemingly atypical concatenation of talents in a subset of families? What are the origins of these early personal and parental competencies? What are the processes and mechanisms that are implicated in parents' and children's positive responses to powerful risk factors? Are there critical points in development that set the trajectories for continued future growth and maintained competence? What resources do children possess that enable them to overcome adversity? What are the roots of these resources? How shall we investigate the processes whereby protection transcends risk?

THE POWER OF LONGITUDINAL RESEARCH

The questions are many, the answers are less forthcoming. However, one can hope that a vital developmental psychopathology research-oriented, clinically sophisticated, equally knowledgeable about normal and abnormal development, interdisciplinary in its sophistication about biological and behavioural sciences, will, in the decades ahead, provide a data base that will advance solutions to these vital questions.

The consequences that would ensue from such a knowledge base would advance the cause of children's adaptation to stress and in doing so would bring untold benefits to the well-being of society. A word about method in achieving such a goal is in order and it can best be set forth by acknowledging the power of Werner's study of the children of Kuaia. For it is through the power of her 30-year longitudinal study that we have been able to perceive differential outcomes in a cohort at risk, studied pre-natally and at multiple age points that carried the knowledge base into adulthood. Only in this manner has Werner been enabled to relate past events to present adaptations. Therein lies the power of longitudinal research. How else would it have been possible to know of the interrelatedness she observed of early experience, family and personality contexts, stressful life events and differential outcomes observed in adulthood?

Similarly Sameroff and other investigators who have studied children born to schizophrenic mothers have maximized our knowledge of outcomes in adolescence and adulthood by studying these children at risk over time and maintaining their efforts to do so into the risk years of adolescence and early adulthood.

Adolf Meyer sought the solution to understanding mental breakdown via retrospection and recall. He provided a milestone, albeit a limited one because of the difficulty of recreating the past. On the current scene other research groups have turned to the longitudinal method to study, over time, children deemed to be at risk not solely with the goal of identifying whether or not they become mentally disordered but rather to observe attributes, adaptations and transitions in the course of growing up.

One recognizes and admires the enormous commitment demanded of such investigators, but it is the most valid method for providing the needed picture of developmental continuities and discontinuities of 'at-risk' children.

A definitive answer to the issue of risk, actualized or not actualized, lies in the longitudinal study of those who are vulnerable to disorder and become ill, contrasted with others who share a similar risk status but remain resilient despite the presence of adversity. Therein lies the power of longitudinal study.

REFERENCES

Achenbach, T. M. (1990). Conceptualization of developmental psychopathology. In M. Lewis and S. M. Miller (eds.) *Handbook of developmental psychopathology*, pp. 3–14. New York: Plenum Press.

Anthony, E. J. & Cohler, B. J. (eds.) (1987). *The invulnerable child.* New York: Guilford.

Attie, I., Brooks-Gunn, J. & Petersen, A. (1990). A developmental perspective on eating disorders and eating problems. In M. Lewis & S. M. Miller (eds.) *Handbook of developmental psychopathology*, pp. 409–420. New York: Plenum Press.

Beardslee, W. R., Bemporad, J. Keller, M. B. & Klerman, G. L. (1983). Children of parents with major affective disorder: a review. *American Journal of Psychiatry*, **140**, 825–32.

Billings, A. G. & Moos, R. H. (1983). Comparison of children of depressed and non-depressed parents: a social environmental perspective. *Journal of Abnormal Child Psychology*, **11**, 483–6.

Billings, A. G. & Moos, R. H. (1985). Children of parents with bipolar depression: a controlled one-year follow-up. *Journal of Abnormal Child Psychology*, **14**, 149–66.

Birch, H. G. & Gussow, J. D. (1970). *Disadvantaged children: health, nutrition, and school failure*. New York: Harcourt, Brace & World.

Bleuler, M. (1984). A life-span study of children at risk: Different forms of childhood stress and patterns of adult psychiatric outcome. In *Children at risk for schizophrenia*, pp. 535–542. Cambridge: Cambridge University Press.

Bowlby, J. (1951). *Maternal care and mental health*. Geneva: WHO; New York: Columbia University Press.

Bowlby, J. (1953). Some pathological processes set in train by early mother–child separation. *Journal of Mental Science*, **99**, 265–72.

Bowlby, J. (1960a). Separation anxiety. *International Journal of Psychoanalysis*, **41**, 89–113.

Bowlby, J. (1960b). Grief and mourning in infancy and early childhood. *Psychoanalytic Study of the Child*, **15**, 9–52.

Bowlby, J. (1973). *Attachment and loss: Separation* (Vol II). New York: Basic Books.

Bowlby, J. (1979). *The making and breaking of affectional bonds*. London: Tavistock Publications.

Bowlby, J. (1980). *Attachment and loss: loss* (Vol II). New York: Basic Books.

Bowlby, J. (1982). *Attachment and loss: attachment*. (2nd edn), vol I, New York: Basic Books.

Bowlby, J. (1988). Developmental psychiatry comes of age. *American Journal of Psychiatry*, **145**, 1–10.

Burton, R. (1621). *The Anatomy of Melancholy* F. Dell and P. Jourdan-Smith (ed), vol II, London: J. M. Dent and Sons, 1961.

Campbell, R. J. (1989). *Psychiatric dictionary* (6th edn.). New York: Oxford University Press.

Cicchetti, D. (1984). The emergence of developmental psychopathology. *Child Development*, **55**, 1–7.

Cicchetti, D. (1989). Developmental psychopathology: Past, present, and future. In D. Cicchetti (ed), *The emergence of a discipline: Rochester symposium on developmental psychopathology*, pp. 1–12. Hillsdale, NJ: Lawrence Erlbaum Associates.

Clark, R. M. (1983). *Family life and school achievement: why poor black children succeed or fail*. Chicago: University of Chicago Press.

Cohn, J. F., Campbell, S., Matias, R. & Hopkins, J. (1990). Face-to-face interactions of postpartum depressed and non-depressed mother–infant pairs at 2 months. *Developmental Psychology*, **26**, 15–23.

DSM III-R. (1987). *Diagnostic and statistical manual of mental disorders* (3rd edn, revised). Washington, DC: American Psychiatric Association.

Dodge, K. A. (1990). Developmental psychopathology in children of depressed mothers. *Developmental Psychology*, **26**, 3–6.

Downey, G. & Coyne, J. C. (1990). Children of depressed parents: An integrative review. *Psychological Bulletin*, **108**, 50–76.

Eisenberg, L. (1977). Development as a unifying concept in psychiatry. *British Journal of Psychiatry*, **131**, 225–37.

Elder, G. H. (1974). *Children of the great depression: social change in life experience*. Chicago:

University of Chicago Press.

Erlenmeyer-Kimling, L., Marcuse, Y., Cornblatt, B., Friedman, D., Rainer, J. D. & Rutschmann, J. (1984). The New York High-Risk Project. In N. F. Watt et al. (eds.) *Children at risk for schizophrenia*, pp. 167–239. Cambridge: Cambridge University Press.

Fendrich, M., Warner, V. & Weissman, M. M. (1990). Family risk factors, parental depression, and psychopathology in offspring. *Developmental Psychology*, **26**, 40–50.

Festinger, T. (1983). *No one ever asked us . . . a postscript to foster care*. New York: Columbia University Press.

Freud, S. (1955). The psychogenesis of a case of homosexuality in a woman. In J. Strachey (ed.), *The standard edition of the complete psychological works of Sigmund Freud*, vol 18, (1920–1922), pp. 146–172. London: The Hogarth Press and the Institute of Psychoanalysis.

Freud, A. (1965). *Normality and pathology in development: assessments of development*. New York: International Universities Press.

Freud, A. (1976). Psychopathology as seen against the background of normal development. *British Journal of Psychiatry*, **129**, 401–6.

Garmezy, N. (1974). Children at risk: the search for the antecedents of schizophrenia – Part II: Ongoing research programmes, issues and intervention. *Schizophrenia Bulletin*, **9**, 55–125.

Garmezy, N. (1982). The case for the single case in research. In A. E. Kazdin & A. H. Tuma (eds.), *New directions for methodology of social and behavioral sciences: Single-case research designs*, vol. 13, pp. 5–17. San Francisco: Jossey-Bass.

Garmezy, N. (1985). Stress-resistant children: the search for protective factors. In J. E. Stevenson (ed.), *Recent research in developmental psychopathology. Journal of Child Psychology and Psychiatry Book Supplement*, No. 4, pp. 213–233. Oxford: Pergamon Press.

Garmezy, N. & Masten, A. S. (1991). The protective role of competence indicators in children at risk. In E. M. Cummings (ed.), *Life-span developmental psychology: Perspective on stress and coping*. Hillsdale, NJ: Lawrence Erlbaum.

Garmezy, N. & Streitman, S. (1974). Children at risk: the search for the antecedents of schizophrenia – Part I: Conceptual models and research methods. *Schizophrenia Bulletin*, **8**, 14–90.

Goertzel, V. & Goertzel, M. G. (1962). *Cradles of eminence*. Boston: Little, Brown and Company.

Goldstein, M. J. & Tuma, A. H. (eds.) (1987). High-risk research. *Schizophrenia Bulletin*, **13**, (3) (entire issue), 367–530.

Goodman, S. H. & Brumley, H. E. (1990). Schizophrenic and depressed mothers: relational deficits in parenting. *Developmental Psychology*, **26**, 31–9.

Hans, S. & Marcus, J. (1987). A process model for the development of schizophrenia. *Psychiatry*, **50**, 361–70.

Hetherington, E. M. & Furstenberg, F. F. Jr. (1989). *Readings*, **4**, 4–8.

Hunter, R. & Macalpine, I. (1963). *Three hundred years of psychiatry 1535–1860*. Oxford: Oxford University Press.

Illingworth, R. S. & Illingworth, C. M. (1966). *Lessons from childhood: some aspects of the early life of unusual men and women*. London: E & S Livingstone Ltd.

Lewis, M. (1990). Models of developmental psychopathology. In M. Lewis and S. M. Miller (eds.) *Handbook of developmental psychopathology*, pp. 15–27. New York: Plenum Press.

124   N. GARMEZY

Lewis, M. & Miller, S. M. (eds.) (1990). *Handbook of developmental psychopathology*. New York: Plenum Press.
Lief, A. (1948). *The commonsense psychiatry of Dr Adolf Meyer: The Life Chart*, pp. 418–422. New York: McGraw-Hill.
Long, J. V. F. & Vaillant, G. E. (1984). Natural history of male psychological health. XI: escape from the underclass. *American Journal of Psychiatry*, **141**, 341–6.
Marcus, J., Hans, S. L., Nagler, S., Auerbach, J. G., Mirsky, A. F. & Aubrey, A. (1987). Review of the NIMH Israeli Kibbutz-City Study and the Jerusalem Infant Development Study. *Schizophrenia Bulletin*, 13(3), 425–38.
Masten, A. S., Best, K. M. & Garmezy, N. (1990). Resilience and development: contributions from the study of children who overcome adversity. *Development and Psychopathology*, **2**, 425–44.
Mednick, S. A. & Schulsinger, F. (1968). Some premorbid characteristics related to breakdown in children with schizophrenic mothers. *Journal of Psychiatric Research* (Suppl. 1) **6**, 354–62.
Mednick, S. A., Cudeck, R., Griffith, J. J., Talovic, S. A. & Schulsinger, F. (1984). The Danish high-risk project. In N. F. Watt, E. J. Anthony, L. C. Wynne, and J. E. Rolf (eds.) *Children at risk for Schizophrenia*, pp. 19–70. Cambridge: Cambridge University Press.
Meyer, A. (1919). The Life Chart. In *Contributions to medical and biological research*. New York: Paul B. Hoeber.
Mirsky, A. F., Quinn, O. W., Schwerdt, P. & Buchsbaum, M. S. (1987). The Genain Quadruplets: A 25-year follow-up of four monozygous women discordant for the severity of schizophrenic illness. In N. E. Miller and G. D. Cohen (eds.) *Schizophrenia and aging*, pp. 83–94. New York: Guilford.
Orvaschel, H., Walsh-Allis, G. & Weijai, Y. (1988). Psychopathology in children of parents with recurrent depression. *Journal of Abnormal Child Psychology*, **16**, 17–28.
Piaget, J. (1975). Foreword. In E. J. Anthony (ed.), *Explorations in child psychiatry*, pp. vii–ix. New York: Plenum Press.
Phillips, L. (1968). *Human adaptation and its failures*. New York: Academic Press.
Radke-Yarrow, M., Cummings, E. M., Kuczynski, L. & Chapman, M. (1985). Patterns of attachment in two- and three-year-olds in normal families and families with parental depression. *Child Development*, **56**, 884–93.
Rodnick, E. H. & Goldstein, M. J. (1974). Premorbid adjustment and the recovery of mothering function in acute schizophrenic women. *Journal of Abnormal Psychology*, **83**, 623–8.
Rosenthal, D. (1963). *The Genain Quadruplets*. New York: Basic Books.
Rutter, M. (1966). *Children of sick parents: an environmental and psychiatric study*. London: Oxford University Press.
Rutter, M. (1979). Maternal deprivation, 1972–1978: New findings, new concepts, new approaches. *Child Development*, **50**, 283–305.
Rutter, M. (ed.) (1980*b*). *Scientific foundations of developmental psychiatry*. London: William Heinemann Medical Books Ltd.
Rutter, M. (ed.) (1983). *Developmental neuropsychiatry*. New York: Guilford Press.
Rutter, M. (1984*a*). Psychopathology and development: I. Childhood antecedents of adult psychiatric disorder. *Australian and New Zealand Journal of Psychiatry*, **18**, 225–34.
Rutter, M. (1984*b*). Psychopathology and Development: II. Childhood experiences and personality. *Australian and New Zealand Journal of Psychiatry*, **18**, 314–27.

Rutter, M. (1985). Resilience in the face of adversity: protective factors and resistance to psychiatric disorder. *British Journal of Psychiatry*, **147**, 598–611.

Rutter, M. (1986). Child psychiatry: the interface between clinical and developmental research. *Psychological Medicine*, **16**, 151–69.

Rutter, M. (1987*b*). Psychiatric disorder in parents as a risk factor in children. In R. E. Hales and A. J. Frances (eds.) *American Psychiatric Association's Annual Review*, vol. 6, pp. 647–663. Washington, DC: American Psychiatric Association.

Rutter, M. (1988*a*). Epidemiological approaches to developmental psychopathology. *Archives of General Psychiatry*, **45**, 486–500.

Rutter, M. (1988*b*). Longitudinal data in the study of causal processes: some uses and some pitfalls. In M. Rutter (ed.) *Studies of psychosocial risk: the power of longitudinal data*. pp. 1–28. Cambridge: Cambridge University Press.

Rutter, M. (1989). Psychosocial risk trajectories and beneficial turning points. In S. Doxiadis (eds.) *Early influences shaping the individual*, pp. 229–239. New York: Plenum.

Rutter, M. (1990). Commentary: some focus and process considerations regarding effects of parental depression on children. *Developmental Psychology*, **26**, 60–7.

Rutter, M. & Garmezy, N. (1983). Development psychopathology. In P. H. Mussen (ed.), *Handbook of child psychology – vol IV: Socialization, personality, and social development*. E. M. Hetherington (vol. ed.), pp. 775–911. New York: Wiley.

Rutter, M. & Hersov, L. (1985). *Child and adolescent psychiatry* (2nd edn.). Oxford: Blackwell Scientific Publications.

Sameroff, A. J. (1989). Models of developmental regulation: The environtype. In D. Cicchetti (ed.) *The emergence of a discipline*, pp. 41–68. Hillsdale, NJ: Lawrence Erlbaum Associates.

Sameroff, A. J., Barocas, R. & Seifer, R. (1984). The early development of children born to mentally ill children. In N. F. Watt, E. J. Anthony, L. C. Wynne and J. E. Rolf (eds.) *Children at risk for schizophrenia*. pp. 482–514. Cambridge: Cambridge University Press.

Sameroff, A. J., Seifer, R., Baldwin, A., & Baldwin, C. (1993). Stability of intelligence from preschool to adolescence: the influence of family risk factors. *Child Development*, **64**, 80–97.

Sameroff, A. J., Seifer, R. & Zax, M. (1982). Early development of children at risk for emotional disorder. *Monographs of the Society for Research in Child Development*, **47**, (7), Serial No. 199. Chicago: University of Chicago Press.

Sroufe, L. (1989). Pathways to adaptation and maladaptation: Psychopathology as developmental deviation. In D. Cicchetti (ed.), *The emergence of a discipline*. pp. 13–40. Hillsdale, NJ: Lawrence Erlbaum Associates.

Sroufe, L. A. & Rutter, M. (1984). The domain of developmental psychopathology. *Child Development*, **55**, 17–29.

Stone, A. A. & Onque, G. C. (1959). *Longitudinal studies of child personality*. New York: The Commonwealth Fund.

Theis, S. V. S. (1924). *How foster children turn out*. (Publ. 165) New York State Charities and Associate (cited in Stone & Onque, #273).

Watt, N. F., Anthony, E. J., Wynne, L. C. & Rolf, J. E. (eds.) (1984). *Children at risk for schizophrenia: A longitudinal perspective*. Cambridge: Cambridge University Press.

Weissman, M. M., Gammon, G. D., John, K., Merikangas, K. R., Warner, V., Prusoff, B. A., Sholomskas, D. (1987). Children of depressed mothers. *Archives of General Psychiatry*, **44**, 847–53.

Werner, E. E. (1989). High-risk children in young adulthood: a longitudinal study from birth to 32 years. *American Journal of Orthopsychiatry*, **59**, 72–81.

Werner, E. E. & Smith, R. S. (1982). *Vulnerable but invincible: a study of resilient children.* New York: McGraw-Hill.

Werner, E. E. & Smith, R. S. (1992). *Overcoming the odds: high risk children from birth to adulthood.* Ithaca, NY Cornell University Press.

Zigler, E. (1989). Foreword. In D. Cicchetti (ed.), *The emergence of a discipline: Rochester symposium on developmental psychopathology*, pp. ix–xii. Hillsdale, NJ: Lawrence Erlbaum Associates.

7 Developmental psychopathology as a research perspective

MICHAEL RUTTER

Traditionally, developmental psychology and psychiatry have constituted very separate enterprises with distinctive and different styles of research. For the most part, the focus of developmental psychology has been on the universals of developmental processes. It is no accident that most of the 'big' theories of development have been expressed in stage terms. The content of the stages has, of course, varied across theories: psychosexual stages in psychoanalytic theory; cognitive structures in Piagetian theory; psychosocial tasks in Erikson's theory; and age periods (such as the supposed mid-life crisis) in some life-span theories. Nevertheless, in each case, the emphasis has been on a consistent age-dependent progression followed by all individuals. Research findings have failed to support many of the tenets that are central to stage theories, and modern concepts of development have come to include a much greater attention to individual differences, to the effects of social context, to the interplay between persons and their environments, and to people's overall pattern of functioning, as well as continuities and discontinuities in the expression of particular psychological traits (Rutter & Rutter, 1993). As a consequence, developmentalists have necessarily been forced to consider possible continuities and discontinuities between normality and psychopathology, and to recognize that individuals may follow developmental paths that diverge from each other in certain important respects. These considerations have also led to an extension of developmental research to age periods after childhood and thus to a consideration of life-span concepts.

At the same time, psychiatric research (especially that from an epidemiological perspective) has indicated that so-called traditional models of unitary diseases with single causes have a quite limited application in the field of mental disorders. It is possible that such models may apply to severe, qualitatively abnormal, conditions such as autism, schizophrenia and bipolar affective disorders, although even in these cases that is quite uncertain. Enthusiastic claims of the localization of causal single genes have not been replicated and have had to be withdrawn (Plomin, 1991). Social scientists have sometimes viewed single-cause unitary-disease approaches as typical of medical models; however, that is a serious misconception. Person–environment interactions of various sorts are widely operative and generally recognized as important in medicine (Rutter & Pickles, 1991). Moreover, it has come to be appreciated that childhood environments may bring about effects that carry strong implications for health and ill-health in adult life (Bock & Whelan, 1991). A developmental perspective is useful in the whole of medicine, although perhaps it is especially so in psychiatry (Rutter, 1989a). However, that is not just because risk and protective factors for psychiatric disorders manifest in adult life may operate in childhood or adolescence, but also because many mental disorders may represent distortions or exaggerations of normal developmental processes (Plomin, 1991). Factors that influence normal development may also determine abnormal development.

It might be thought that this extension of developmental approaches to encompass aspects of psychopathology, and of psychiatry to include developmental considerations, would simply require a slight broadening of traditional concepts. However, that is to miss the essence of developmental psychopathology. The key point is that this conjunction carries with it very important research advantages for the investigation of causal mechanisms and processes. The preceding chapter by Garmezy provides the historical background and current context of developmental psychopathology; this chapter considers some of the research implications that follow adoption of this perspective.

STUDY OF UNDERLYING PROCESSES

Developmental research strategies have contributed greatly to the study of underlying processes in psychopathology in several different ways which may be illustrated through the use of the three rather different examples of autism, dyslexia and conduct disorder. Although Kanner's (1943) original description of autism expressed the disorder rather differently, it soon came to be viewed as an infantile psychosis, probably an unusually early variety of schizophrenia. There were many problems with this concept (Rutter, 1972) but the way forward was shown best by Hermelin and O'Connor's (1970) application of developmentally derived experimental psychological strategies. Rather than approach autism through the study of symptoms, they examined the possibility that cognitive deficits might underlie the social and behavioural abnormalities. A series of well-planned studies, controlling for mental age level, showed that autistic children differed markedly from mentally retarded controls in their cognitive patterns, especially in their failure to use meaning in their memory of words. It was argued that an intrinsic cognitive deficit in abstraction, coding and sequencing might constitute the basis for autism. Research of this type was crucial in changing the concept of autism from an infantile psychosis to a pervasive developmental disorder (Rutter & Schopler 1988, 1992).

More recently, studies of children's ability to appreciate what other people might be thinking (so-called 'theory of mind') have taken the matter much further. This field of research was set off by a study undertaken by Wimmer and Perner (1983) showing that, at about the age of 4 years, children first began to understand that other people's thought processes might be different from their own. The research paradigm involved the possibility of false beliefs in a scenario in which a person saw an object put in place 'A'. While that person was out of the room the object was transferred to place 'B'. The child is then asked where the person will look for the object on returning to the room: place 'A' (where the person should think the object is because she saw it put there) or in place 'B' (where, as the child knows, it actually is, because it was moved while the person was absent). Very young children tend to say 'B', not realizing the difference in perspective between themselves and the person in the experiment; whereas older children tend to say 'A', appreciating that the other person's thoughts would have been determined by what they themselves saw, rather than by what only the child knows. Baron-Cohen, Leslie and Frith (1985) were quick to realize the utility of applying this approach in autism (see Frith, 1989) and went on to show that even older autistic individuals were seriously lacking in this ability to understand what other people were likely to be thinking. The consequence has been a veritable explosion of studies (see Astington, Harris & Olson, 1988; Whiten, 1991) of both normal and autistic children, which have been enormously informative regarding both normal and abnormal development. The results have served to confirm an impaired 'theory of mind' as part of the cognitive deficit in autism. In addition, they have been important in using autism as an experimental group that differs from normal in its cognitive pattern in order to understand better the links in normal children between cognition and the development of social relationships.

The research has also been crucial in raising questions about the precursors of 'theory of mind' in ordinary development and about the meaning of apparently normal social development in the first 18 to 24 months in some autistic individuals. The first issue has highlighted the need to view the acquisition of 'theory of mind', not in sudden stage-like acquisition terms, but rather in the broader context of a range of cognitive processes beginning to come into operation at ages much earlier than 4 years (Rogers & Pennington, 1991). The second issue has served as an important reminder that when a brain disorder is acquired and when its functional consequences become manifest are far from synonymous. That is both because, as development proceeds, the brain areas subserving a particular psychological function may change (see Goldman-Rakic et al., 1983), and also because the experiential input 'driving' these functions varies with age. Thus, auditory input is not required for normal babble in infancy but it is necessary from age 6 months or so onwards. As a result, the babble of deaf children appears unexceptional to begin with, and then in the second half of the first year acquires its typically abnormal features. Similarly, the sensory discrimination of different voice sound is not dependent on language experience in infancy but it is in later childhood (Aslin, Pisoni & Jusczyk, 1983). Goodman (1991) has argued that considerations of this kind may explain why some cases of autism appear to have a later onset, even though the underlying brain disorder is likely to have been present from before birth.

Developmental considerations have also been important in making sense of the apparent paradox that, although twin data indicate a very high heritability for autism (Rutter, 1991a), obstetric complications differentiate autistic from non-autistic siblings or co-twins. The latter finding led Steffenberg et al. (1989) to argue that environmentally determined perinatal damage played an important causal role in autism. Bailey et al.'s (1991) twin study has pointed to a possible resolution of the paradox through its finding that the link between obstetric complications and autism seemed to be mediated by congenital anomalies of a type likely to have been acquired in the first third of pregnancy. The implication is that the anomalies and the obstetric complications are both the result of a genetically abnormal fetus (a well-demonstrated effect with other genetic anomalies – Goodman, 1990) or, more speculatively, that the genetic abnormality creates an unusual vulnerability to the ever-present vagaries of development.

Dyslexia, or developmental disorders of reading/spelling, provide a rather different example of how developmental perspectives have contributed to an understanding of the basis of psychopathology. Once again, the first step was an appreciation that it was likely to be useful to examine the cognitive processes important in normal development – in this instance, phonological coding and the appreciation of rhyme and alliteration (Goswami & Bryant, 1990). However, because the reading skills of even dyslexic children improve with age, it became both necessary and possible to use several other research tactics to challenge and test the causal hypothesis. First, Bradley and Bryant (1985) argued that it was necessary to control for reading age (and not just overall mental age) to rule out the possibility that the phonological deficit derived from the lack of reading experiences, rather than the other way around. Secondly, it was necessary to determine whether phonological deficits at an early age predicted reading difficulties at a later age (and, equally, that they did not predict other scholastic skills, such as mathematics). Third, the hypothesized causal connection was tested by determining whether experimental interventions designed to improve rhyming and alliteration skills would lead also to improved reading performance at a later age. The findings showed that they did. Two further steps in the research process involved a return to abnormal groups to provide investigative 'leverage'. Thus, one group of investigators showed that the phonology-reading link still held in deaf individuals in whom it might be thought that it would play a much reduced role (see Shankweiler & Leiberman, 1989). Most crucially, twin research has shown a close genetic link between phonological deficits and reading difficulties in a dyslexic sample (Olson, Wise & Rack, 1989). As with autism, a range of questions has still to be answered, but the combination of developmental and psychopathological research strategies has been extremely effective in providing rigorous tests of causal hypotheses. As with autism, it should be noted that the developmental psychopathology perspective has been equally useful in throwing light on dyslexia and on normal development.

Conduct disorders provide yet a further disparate example. Psychopathologists have tended to view this large group of disorders as generally homogeneous, with antisocial behaviour as the unifying feature, and with antisocial personality disorder as the typical outcome in adult life (Robins, 1966, 1978). Developmental perspectives have been important in three separate connections. First, longitudinal studies have shown that conduct disorders with an unusually early onset are particularly likely to persist into adult life and that these early onset, highly persistent, disorders tend to be associated with hyperactivity, inattention, poor peer relationships, and low autonomic reactivity (Farrington, Loeber & Van Kammen, 1990*a*; Magnusson & Bergman, 1990). Thus, longitudinal data have been helpful in pointing to possible heterogeneity within conduct disorders. Secondly, developmental studies have shown the importance of social attributional biases in anti-social children and have raised the important possibility that the conduct problems may have their basis in social deficits (Dodge et al., 1986). This possibility is also raised by the data indicating that conduct disorders in childhood lead on to pervasive social malfunction in adult life of a kind not confined to antisocial personality disorder (Zoccollilo et al., 1992). Thirdly, twin study findings suggest that, whereas juvenile delinquency has only a quite minor genetic argument, genetic factors are more important in adult criminality (McGuffin & Gottesman, 1985). The implication is that genetic influences may be more important in conduct disorders persisting from childhood into adult life than in those confined to the period of childhood and adolescence. Researchers in the field of conduct disorders have come to appreciate the research leverage afforded by attention to age of onset and to continuities/discontinuities across the life span (Farrington et al., 1990*b*).

These examples illustrate the value of developmental approaches to psychopathology but they also show the utility of studying disorders to understand developmental processes. The experimental method is fundamental in the investigation of causal questions. It relies on testing for within-individual change over-time in relation to some hypothesized causal variable (Farrington, 1988). For obvious reasons, laboratory experiments are not possible for many developmental questions – because there is a need to study change over very long time spans, because the hypothesized causal factor is not open to experimental manipulation for ethical or practical reasons, or because the hypothesized mechanisms rely on social context for their effects. Naturalistic studies overcome those problems, but usually suffer greatly from the extreme difficulty of separating one influence from another. In that situation, investigators need to search for 'experiments of nature' in which special groups or special circumstances allow variables that ordinarily go together to be separated (Rutter, 1981*a*). Individuals with some disorder, or who are psychopathologically unusual in some way, may provide just such an opportunity. The already mentioned examples of autism and of dyslexia do so because social and reading skills (respectively), which ordinarily are fairly strongly associated with mental age are not so linked in these groups. Deaf and blind individuals (O'Connor &

Hermelin, 1978) and idiots savants (Hermelin & O'Connor, 1986) have been similarly used to study cognitive processes.

DIVERSITY OF RISK OUTCOMES

A disease orientation leads to research focusing on possible causes of particular diseases. Epidemiological findings in medicine generally, however, made it apparent long ago that a single risk factor may predispose to a heterogeneous range of diseases. Thus, smoking is a risk factor, not only for lung cancer but also for coronary heart disease, osteoporosis, and chronic bronchitis. Similarly, obesity creates an increased risk for coronary artery disease, diabetes and osteoarthritis. The same considerations apply in psychiatry. The important research implication is that longitudinal data are essential in order to determine the full risks associated with any one risk factor (Rutter, 1988). However, it is not enough to consider risks just in relation to specified disease outcomes. That is because the main risk may lie in some specific or general disturbance in psychological functioning, rather than in a raised rate of one or more disorders. For example, Hodges and Tizard's (1989a, b) follow-up at 16 years of children who spent their first few years in a residential nursery indicated that at least half showed a distinctive pattern of peer relationships characterized by a lack of depth and of selectivity and a tendency not to use friends for emotional support. The findings are relevant for an understanding of the possible role of early attachment relationships for the development of close friendships in later life, as well as for a risk outcome that does not fit easily into current psychiatric concepts. Somewhat similar issues derive from Rutter and Mawhood's (1991) follow-up into adult life of boys with a severe development disorder of receptive language. Almost all acquired conversational speech but about half failed to develop close mutual friendships or love relationships, although they did not show any psychiatric disorder as usually conceptualized.

Follow-up studies extending into middle childhood of very low birth weight babies have suggested that there is a raised rate of clumsiness and of behaviour difficulties (Casaer, de Vries & Marlow, 1991). Again, the sequelae seem to involve clinically important impaired functioning but the impairments found do not coincide with currently recognized diagnostic categories. A developmental psychopathology perspective requires that longitudinal studies of high-risk groups examine outcomes in terms of effects on psychological development as well as on disease or disorder categories. The nature and extent of continuities between normality and psychopathology constitutes a main focus for investigation, rather than something that is assumed to be present or absent. Of course, the findings may sometimes lead to the need for a reconceptualization of disorders. That is happening, currently, with respect to the creation, in both DSM-III-R (American Psychiatric Association, 1987) and ICD-10 (World Health Organization, 1992) of attachment disorder categories to cover the psychopathological patterns that seem to be associated with grossly abnormal patterns of upbringing involving severe abuse or neglect. The nosological validity of these categories is still uncertain but it is clear that previous diagnostic concepts do not provide what is needed and hence that some change is required.

PHENOTYPIC DEFINITION

It might be thought that the problems involved in defining psychopathological categories mainly apply to the outcomes associated with complex risk experiences involving many facets. However, that is not so, as is clear, for example, from psychiatric genetic studies. One of the major difficulties in applying molecular genetic strategies to psychiatric disorders has been the uncertainty about how to define the phenotype. There is good agreement on what constitutes 'core' schizophrenia or bipolar affective psychosis but great controversy on how widely to extend the diagnostic boundaries. Thus, it seems clear that the schizophrenia phenotype includes some varieties of personality disorder (so-called 'schizotypy') but there is much uncertainty on how to define such disorders. Similar issues arise with respect to autism (Rutter, 1991*a*).

Several rather different possibilities need to be considered. First, it is known that some single gene disorders have a very wide and variable range of expression. Thus, neurofibromatosis may be manifest by gross deformities associated with nerve tumours (as shown in the film 'The Elephant Man') or just some 'café au lait' spots on the skin that require an expert to notice them. Secondly, genes may lead, not to a single disease, but rather to a range of sequelae that do not cluster into any single disease category – so-called 'pleiotropy' (Plomin, 1991). Thirdly, the proneness or liability to the 'illness' (e.g. schizophrenic psychosis) may lie in some form of personality disorder that is much more common than the 'illness' itself. Such personality disorders may themselves constitute either qualitatively distinct categories or classes or they may represent the extreme of normally distributed personality variations. Equally, multi-factorial genetic models of psychiatric disorder are based on the assumption that there is some underlying, normally distributed, 'liability', with the overt disorder being manifest only above some particular threshold.

In addition, there are many psychiatric disorders that seem to have close parallels within the range of normal variations (Rutter & Sandberg, 1985): for example, anorexia nervosa and adolescent dieting, alcoholism and heavy drinking, depressive disorder and 'normal' feelings of misery, 'dyslexia' and normally distributed reading skills, development language disorders and normal variations in the timing of language acquisition – to mention but a few. Are the disorders qualitatively distinct from normality, or do they represent extremes of the normal distribution? All of these possibilities require that continuities and discontinuities between normality and disorder be the subject of empirical study – a key feature of developmental psychopathology. Until recently, the means to test these notions empirically were lacking but advances in statistical modelling and, especially, in behaviour genetics have opened up a range of possibilities. Thus, Lenzenweger and Moldin (1990) used admixture analyses (based on a latent class approach) to examine perceptual aberrations as an index of a liability to schizophrenia; Eaves et al. (1987) used a latent trait analysis to compare multiple gene and single gene models for affective disorder; and De Fries and Fulker (1985, 1988) have devised a multiple regression approach to determine whether disorders are genetically continuous with variations in the normal distribution. An application of the last approach to intelligence showed that severe retardation was discontinuous with the normal range of intelligence, whereas much of mild retardation probably did represent the extreme of normal variation (Plomin, 1991).

HETEROTYPIC CONTINUITY

Until very recently, most of the longitudinal studies of psychological traits have been based on correlations over time for characteristics (such as aggressivity or fearfulness) defined in the same way for all ages across the developmental time span covered by the study. The results have generally shown rather modest individual consistency, especially from the preschool years (Brim & Kagan, 1980). It has become clear, both for psychopathology, and for normally distributed characteristics, that it cannot be assumed that a single underlying trait will be manifest in the same way at all age periods. This became apparent in the case of schizophrenia some years ago (Rutter and Garmezy, 1983). Thus, longitudinal data showed that, although schizophrenia, as a psychotic disorder, usually did not become manifest until late adolescence or adult life, it had been preceded by abnormalities in childhood in about half the cases. Usually, this took the form of social difficulties, neurodevelopmental immaturities and attentional deficits involving poor signal/noise discrimination. Hanson, Gottesman and Heston's (1976) data on the offspring of parents with schizophrenia are important in their demonstration that the constellation that combines these features is a much better differentiator than any of the characteristics considered in isolation. The features are not sufficiently clear-cut for the behaviour of any individual child to be reliably diagnosed as preschizophrenic, but there is no doubt that this childhood pattern does constitute a precursor for the later development of a schizophrenic psychosis. The form of the behaviour changes with age but the underlying construct remains the same.

The need, in many psychopathological instances, to focus on constellations of behaviour, rather than individual traits, has also been well demonstrated in Magnusson and Bergman's (1988, 1990) analysis of the Stockholm longitudinal study data. Like other investigators, they found that aggressivity in childhood predicted criminality in adult life. However, what was new, and important, in their analysis was the demonstration that the predictive power lay in the combination of aggressivity, hyperactivity, inattention and poor peer relationships. When this multiple-problem group was removed from the sample, aggressivity lost its predictive power. Similarly, poor peer relationships predicted adult criminality only when it occurred in association with other 'problem' behaviours. As Magnusson and Bergman emphasized, the implication is that variables may change their meaning according to whether or not they occur in conjunction with other variables. Their 'person-oriented' approach provides one good way of examining this possibility. Of course, interactions can be looked for in dimensional variable-orientated analyses but they have their limitations for this purpose and it needs to be appreciated that a statistically significant 'main' effect does not necessarily mean that the variable in question has a significant effect when it occurs in isolation from other variables (Rutter, 1983a; Rutter & Pickles, 1991).

The issues are closely comparable to those involved in the study of comorbidity – the association between two supposedly different disorders (Caron & Rutter, 1991). It is evident that in some instances the meaning of a 'disorder' changes when it occurs in association with some other 'disorder'. Thus, depression in association with conduct disorder does not seem to have the same correlates or outcome as depression occurring on its own (Angold & Rutter, 1992; Harrington et al., 1991; Puig-Antich et al., 1989); and hyperactivity in conjunction with anxiety seems not to respond to stimulant medication in the fashion typical of hyperactivity on its own (Taylor et al., 1987; Pliszka, 1989).

Comorbidity and heterotypic continuity come together in findings that one disorder in childhood leads to an apparently different disorder in adult life. This seems to be the case, for example, in the observation that conduct disorder in childhood predisposes to depressive symptomatology in adult life (Robins, 1986; Rutter, 1991b), and to a range of personality disorders that are not confined to those involving antisocial behaviours (Zoccolillo et al., 1992). These results force a reconsideration of traditional psychiatric concepts, but it is important to appreciate that the fact that disorder 'A' commonly leads on to disorder 'B' does not necessarily mean that both represent the same latent disorder construct. That constitutes but one possibility among several that need to be put to the empirical test. Genetic designs that incorporate a long-term longitudinal follow-up provide one essential strategy for this purpose. Thus, using an adoptive design, Cadoret et al. (1990) found that anti-social disorder in parents was genetically associated with antisocial disorder in the away-adopted offspring but not with depressive symptoms. On the other hand, anti-social disorder was associated with a markedly elevated, environmentally mediated, risk of depressive symptoms in the same individual. The implication was that the association over time between conduct disorder and depression did not represent heterotypic continuity, but rather an example of one disorder creating a risk factor for another. On the other hand, it is possible that the connection between conduct disorder in childhood and non-antisocial varieties of personality disorder in adult life may constitute heterotypic continuity. Genetic designs (both twin and adoptee) would help test that suggestion. The available data are far too few for any conclusions. However, the point is that longitudinal data have been important in posing the question and research strategies associated with a developmental psychopathology perspective are valuable in testing competing hypotheses on the meaning of the findings.

Heterotypic continuity also needs to be considered in relation to normal psychological development. Infant cognition and intelligence in later childhood and adult life constitutes a striking and important example. Numerous studies have shown that developmental quotients in the first two or three years of life have a negligible correlation with later IQ. It has also been found that the heritability of developmental quotients is much lower than that of later IQ (Plomin, 1986). Accordingly, it came to be assumed that cognitive skills in infancy have only a very weak connection with cognitive skills later in life. It is now clear that this was a mistaken assumption (Bornstein & Sigman, 1986; Slater et al., 1989). The change in view stemmed from well-replicated evidence that measures of attention and habituation in infancy did show substantial correlations with later IQ. Of course, in itself, this does not demonstrate heterotypic continuity but the finding that, in adoptees attentional measures, unlike developmental quotients, also correlate with the IQ of the biological parents suggests that this may well be the correct explanation (DiLalla et al., 1990).

With several of the issues discussed so far, it has been apparent that genetic research strategies are very useful in tackling key issues with respect to developmental psychopathology. Non-geneticists still tend to assume that the main purpose of genetics in psychology is to assess the degree of heritability of some trait. This is a seriously mistaken notion both because genetic strategies are crucial for the testing of environmental risk hypotheses and because they provide considerable opportunities for the study of developmental and psychopathological processes and mechanisms (Rende & Plomin, in press; Rutter, 1991*c*).

ORIGINS OF LIFE EXPERIENCES

One of the key questions in the study of psychosocial risk factors, but one of the least investigated, concerns their origins. It is obvious that psychosocial stresses and adversities are far from randomly distributed; some individuals experience many serious hazards whereas others experience very few. Scarr (Chapter 2, this volume) puts the case for the role of genetic factors in people's behaviour that serves to shape and select their environments. Plomin and Bergeman (1991) make the same point that genetic factors influence the distribution of risk experiences but also note that some supposedly environmental measures may actually reflect genetic influences more than environmental ones. Thus, the ways in which parents talk and play with their children reflects an important part of children's experiences but, of course, they also reflect the qualities of the parents as individuals. Often, much of the parental effect on children's psychological development derives from the shared genes rather than the provided environment.

These genetic considerations are important but it is crucial to appreciate that the question of the origins of life experiences is far broader than $G \rightarrow E$ effects (Rutter & Rutter, 1993). Thus, it is clear that people's role in shaping and selecting their environments goes well beyond genetic determinants. For example, Robins (1966), in her long-term follow-up of boys with conduct disorders, showed that, as adults, compared with general population controls, they had much higher rates of unemployment, disrupted friendships, marital breakdowns, lack of social support, and poor living conditions. In her discussion of these findings, the outcome was conceptualized in terms of personality disorder as a continuation of the conduct disorder evident in childhood. That is an entirely appropriate way of viewing the findings but it is also the case that these adult features constitute the risk environments much studied in relation to adult depression. Genetic factors may play a part in the process, but in view of the modest heritability of conduct disorder (DiLalla & Gottesman, 1989), it is unlikely that they predominate. Similarly, Quinton and Rutter's (1988) follow-up of girls reared in group foster homes showed that they had a much increased rate of teenage pregnancies and marriage, and a much greater tendency to make unhappy disrupted marriages with deviant men. Again, this tendency is both a reflection of continuing psychosocial problems and the creation of new stressful environments. The developmental psycho-pathology perspective is important in suggesting the need to treat adult environments as both a dependent variable (in relation to childhood risk factors) and an independent one (in relations to risk effects for adult behaviour).

Traditionally, causal questions have usually been posed in terms of individual differences, such as why 'A' is unemployed or depressed, whereas 'B' is not. However, that is only one of several different sorts of causal questions (Rutter, in press). For example, it is equally important to consider cause in relation to levels, as they vary over time, or by geography, or age group. Thus, we may ask why the average height of London school boys increased by some 10 centimetres in the first half of this century (Tizard, 1975) or why unemployment and homelessness have risen so greatly over the last dozen years of Tory rule in Britain. The answer to the former is probably to be found in improved nutrition and to the latter in socio-political factors. However, what emerges from a consideration of influences is that society-wide influences play an important role in determining both the level and distribution of risk environments. With respect to uneven distribution, it is evident, for example, that the unemploy-ment rate in black youths in the UK is much higher than that in white youths, and that this is mainly attributable to racial discrimination (White & McRae, 1989).

Another aspect of variability in people's experience of risk environments stems from their vulnerability to the risks. With most environmental hazards, physical or psychosocial, there is considerable variability in people's response (Rutter & Pickles, 1991). Quantitative geneticists have found very few replicated examples of gene–environment interactions but person–environment interactions are widespread in both biology and medicine. This paradox, sometimes known as the Plomin's paradox because of Plomin's influential writings on the topic (see Wachs & Plomin, 1991; Plomin, de Fries & Fulker, 1988) is probably due to several different factors. These include both statistical considerations (e.g. many interactions apply only to sub-groups of the population, also many statistical tests for interactions lack adequate power – Wahlsten, 1990) and conceptual issues (e.g. the person effects may not be genetically determined and the interaction may require specification and measurement of the relevant aspect of the environment if it is to be assessed).

A key developmental consideration in relation to the interplay between persons and their environments is that the individual variability in susceptibility to particular environments may derive from earlier experiences (Bock & Whelan, 1991). For example, sub-nutrition in infancy is known to be associated with a much increased risk of coronary heart disease in adult life (Barker, 1991) – possibly as a result of an increased vulnerability to unduly rich diets. Also, animal studies have shown that acute physical stressors in infancy are followed by a lasting neuroendocrine change that is associated with an enhanced resistance to later stress (Hennessy & Levine, 1979). Conversely, chronically adverse parental care in childhood is associated with an increased risk of depression in adult life – probably in part because it creates a greater vulnerability to stress in adult life (Harris, Brown & Bifulco, 1990).

Most of the classic developmental theories were expressed in universal individualistic terms with little more than lip service to the role of social context. However, psychopathological studies have indicated that the developmental implications of both individual behaviours and experiences often vary by gender and that this may be explicable, at least in part, by social context effects. For example, the adult follow-up of children reared in Group Homes undertaken by Quinton and Rutter (1988) showed that whereas girls tended to seek escape from stressful family circumstances through teenage pregnancy and marriage, boys were much less likely to do so (Rutter et al., 1990). Also, whereas conduct disordered girls tended to marry boys with similar problems, this was not so for conduct disordered boys (Zoccolillo et al. 1992). To an important extent, this gender difference reflected the fact that conduct disordered boys tended to marry at a much older age. Another example of gender differences is provided by shyness, where several studies have shown that this tends to be associated with negative social interactions in boys but positive ones in girls (Stevenson-Hinde, 1986; Rubin & Asendorpf, in press). The explanation is not known but it may well lie in the different social expectations for boys and girls.

RISK MECHANISMS

In his review, Garmezy (Chapter 6, this volume) notes that psychiatric high risk studies were dominated for many years by longitudinal investigations of children born to, and reared by, schizophrenic mothers. The studies were informative in various ways but what is striking with the benefit of hindsight is the developmental naivety of the assumption that parental schizophrenia constituted the one essential risk factor and that schizophrenia in the children represented the one key psychopathological outcome. Thus, very few studies included any comparison group with some other form of parental mental disorder or with psychosocial risk factors outside of mental illness. Also, there was very little appreciation of the need to take into account that the psychological functioning of the children in high risk groups will vary over time. As Erlenmeyer-Kimling et al. (1990) observed in their thoughtful analysis of their own long term follow-up findings: 'for subjects with erratic courses, their status as dysfunctional versus non-dysfunctional is very much a question of when the classification is made . . . This is the dilemma . . . of defining what constitutes 'outcome' and deciding when outcome occurs' (p. 362). Research findings have now made clear that parental mental disorder is a risk indicator that involves a quite diverse range of risk mechanisms and of risk outcomes (Rutter, 1989*b*, 1990*a*). Indeed, so far as affective disorder in parents is concerned, the main risk seems to stem from the often associated family discord and problems in parenting rather than from the disorder per se (Downey & Coyne, 1990). This is true to some extent, too, with parental schizophrenia although the specific genetic risk is more evident than with parental depression.

These psychiatric 'high risk' studies were based on oversimplified risk expectations but they have been informative in shedding light on risk mechanisms, albeit not the ones that constituted the basis for the original design. What the studies do illustrate, however, is the value of taking (relatively) extreme risk situations to study developmental processes. The findings also bring out the important advantage of prospective longitudinal designs in that they allow detailed study of the different elements of the risk situation and hence that they enable competing hypotheses on risk mechanisms to be put to the test. This is evident in the parental depression-discord example just given but there are numerous other instances – such as the finding that early parental loss is a risk factor for depressive disorder in adult life only when it is accompanied by poor parental care (Brown, Harris & Bifulco, 1986).

Four other general issues require particular mention in relation to 'high risk' designs. First, as already noted, prospective longitudinal studies have been crucial in demonstrating the diversity of psychopathological outcomes. Thus, parental mental disorder leads not only to an increased risk for the same type of psychiatric condition in the children but also to a raised risk for a wide range of other psychopathology (Rutter, 1989*b*). This is not so easily identified in retrospective studies. Second, longitudinal data are needed for the adequate study of 'escape' from risk. With virtually all risk factors, it has been found that a substantial proportion of children exposed to the risk survive without serious psychopathological sequelae. This does not necessarily mean that they have been unaffected by their experiences, or that there are not subtle sequelae, but relatively speaking they have 'escaped' serious damage. That is a most important observation from both theoretical and practical perspectives. It raised questions about individual differences in susceptibility and also it highlights the need to study possible protective, as well as risk, factors (Garmezy, 1985; Masten and Garmezy, 1985; Rutter, 1990*b*; Jenkins & Smith, 1990). Both developmental and clinical considerations shape research into such protective and risk processes. To begin with, medical analogies make it clear that it would be most unwise to assume that protective effects have to be found in hedonically positive experiences. Often, controlled exposure to the risk factor is required for resistance to develop. This is obvious in relation to acquired immunity to infectious agents but probably there are psychological equivalents (Rutter, 1990*b*); this notion underlies the concept of stress inoculation training (Meichenbaum, 1985). Possibly, Elder's (Elder, Liker & Jaworski, 1984) finding that disadvantaged children who had to take on increased responsibilities during the Great Economic Depression, and who did so successfully, fared better than other children in the long run is an example of this type. It seems that protective mechanisms may derive as much from preceding or succeeding circumstances from those operating at the time of risk exposure. Longitudinal data are crucial for examination of this possibility.

In that connection, it is relevant to note that risk mechanisms, too, often involve indirect chain effects of one kind or another – the third general issue to underline. Thus, early parental loss that leads to poor parenting seems to create a risk for adult depression in part because it is associated with an increase in vulnerability to the ill-effects of acute stress experiences in adult life (Harris et al., 1990). The same may apply to a broader range of childhood vulnerability factors (Rodgers, 1990). Similarly, an institutional rearing (together with the multiplicity of psychosocial risks that it indexes) seems to predispose to poor social functioning in adult life in part because it increases the risk of teenage marriage to a deviant spouse (and associated teenage motherhood) and because it increases susceptibility to adverse circumstances in adult life (Quinton & Rutter, 1988; Rutter, 1991*b*). Another example is provided by the sequelae of poor schooling in which the long-term risks seem to reside in the chain effects associated with poor school attendance and early drop-out from education, making it likely that the young people will lack educational qualifications and so land up in unskilled jobs with an increased risk of unemployment (Gray, Smith & Rutter, 1980; White & McRae, 1989). It is important that high-risk studies use longitudinal research designs to delineate these various indirect chain-effect risk processes.

Such processes include so-called turning point effects (Pickles & Rutter, 1991) in which risky life trajectories may change direction onto a more adaptive path, or vice versa – the fourth general issue to note. Often turning points tend to be thought of in negative terms, with the focus on stress events that create a psychiatric risk in people whose previous psychological development has been unremarkable. However, this is probably a rather misleading way of thinking about the phenomenon, if only because stress experiences tend to emphasize or accentuate pre-existing characteristics rather than alter their pattern – what Elder and Caspi (1990) have termed the 'accentuation principle'. The point brings out the important consideration that life experiences may serve to increase continuities, as well as bring about change. Biologically speaking, developmental continuities and discontinuities are to be expected, and stress or adversity may work in either direction.

However, most psychosocial turning points probably should not be conceptualized in stress terms at all. Rather, they alter life trajectories because they open up (or close down) important opportunities, because they are accompanied by a lasting change in the environment, because they influence people's selection or shaping of their environment, or because they affect people's control over their lives. Thus, Elder (1986) found that, for young men from a disadvantaged background, early entry into the Armed Forces proved to be a protective factor in relation to adult outcomes. That seemed to come about because entering the Army enabled them to continue their education and also allowed them to postpone marriage to a time when they were more mature and also were in contact with a wider social network than that prevailing in their earlier disadvantaged circumstances. Similarly, Quinton and Rutter (1988) found that a harmonious marriage with a non-deviant spouse was a protective factor for institution-reared girls. At an earlier point, positive school experiences seemed to make it more likely that the girls would exert planning in their lives, which, in turn, increased the likelihood of a harmonious marriage to a non-deviant spouse.

It is noteworthy that many of the turning points that bring with them enhanced resilience occur in adult life and few of them are of a type that bring their benefits through experiences that are characterized by being especially happy-making. The bringing together of developmental and clinical research perspectives emphasizes the wide range of psychological processes that affect normal and abnormal development; only a few operate through the pleasantness or unpleasantness of their effects.

AGE-RELATED VULNERABILITIES

One key element in a developmental approach to psychopathology is the recognition that the nature or extent of risks may be affected by the age at which they impinge. Thus, it is well known that an uncorrected strabismus in infancy leads to a failure to develop binocular vision, because visual input in the early years is necessary for the normal maturation and functioning of the visual cortex (Blakemore, 1991). Although the evidence is much less satisfactory, it is possible that transient hearing loss (as a result of secretory otitis media; so-called 'glue ear') during the phase of language acquisition may be associated with some persistent verbal deficits (Haggard & Hughes, 1991). It may be, too, that a regular lack of selective attachments in the preschool years (perhaps as a result of an institutional upbringing) is associated with a lasting, although not immutable, impairment in close friendships and love relationships (Rutter, 1991d). Developmentalists have had to reject the concept of fixed 'critical periods' with respect to most aspects of development, but nevertheless it seems likely that psychological functions may mature more readily if the right conditions are present during a particular 'sensitive period'. The challenge for the future is to design research that can test such hypotheses and delineate the circumstances and limits of their operation.

Of course, age-related vulnerabilities are by no means confined to the particular sort of sensitive period effect by which optimal development is (partially) reliant on certain experiences occurring at a particular age or phase. At least, six other types are known to occur. First, sensitivity to the immediate effects of particular experiences may vary with age. Thus, pre-school children above the age of 6 months or so are those most likely to be adversely affected by stressful separation experiences (such as admission to hospital or a residential nursery). Presumably, this is because they have reached the age at which selective attachments are important but are still not old enough for them easily to maintain relationships during the course of a separation (Rutter, 1981b). Secondly, recovery from damage may be greater when continuing maturational processes in the brain are associated with greater plasticity. Thus, damage to the left hemisphere in adult life usually results in aphasia, with some lasting persistence of language abnormalities; by contrast, comparable damage in infancy has both different, and lesser, effects usually followed by near-normal acquisition of language (Goodman, 1987, 1991). It seems that, when the left hemisphere is seriously damaged in very early life, language functions can be taken over by the right hemisphere. Thirdly, lasting sequelae from early damage to the brain may sometimes be greater than from later damage, either because the brain deficit interferes with new learning or because neuronal reorganization leads to anomalous misconnections from faulty 'rewiring' (Goodman, 1991; Rutter, 1983b). Thus, early bilateral damage is more likely to lead to a general lowering of intellectual performance. Also, cognitive deficits following early brain damage are more strongly associated with the occurrence of epilepsy (reflecting brain malfunction rather than non-function) than with the side of the lesion (Vargha-Khadem et al., 1992).

Fourthly, young people may be affected by the timing of their development being 'out-of-step' with that of their peer group. Thus, girls who reach their menarché unusually early are more likely than other girls of the same age to engage in norm-breaking behaviour (Stattin & Magnusson, 1990). The phenomenon is a consequence of being 'out-of-step' in a culturally negative direction only; very late puberty does not have comparable negative effects (Caspi & Moffitt, 1991; Caspi et al., unpublished observations). The behavioural effect is mediated by the social consequences of the physiological charge; the increase in norm-breaking behaviour occurs only in early maturing girls who associate with a much older peer group. Also, in most respects, the negative effects of very early puberty proved to be transient. By the age of 25 years, early maturing girls in the Stockholm study no longer stood out as different from their contemporaries in rule-breaking behaviour. However, they did remain different in educational qualifications. This was not because early puberty led to any lasting change in personality but rather because early drop-out from schooling required positive steps to re-enter education if the immediate consequences were not to persist. The finding emphasizes that psychological continuities may reside in social, rather than in intra-psychic, effects.

Fifthly, there may be effects from physical changes associated with physiological maturation. Thus, Attie and Brooks-Gunn (1989) found that undue weight gain in adolescent girls was important in precipitating disturbed eating patterns. Interestingly, however, the persistence of such patterns between 14 and 16 years was more strongly associated with depressed mood and disturbed family relationships, a finding that serves as a reminder that the mechanisms involved in continuation of a behaviour may not be identical with those involved in its onset.

Lastly, the correlates and consequences of psychopathology may vary with the timing of its onset. Thus, unusually early onset conduct disturbance is particularly likely to be associated with hyperactivity and carries an especial risk of persistence into adult life (Farrington et al., 1990a). Conversely, late onset delinquency and conduct disturbance differs from comparable disorders beginning in earlier childhood in not having an association with reading difficulties (Rutter, Tizard & Whitmore, 1970).

DISAGGREGATING AGE EFFECTS

As is evident from these few examples of age-related vulnerabilities, chronological age indexes a wide variety of features – physiological, psychological, and social – and in itself it provides no explanation (Rutter, 1989c). The task for the developmental psychopathology investigator is to search for appropriate 'experiments of nature' in which the individual aspects of age are teased apart (Rutter, 1981a). Fortunately, these abound in prevailing life circumstances. A 'flavour' of the range of diverse research strategies may be provided by a sample of rather different examples. One necessary contrast is between age as a reflection of biological maturation and as an index of key experiences. Cahan and Cohen (1989) recognized the importance of this distinction with respect to children's intellectual development. Most school systems provide the necessary experiment because all children tend to start school at the beginning of the academic year (rather than at a fixed age). The consequence is that the 12-month age spread within any one class reflects biological differences (on the assumption that birth dates are more or less randomly distributed), whereas the 12-month age difference between one class and the next reflects duration of schooling. The contrast showed both biological age and schooling effects but for most intellectual functions, the latter tended to be stronger.

A somewhat similar issue concerns the peak age of delinquency in adolescence. Farrington (1986) argued that, if this reflected biological age influences, it should remain invariant over time, whereas, if it reflected some experimental factor such as age of leaving school, it might well vary over time. Secular trend analyses showed that the peak in males had gone up over time, more or less reflecting rises in the school leaving age. Curiously, the trend in females went in the oppositie direction, suggesting that some other factor must be operating.

Comparable issues apply at the other end of the age span, as three very different examples illustrate. It has long been realized that suicide rates increase with age, usually reaching a peak only in advanced old age. Although it may seem likely that this reflects degenerative biological processes, it is evident that this is not the main explanation. Marital dissolution, either through divorce or widowhood, also increases with age, and Kreitman's (1988) analyses clearly showed that it is such dissolution that carries the main association with suicide. When marital status is taken into account, the association between age and suicide is largely lost. Osteoporosis would seem an even stronger candidate for a consequence of inevitable biological 'wearing out'. However, comparisons within age groups according to level of exercise and (in women) use of hormone replacement therapy (HRT) shows that hormone levels and exercise account for much of the effect (Quigley et al., 1987; Lane et al., 1986, 1987). Bone density in women on HRT, and in adults of both sexes who take regular vigorous exercise, shows much less diminution with age than that seen ordinarily. Diminishing fertility with age in women provides a third example. The query here is whether the reduction in fertility is a consequence of diminishing sexual activity or anxiety over 'time running out' or biological changes in the ova. In this case, the in vitro fertilization of eggs from donor semen provided the necessary experiment – with findings supporting the biological change hypothesis (Schwartz & Mayaux, 1982).

The marked individual differences in the timing of puberty provide an opportunity for separating endocrine effects from other facets of chronological age. Angold and Rutter (1992) found that the rise in depression with increasing age in a clinic sample of some 3500 children and adolescents could not be accounted for by puberty. The finding so far is based on cross-sectional data and needs to be checked using a longitudinal design in which causal influences can be tested through the examination of intra-individual change over time (Farrington, 1988). Also, it remains to be determined which facet of age, other than puberty, is responsible for the increase in depressive type problems during adolescence. The point of these examples is not to indicate all the various research strategies that may be used to tease apart the different facets of age (that would require a chapter of its own), but rather to show that this separation is possible if the researcher seeks out the appropriate real life circumstances. Such quasi-experimental testing is crucial – as already discussed.

CONCLUSIONS

In the preceding chapter, Garmezy made clear that: 'The focus of developmental psychology is on the research enterprise'. He went on to note that the bringing together of developmental and clinical perspectives went well beyond the prediction of maladaptive behaviour, was by no means confined to psychology, and included adult life as well as childhood. Both that chapter and this one have been explicit that developmental psychopathology is not a theory or a model. Moreover, the conjunction of the two approaches is as important in the light that the study of extremes may throw on normal development, as in the understanding of the processes underlying psychopathology. As a research enterprise, it necessarily borrows or adopts concepts and strategies from many other fields – genetics, epidemiology, experimental and developmental psychology, neurobiology, and sociology to mention but a few. It makes no claim to provide the best approach to the study of all aspects of all types of psychiatric disorder. Nevertheless, it does argue that the combination of developmental and clinical research perspectives provides a most useful means of research leverage. A few examples have been given in this chapter to illustrate some of the investigative paths that seem to lead ahead. While these rely heavily on longitudinal methods of one kind or another, they exemplify a wide diversity of longitudinal strategies and tactics, most of which make use of contrasting groups in order to focus on underlying mechanisms and processes and to test competing hypothesis on which these may be.

REFERENCES

American Psychiatric Association (1987). *Diagnostic and statistical manual of mental disorders (DSM-III)*. Washington, DC: American Psychiatric Association.

Angold, A. & Rutter, M. (1992). The effects of age and pubertal status on depression in a large clinical sample. *Development and Psychopathology*, **4**, 5–28.

Aslin, R. N., Pisoni, D. B. & Jusczyk, P. W. (1983). Auditory development and speech perception in infancy. In M. M. Haith & J. J. Campos (eds.) *Infancy and Developmental psychobiology, Vol. 2, Mussen's Handbook of child psychology (4th ed)*, pp. 573–687, New York: Wiley.

Astington, J. W., Harris, P. L. & Olson, D. R. (eds.) (1988). *Developing theories of mind*. Cambridge: Cambridge University Press.

Attie, I. & Brooks-Gunn, J. (1989). Development of eating problems in adolescent girls:

a longitudinal study. *Developmental Psychology*, **25**, 70–9.

Bailey, A. J., Le Couteur, A., Rutter, M., Pickles, A., Yuzda, E., Schmidt, D. & Gottesman, I. (1991). Obstetric and neurodevelopmental data from the British twin study of autism. *Psychiatric Genetics*, **2**, Abstract S7A/1.

Barker, D. J. P. (1991). In G. R. Bock & J. Whelan (eds.). *The childhood environment and adult disease*. Ciba Foundation Symposium No. 156. Chichester: Wiley.

Baron-Cohen, S., Leslie, A. M. & Frith, U. (1985). Does the autistic child have a 'theory of mind'? *Cognition*, **21**, 37–46.

Blakemore, C. (1991). Sensitive and vulnerable periods in the development of the visual system. In G. R. Bock & J. Whelan (eds.) *The childhood environment and adult disease*. Ciba Foundation Symposium No. 156. pp. 129–147, Chichester: Wiley.

Bock, G. R. & Whelan, J. (eds.) (1991). *The childhood environment and adult disease*. Ciba Foundation Symposium No. 156. Chichester: Wiley.

Bornstein, M. H. & Sigman, M. D. (1986). Continuity in mental development from infancy. *Child Development*, **57**, 251–74.

Bradley, L. & Bryant, P. (1985). *Rhyme and reason in reading and spelling*. International Academy for Research in Learning Disabilities Monograph Series No. 1. Ann Arbor: University of Michigan Press.

Brim, Jr. O. G. & Kagan, J. (eds.) (1980). *Constancy and change in human development*. Cambridge, Mass.: Harvard University Press.

Brown, G. W., Harris, T. O. & Bifulco, A. (1986). Long-term effects of early loss of parent. In M. Rutter, C. E. Izard and P. B. Read (eds.), *Depression in young people: Developmental and clinical perspectives*, pp. 251–296, New York: Guilford Press.

Cadoret, R. J., Troughton, E., Merchant, L. M. & Whitters, A. (1990). Early life psychosocial events and adult affective symptoms. In L. Robins and M. Rutter (eds.), *Straight and devious pathways from childhood to adulthood*. pp. 300–313, New York: Cambridge University Press.

Cahan, S. & Cohen, N. (1989). Age versus schooling effects on intelligence development. *Child Development*, **60**, 1239–49.

Caron, C. & Rutter, M. (1991). Comorbidity in child psychopathology: concepts, issues and research strategies. *Journal of Child Psychology and Psychiatry*, **32**, 1063–80.

Casaer, P., de Vries, L. & Marlow, N. (1991). Prenatal and perinatal risk factors for psychosocial development. In M. Rutter & P. Casaer (eds.), *Biological risk factors for psychosocial disorders*. pp. 139–174, Cambridge: Cambridge University Press.

Caspi, A. & Moffitt, T. E. (1991). Individual differences are accentuated during periods of social change: the sample case of girls at puberty. *Journal of Personality and Social Psychology*, **61**, 157–168.

DeFries, J. C. & Fulker, D. W. (1985). Multiple regression analysis of twin data. *Behavior Genetics*, **15**, 467–73.

DeFries, J. C. & Fulker, D. W. (1988). Multiple regression analysis of twin data: etiology of deviant scores versus individual differences. *Acta Geneticae Medicae et Gemellologiae*, **37**, 205–16.

DiLalla, L. F. & Gottesman, I. I. (1989). Heterogeneity of causes for delinquency and criminality: lifespan perspective. *Development and Psychopathology*, **1**, 339–49.

DiLalla, L. F., Thompson, L. A., Plomin, R., Phillips, K., Fagan III, J. F., Haith, M. M., Cyphers, L. H. & Fulker, D. W. (1990). Infant predictors of preschool and adult IQ: a study of infant twins and their parents. *Developmental Psychology*, **26**, 759–69.

Dodge, K. A., Pettit, G. S., McClaskey, C. L. & Brown, M. (1986). Social competence in children. *Monographs of the Society for Research in Child Development*, **51** (2, Serial No. 213).

Downey, G. & Coyne, J. C. (1990). Children of depressed parents: An integrative review. *Psychological Bulletin*, **108**, 50–76.

Eaves, L. J., Martin, N. G., Heath, A. C. & Kendler, K. S. (1987). Testing genetic models for multiple symptoms: an application to the genetic analysis of liability to depression. *Behavior Genetics*, **17**, 331–41.

Elder Jr., G. H. (1986). Military times and turning points in men's lives. *Developmental Psychology*, **22**, 233–45.

Elder Jr., G. H. & Caspi, A. (1990). Studying lives in a changing society: sociological and personological explorations. In A. I. Rabin, R. A. Zucker, S. Frank & R. A. Emmons (eds.) *Studying persons and lives*. New York: Springer.

Elder Jr., G. H., Liker, J. K. & Jaworski, B. J. (1984). Hardship in lives: historical influences from the 1930s to old age in postwar America. In K. McCluskey and H. Reese (eds.) *Life-span development psychology: Historical and cohort effects*. New York: Academic Press.

Erlenmeyer-Kimling, L., Cornblatt, B. A., Bassett, A. S., Moldin, S. O., Hilldoff-Adamo, U. & Roberts, S. (1990). High-risk children in adolescence and young adulthood: course of global adjustment. In L. Robins & M. Rutter (eds.) *Straight and devious pathways from childhood to adulthood*. pp. 351–364, New York: Cambridge University Press.

Farrington, D. P. (1986). Age and crime. In M. Tonry and N. Morris (eds.). *Crime and justice*, vol. 7, Chicago: Chicago University Press.

Farrington, D. P. (1988). Studying changes within individuals: The causes of offending. In M. Rutter (ed.). *Studies of psychosocial risk: the power of longitudinal data*. pp. 158–183, Cambridge: Cambridge University Press.

Farrington, D. P., Loeber, R. & Van Kammen, W. B. (1990*a*). Long-term criminal outcomes of hyperactivity–impulsivity–attention deficit and conduct problems in childhood. In L. Robins & M. Rutter (eds.). *Straight and devious pathways from childhood to adulthood*. pp. 62–81, New York: Cambridge University Press.

Farrinton, D. P., Loeber, R., Elliott, D. S., Hawkins, J. D., Kandel, D. B., Klein, M. W., McCord, J., Rowe, D. C. & Tremblay, R. E. (1990*b*). Advancing knowledge about the onset of delinquency and crime. In B. B. Lahey & A. E. Kazdin (eds.) (1990). *Advances in clinical child psychology*, vol. 13, pp. 283–342, New York: Plenum.

Frith, U. (1989). *Autism: explaining the enigma*. Oxford: Basil Blackwell.

Garmezy, N. (1985). Stress resistant children: the search for protective factors. In J. Stevenson (ed.). *Recent research in developmental psychology*. Book Supplement to the *Journal of Child Psychology and Psychiatry*, No. 4. Oxford: Pergamon Press.

Goldman-Rakic, P. S., Isseroff, A., Schwartz, M. L. & Bugbee, N. M. (1983). The neurobiology of cognitive development. In M. M. Haith and J. J. Campos (eds.). *Infancy and developmental psychobiology, Vol. 2, Mussen's Handbook of child psychology* (4th ed.), pp. 281–344, New York: Wiley.

Goodman, R. (1987). The developmental neurobiology of language. In W. Yule & M. Rutter (eds.). *Language development and disorders*. Clinics in Developmental Medicine No. 101/102. London/Oxford: Mac Keith Press/Blackwell Scientific; Philadelphia: Lippincott.

Goodman, R. (1990). Technical note: are perinatal complications causes or consequences of autism? *Journal of Child Psychology and Psychiatry*, **31**, 809–12.

Goodman, R. (1991). Developmental disorders and structural brain development. In M. Rutter & P. Casaer (eds.). *Biological risk factors for psychosocial disorders.* pp. 20–49, Cambridge: Cambridge University Press.

Goswami, U. & Bryant, P. (1990). *Phonological skills and learning to read.* Hove, East Sussex: Erlbaum.

Gray, G., Smith, A. & Rutter, M. (1980). School attendance and the first year of employment. In L. Hersov & I. Berg (eds.). *Out of school: Modern perspectives in truancy and school refusal.* pp. 343–370, Chichester: Wiley.

Haggard, M. P. & Hughes, E. A. (1991). *Screening children's hearing: a review of the literature and implications of otitis media.* London: HMSO.

Hanson, D. R., Gottesman, I. I. & Heston, L. L. (1976). Some possible childhood indicators of adult schizophrenia inferred from children of schizophrenics. *British Journal of Psychiatry*, **129**, 142–54.

Harrington, R., Fudge, H., Rutter, M., Pickles, A. & Hill, J. (1991). Adult outcomes of childhood and adolescent depression. II. Links with antisocial disorder. *Journal of the American Academy of Child and Adolescent Psychiatry*, **30**, 434–9.

Harris, T., Brown, G. W. & Bifulco, A. (1990). Loss of parent in childhood and adult psychiatric disorder: attentative overall model. *Development and Psychopathology*, **2**, 311–28.

Hennessy, J. W. & Levine, S. (1979). Stress, arousal, and the pituitary-adrenal system: a psychoendocrine hypothesis. In J. M. Sprague and A. N. Epstein (eds.). *Progress in psychobiology and physiological psychology.* New York: Academic Press.

Hermelin, B. & O'Connor, N. (1970). *Psychological experiments with autistic children.* Oxford: Pergamon.

Hermelin, B. & O'Connor, N. (1986). Idiot savant calendrical calculators: rules and regularities. *Psychological Medicine*, **16**, 885–93.

Hodges, J. & Tizard, B. (1989a). IQ and behavioural adjustment of ex-institutional adolescents. *Journal of Child Psychology and Psychiatry*, **30**, 53–75.

Hodges, J. & Tizard, B. (1989b). Social and family relationships of ex-institutional adolescents. *Journal of Child Psychology and Psychiatry*, **30**, 77–97.

Jenkins, J. M. & Smith, M. A. (1990). Factors protecting children living in disharmonious homes: maternal reports. *Journal of the American Academy of Child and Adolescent Psychiatry*, **29**, 60–9.

Kanner, L. (1943). Austistic disturbances of affective contact. *Nervous Child*, **13**, 43–56.

Kreitman, N. (1988). Suicide, age and marital status. *Psychological Medicine*, **18**, 121–8.

Lane, N. E., Bloch, D. A., Jones, H. H., Marshall, W. H., Wood, P. D. & Fries, J. F. (1986). Long-distance running, bone density, and osteoarthritis. *Journal of the American Medical Association*, **255**, 1147–51.

Lane, N. E., Bloch, D. A., Wood, P. D. & Fries, J. F. (1987). Aging, long-distance running and the development of musculoskeletal disability: a controlled study. *American Journal of Medicine*, **82**, 722–80.

Lenzenweger, M. F. & Moldin, S. O. (1990). Discerning the latent structure of hypothetical psychosis proneness through admixture analysis. *Psychiatry Research*, **33**, 243–57.

Magnusson, D. & Bergman, L. R. (1988). Individual and variable-based approaches to longitudinal research on early risk factors. In M. Rutter (ed.). *Studies of psychosocial risk: the power of longitudinal data.* pp. 45–61, Cambridge: Cambridge University Press.

Magnusson, D. & Bergman, L. R. (1990). A pattern approach to the study of pathways from childhood to adulthood. In L. Robins & M. Rutter (eds.). *Straight and devious pathways from childhood to adulthood.* pp. 101–115, New York: Cambridge University Press.

Masten, A. S. & Garmezy, N. (1985). Risk, vulnerability, and protective factors in developmental psychopathology. In B. B. Lahey & A. E. Kazdin (eds.). *Advances in clinical child psychology,* vol. 8, pp. 1–52, New York: Plenum Press.

McGuffin, P. & Gottesman, I. I. (1985). Genetic influences on normal and abnormal development. In M. Rutter & L. Hersov (eds.). *Child and adolescent psychiatry: modern approaches* (2nd edn.). pp. 17–33, Oxford: Blackwell Scientific.

Meichenbaum, D. (1985). *Stress Inoculation Training.* Oxford: Pergamon Press.

O'Connor, N. & Hermelin, B. (1978). *Seeing and hearing and space and time.* London: Academic Press.

Olson, R. K., Wise, B. W., & Rack, J. P. (1989). Dyslexia: deficits, genetic aetiology, and computer-based remediation. *Irish Journal of Psychology,* 10, 494–508.

Pickles, A. & Rutter, M. (1991). Statistical and conceptual models of 'turning points' in developmental processes. In D. Magnusson, L. R. Bergman, G. Rudinger & B. Törestad (eds.). *Problems and methods in longitudinal research: stability and change.* Cambridge: Cambridge University Press.

Pliszka, S. (1989). Effect of anxiety on cognition, behaviour, and stimulant response in ADHD. *Journal of the American Academy of Child and Adolescent Psychiatry,* 28, 882–7.

Plomin, R. (1986). *Development, genetics and psychology.* Hillsdale, NJ: Erlbaum.

Plomin, R. (1991). Genetic risk and psychosocial disorders: links between the normal and abnormal. In M. Rutter & P. Casaer (eds.). *Biological risk factors for psychosocial disorders.* pp. 101–138, Cambridge: Cambridge University Press.

Plomin, R. & Bergeman, C. S. (1991). The nature of nurture: genetic influence on 'environmental' measures. *Behavioral and Brain Sciences,* 14, 373–86.

Plomin, R., DeFries, J. C. & Fulker, D. W. (1988). *Nature and nurture during infancy and early childhood.* New York: Cambridge University Press.

Puig-Antich, J., Goetz, D., Davies, M., Kaplan, T., Davies, S., Ostrow, L., Asnis, L., Twomey, J., Iyengar, S. & Ryan, N. D. (1989). A controlled family history study of prepubertal major depressive disorder. *Archives of General Psychiatry,* 46, 406–18.

Quigley, M. E. T., Martin, P. L., Burnier, A. M. & Brooks, P. (1987). Estrogen therapy arrests bone loss in elderly women. *American Journal of Obstetrics & Gynecology,* 156, 1516–23.

Quinton, D. & Rutter, M. (1988). *Parenting Breakdown: the making and breaking of inter-generational links.* Aldershot: Avebury.

Rende, R. & Plomin, R. (in press). Genetic influences on behavioural development. In M. Rutter & D. Hay (eds.). *Developmental principles and clinical issues in psychology and psychiatry.* Oxford: Blackwell Scientific.

Robins, L. (1966). *Deviant children grown up.* Baltimore: Williams and Wilkins.

Robins, L. (1978). Sturdy childhood predictors of adult antisocial behaviour: replications from longitudinal studies. *Psychological Medicine,* 8, 611–22.

Robins, L. (1986). The consequences of conduct disorder in girls. In D. Olweus, J. Block & M. Radke-Yarrow (eds.). *Development of antisocial and prosocial behaviour: Research, theories, and issues.* pp. 385–414, Orlando, Fla: Academic Press.

Rodgers, B. (1990). Influences of early-life and recent factors on affective disorder in women: An exploration of vulnerability models. In L. Robins & M. Rutter (eds.). *Straight and devious pathways from childhood to adulthood.* pp. 314–327, New York:

Cambridge University Press.

Rogers, S. J. & Pennington, B. F. (1991). A theoretical approach to the deficits in infantile autism. *Developmental Psychology*, **3**, 137–62.

Rubin, K. & Asendorpf, J. S. (in press). *Shyness, inhibition and social withdrawal.* Chicago: University of Chicago Press.

Rutter, M. (1972). Childhood schizophrenia reconsidered. *Journal of Autism and Childhood Schizophrenia*, **2**, 315–37.

Rutter, M. (1981*a*). Epidemiological/longitudinal strategies and causal research in child psychiatry. *Journal of the American Academy of Child Psychiatry*, **20**, 513–44.

Rutter, M. (1981b). *Maternal deprivation reassessed* (2nd edn.). Harmondsworth, Middx.: Penguin.

Rutter, M. (1983*a*). Statistical and personal interactions: facets and perspectives. In D. Magnusson & V. Allen (eds.). *Human development: An interactional perspective.* pp. 295–319, New York: Academic Press.

Rutter, M. (1983*b*). Issues and prospects in developmental neuropsychiatry. In M. Rutter (ed.). *Developmental neuropsychiatry.* pp. 577–598, New York: Guilford Press.

Rutter, M. (1988). Longitudinal data in the study of causal processes: some uses and some pitfalls. In M. Rutter (ed.). *Studies of psychosocial risk: the power of longitudinal data.* pp. 1–28, Cambridge: Cambridge University Press.

Rutter, M. (1989*a*). Pathways from childhood to adult life. *Journal of Child Psychology and Psychiatry*, **30**, 23–51.

Rutter, M. (1989*b*). Psychiatric disorder in parents as a risk factor for children. In D. Shaffer, I. Philips & N. B. Enzer (eds.). *Prevention of mental disorders, alcohol and other drug use in children and adolescents.* OSAP Prevention Monograph 2. pp. 157–189, Rockville, Maryland: Office for Substance Abuse Prevention, US Department of Health and Human Services.

Rutter, M. (1989*c*). Age as an ambiguous variable in developmental research: Some epidemiological considerations from developmental psychopathology. *International Journal of Behavioral Development*, **12**, 1–34.

Rutter, M. (1990*a*). Commentary: Some focus and process considerations regarding effects of parental depression on children. *Developmental Psychology*, **26**, 60–7.

Rutter, M. (1990*b*). Psychosocial resilience and proective mechanisms. In J. Rolf, A. Masten, D. Cicchetti, K. Nuechterlein & S. Weintraub (eds.). *Risk and protective factors in the development of psychopathology.* pp. 181–214, New York: Cambridge University Press.

Rutter, M. (1991*a*). Autism as a genetic disorder. In P. McGuffin & R. Murray (eds.). *The new genetics of mental illness.* pp. 225–244, London: Butterworth-Heinemann.

Rutter, M. (1991*b*). Childhood experiences and adult psychosocial functioning. In G. R. Bock & J. Whelan (eds.). *The childhood environment and adult disease.* Ciba Foundation Symposium No. 156. pp. 189–200, Chichester: Wiley.

Rutter, M. (1991*c*). Nature, nurture, and psychopathology: A new look at an old topic. *Development and Psychopathology*, **3**, 125–36.

Rutter, M. (1991*d*). A fresh look at 'maternal deprivation'. In P. Bateson (ed.). *The development and integration of behaviour.* pp. 331–374, Cambridge: Cambridge University Press.

Rutter, M. (in press). Concepts of cause and implications for intervention. In A. C. Petersen & J. Mortimer (eds.). *Youth unemployment and society.* New York: Cambridge University Press.

Rutter, M. & Garmezy, N. (1983). Developmental psychopathology. In E. M. Hetherington (ed.). *Socialization, personality, and social development*, vol. 4. *Mussen's Handbook of child psychology* (4th edn.). pp. 775–911, New York: Wiley.

Rutter, M. & Mawhood, L. (1991). The long-term psychosocial sequelae of specific developmental disorders of speech and language. In M. Rutter & P. Casaer (eds.). *Biological risk factors for psychosocial disorders.* pp. 233–259, Cambridge: Cambridge University Press.

Rutter, M. & Pickles, A. (1991). Person–environment interactions: concepts, mechanisms and implications for data analysis. In T. Wachs & R. Plomin (eds.). *Conceptualization and measurement of organism–environment interaction.* pp. 105–141, Washington, DC: American Psychological Association.

Rutter, M., Quinton, D. & Hill, J. (1990). Adult outcome of institution-reared children: Males and females compared. In L. Robins & M. Rutter (eds.). *Straight and devious pathways from childhood to adulthood.* pp. 135–157, Cambridge: Cambridge University Press.

Rutter, M. & Rutter, M. (1993). *Developing minds: challenge and continuity across the lifespan.* Harmondsworth, Middx.: Penguin; New York: Basic Books.

Rutter, M. & Sandberg, S. (1985). Epidemiology of child psychiatric disorder: Methodological issues and some substantive findings. *Child Psychiatry and Human Development*, **15**, 209–33.

Rutter, M. & Schopler, E. (1988). Autism and pervasive developmental disorders. In Rutter, M., Tuma, A. H. & Lann, I. S. (eds.). *Assessment and diagnosis in child psychopathology.* pp. 408–434, New York: Guilford Press.

Rutter, M. & Schopler, E. (1992). Classification of pervasive developmental disorders: Some concepts and practical considerations. *Journal of Autism and Developmental Disorders* (in press).

Rutter, M., Tizard, J. & Whitmore, K. (eds.) (1970). *Education, health and behaviour.* London: Longmans. (Reprinted, 1981, Krieger, Melbourne, FA).

Schwartz, D. & Mayaux, M. J. (1982). Female fecundity as a function of age. *New England Journal of Medicine*, **306**, 404–6.

Shankweiler, D. & Lieberman, I. Y. (eds.) (1989). *Phonology and reading disability: Solving the reading puzzle.* Ann Arbor: University of Michigan Press.

Slater, A., Cooper, R., Rose, D. & Morison, V. (1989). Prediction of cognitive performance from infancy to early childhood. *Human Development*, **32**, 137–47.

Stattin, H. & Magnusson, D. (1990). *Pubertal maturation in female development.* Hillsdale, NJ: Erlbaum.

Steffenberg, S., Gillberg, C., Hellgren, L. et al. (1989). A twin study of autism in Denmark, Finland, Iceland, Norway and Sweden. *Journal of Child Psychology and Psychiatry*, **30**, 405–16.

Stevenson-Hinde, J. (1986). Individuals in relationships. In R. A. Hinde & J. Stevenson-Hinde (eds.). *Relationships within families: Mutual influences.* pp. 68–80, Oxford: Clarendon Press.

Taylor, E., Schachar, R., Thorley, G., Wieselberg, H. M., Everitt, B. & Rutter, M. (1987). Which boys respond to stimulant medication? A controlled trial of methylphenidate in boys with disruptive behaviour. *Psychological Medicine*, **17**, 121–43.

Tizard, J. (1975). Race and IQ: the limits of probability? *New Behaviour*, **1**, 6–9.

Vargha-Khadem, F., Isaacs, E., van der Werf, S., Robb, S. & Wilson, J. (1992). Development of intelligence and memory in children with hemiplegic cerebral palsy:

the deleterious consequences of early seizures. *Brain*, **115**, 315–29.

Wachs, T. & Plomin, R. (eds.). (1991). *Conceptualization and measurement of organism–environment interaction.* Washington, DC: American Psychological Association.

Wahlsten, D. (1990). Insensitivity of the analysis of variance to heredity–environment interaction. *Behavioral and Brain Sciences*, **13**, 109–61.

White, M. & McRae, S. (1989). *Young adults and long-term unemployment.* London: Policy Studies Institute Publications.

Whiten, A. (ed.) (1991). *Natural theories of mind.* Oxford: Basil Blackwell.

Wimmer, H. & Perner, J. (1983). Beliefs about beliefs: representation and constraining function of wrong beliefs in young children's understanding of deception. *Cognition*, **13**, 103–28.

World Health Organization (1992). ICD-10: The ICD-10 classification of mental and behavioural disorders: clinical descriptions and diagnostic guidelines. Copyright. Geneva: World Health Organization.

Zoccolillo, M., Pickles. A., Quinton, D. & Rutter, M. (1992). The outcome of childhood conduct disorder: implication for defining adult personality disorder & conduct disorder. *Psychological Medicine*, **22**, 971–86.

8 Longitudinal research on human aging: the power of combining real-time, microgenetic, and simulation approaches

ANDREAS KRUSE

ULMAN LINDENBERGER

PAUL B. BALTES

INTRODUCTION

In the present chapter, we proceed from the premise that the study of ontogenesis requires a methodology that is inherently focused on the study of intra-individual change and inter-individual differences in intra-individual change (Baltes, P. B., Reese, & Nesselroade, 1977). We argue, however, that real-time longitudinal studies with single cohorts is not enough. Rather, as outlined already in the 1960s and 1970s in the field of life-span development and aging (Baltes, P. B., 1968; Labouvie, 1980; Nesselroade & Reese, 1973; Schaie, 1965, 1979), the final power of longitudinal research rests in its creative use as a rather heterogeneous category of research strategies including microgenetic and simulation approaches (Baltes, P. B. & Goulet, 1971; Baltes, P. B. et al., 1977; Siegler & Crowley, 1991).

The call for a broad range of longitudinal methods is based on the assumption that behavioural development is the result of a complex, multilevel interaction of factors and mechanisms. It is unlikely that this nexus of biologically, socially and societally determined influences on development can be unravelled by longitudinal designs which are essentially descriptive or quasi-experimental in nature. For example, life-span theory suggests that development and aging are jointly determined by age-graded, history-graded, and non-normative systems of influence (Baltes, P. B., 1987; Baltes, Cornelius, & Nesselroade, 1979; Dannefer, 1987; Elder, 1986; Featherman, 1983; Kruse, 1992; Mayer, 1990). Some processes may exhibit a high correlation with age, whereas others are a reflection of historical change. In addition, some events or changes do not occur universally for all people. These non-normative events may have cumulative effects and may lead to an increase in inter-individual variability with age. Developmental trajectories of individuals of a given cohort always represent specific combinations of age-graded, history-graded, and non-normative influences. Without additional assumptions or data, one does not know whether these trajectories are generalizable to other cohorts. Moreover, without decomposition of age and cohort trends into constituent processes – for example, by intensive single-subject studies or by additional experimentation in the laboratory – it is impossible to identify the operative forces and mechanisms with a sufficient degree of precision and certainty. Thus, the analysis of longitudinal change processes requires a coalition of methodologies to estimate the possible range of intra-individual change trajectories, and to identify possible antecedents of age-related change.

A TAXONOMY OF LONGITUDINAL RESEARCH METHODS

We propose that longitudinal methods fall into three basic categories: real-time, microgenetic, and simulation studies (Baltes, P. B. et al., 1979; Baltes, P. B. & Nesselroade, 1979; cf. Rudinger & Wood, 1990). With respect to real-time studies, a distinction can be made between single-cohort and multiple-cohort designs. The classical one-cohort real-time longitudinal study is well suited for the description of developmental processes, especially if the theory assumes that the processes to be studied are relatively invariant across cultures and historical time. The best examples for such processes are normally found in early childhood (e.g. sensorimotor development), and presumably are under relatively direct genetic control. However, relatively invariant developmental processes are also obtained when society- and socialization-based influences are well standardized as to age and have become stabilized over historical time.

Multiple-cohort studies, especially if they implement a full-blown cohort-sequential design (Baltes, 1968; Baltes et al., 1977; Schaie, 1965), serve to estimate the relative importance of historical change processes for developmental change functions across a given historical period. In contrast to single-cohort studies, cohort-sequential studies are well suited to explore the historical relativity (i.e. context dependence) of developmental change functions (for an example, see Schaie, 1990a). The extent and direction of historical effects alone adds to our knowledge about the possible range of development, and may guide our subsequent search for causal mechanisms.

The main disadvantage of both single- and multiple-cohort real-time longitudinal studies is their relative lack of explanatory power. Despite recent advances in statistical methodology (Collins & Horn, 1991; Magnusson & Bergman, 1990), especially in time series analysis (Gollob & Reichardt, 1991; Jones, 1991) and structural modelling (Muthén, 1991), causal inferences are generally difficult to draw on the basis of real-time longitudinal data, mainly because we lack experimental control over antecedent conditions (cf. Rutter, 1988b).

Therefore, real-time longitudinal methods need to be combined with methods that allow for a better control over antecedent conditions if the goal is to test specific hypotheses regarding variables producing age-related change. We suggest two such methods, microgenetic intervention and developmental simulation.

The microgenetic method (Siegler & Crowley, 1991) is based on the assumption that there are important commonalities underlying changes that occur on different time scales (Werner, 1948). Therefore, the careful analysis of time-compressed change functions may lead to a better understanding of medium- and long-term developmental changes. Put differently, microgenetic intervention may help to explain age-related change functions by a systematic analysis of age differences in the quantity or quality of intra-individual change processes. Microgenetic work often involves the observation of individual subjects, a high density of observations, and intensive data analysis to infer interindividual differences in intra-individual change (Baltes, P. B. et al., 1977; Siegler & Crowley, 1991; cf. Werner, 1948). Good examples for this type of design are cognitive training studies which provide optimal learning conditions to identify age differences in developmental reserve capacity and to explore the boundary conditions of what is possible in principle (Baltes, P. B. & Kliegl, 1992; Baltes, P. B. & Lindenberger, 1988; Kliegl & Baltes, 1987*a*, 1987*b*, Willis, 1987).

Developmental simulation refers to the theory-guided arrangement of experimental conditions that simulate or mimick age-related change for the purpose of explanatory decomposition of age trends observed in real-time studies (Baltes & Goulet, 1971). As a research strategy, the simulation of developmental processes generally involves five steps (cf. Baltes et al., 1977): 1) definition of the developmental phenomenon (i.e. the age-related change function) to be explained; 2) formulation of a set of hypotheses about age-associated variables that might produce the phenomenon; 3) experimental manipulation of these variables; 4) test of the data obtained through simulation against the target phenomenon (isomorphy check); 5) examination of external validity as well as search for alternative causal mechanisms.

Recent research examples of developmental simulation include mathematical models of age differences in skilled memory performance (Kliegl & Lindenberger, 1988; Kliegl, 1992), connectionist models of both stage-like (McClelland, 1989) and more continuous (Siegler, 1988; Hoyer & Hannon, in press) age changes in cognitive functioning, and the simulation of aging-related memory deficits in young adults through the experimental impairment of attentional processing (Nilsson, Bäckman & Karlsson, 1989). An early life-span example is Sjostrom and Pollack's (1971) attempt to understand the differential age trajectories of two types of visual illusions by manipulation of sensory input in different age groups and by application of lenses mimicking age changes in visual acuity.

The combined use of real-time, microgenetic, and simulation approaches is not always possible, mainly because certain developmental processes are difficult to time-compress or simulate in the laboratory. Some developmental factors, some age-associated conditions may not be decomposable into shorter time spans. Despite these difficulties, however, efforts at microgenetic and simulation research are mandatory to achieve a complete understanding of the nature of human development, even if they 'only' demonstrate that a full understanding of the nexus of causal factors and mechanisms involved is not possible.

In the following, to illustrate the power of the expanded view of longitudinal research, we will discuss five prominent issues in the psychological study of human aging: representativeness, inter-individual variability, investigations into limits of functioning (plasticity), the distinction between normal and pathological aging, and the search for mechanisms of successful aging. We do not intend to provide a comprehensive review of any of these issues. Rather, we would like to argue in each case that the acquisition of new knowledge is critically contingent not only upon real-time longitudinal research but also upon the combination of different types of longitudinal methodology. Typical examples from recent research will be used to illustrate this claim.

REPRESENTATIVENESS IN AGING RESEARCH

Representativeness is a generic term referring to individuals, variables, and measurements (Magnusson & Bergman, 1990). In the following, we concentrate our discussion to two threats to representativeness, selective survival and selective sampling. As we would like to argue, problems related to these two issues are especially prominent in aging research. Their examination requires a longitudinal approach.

Selective survival

Chronological age is commonly seen as a marker variable for development, with the goal to replace it by more direct indicators of developmental change processes (Wohlwill, 1970). This also holds true for aging research. In addition, however, chronological age also functions as a marker variable for sample selection (Lawley, 1943–44). In modern Western societies, for instance, about 85% of a birth cohort are alive at age 60 (Dinkel, 1992; Putz & Schwarz, 1984). This percentage is reduced to about 5% at the age of 90. Given that the 5% still alive at age 90 are not randomly selected from the 85% alive at age 60, any direct comparison of 90-year olds with 60-year olds is difficult.

In the case of cross-sectional data, such a comparison will be biased because a highly select sample is compared against a less select sample. More importantly, however, the extent and the direction of the bias cannot be assessed by cross-sectional data because the bias can involve historical changes in the different birth cohorts making up the cross-sectional composition. In the case of real-time longitudinal data, assessment of age-related changes in the parent birth cohorts are possible. However, the results are possibly cohort-specific and the final analyses are increasingly restricted to those individuals who lived long and, in addition, provided data on all measurement occasions (e.g. the biological and longitudinal study survivors). As a consequence, results can only be generalized to a rather small portion of the elderly population.

One way to tackle the problems involved in cross-sectional and real-time longitudinal comparisons of old and very old adults is to carefully analyse the reasons for the existence of selective survival (Manton & Woodbury, 1983; Powell et al., 1990; Siegler & Botwinick, 1979; Cooney, Schaie & Willis, 1988). In analogy to Wohlwill's (1970) line of reasoning, age as a selection variable has to be replaced by other variables that are more direct indicators of interindividual differences in mortality and morbidity (Manton & Woodbury, 1983; cf. Aitken, 1934).

Real-time longitudinal data may lead to a better understanding of selective survival if attempts are intensified to predict who drops out of a sample due to chronic illness and death and who does not. Recent advances in structural modelling techniques with non-random missing data (McArdle & Hamagami, 1991; McArdle et al., 1991; Rovine & Delaney, 1990; Rubin, 1991) may prove to be very useful in this regard. The theoretical rationale for dropout (i.e. selectivity) analyses would be to identify the ensemble of protective and risk factors which contribute to inter-individual differences in longevity. Thus, sample attrition due to selective survival may not be a cause for concern but an opportunity for gaining new insights about the relationship among mortality, morbidity, and age.

Another way to address the problem of selective survival is the increased use of methods with dense spacing of observations or observational formats that are event rather than time driven (Blossfeld, Hamerle & Mayer, 1989). In the extreme case, such a strategy amounts to what we have defined as a microgenetic approach. Especially in the case of very old age, where the average life expectancy is lower than, say, five years, it may be more meaningful to intensively study a small number of individuals over a relatively short period of time than to aim for the implementation of conventional real-time longitudinal designs with fixed intervals of observation.

Selective sampling of the universe of the aging population(s)

Human aging is not well described by a unitary age function that holds true across all individuals and domains; rather, it comprises a multitude of possible trajectories and profiles, both across individuals and domains of functioning (Baltes, 1991; Baltes & Baltes, 1990, 1992; Birren, 1988; Busse & Maddox, 1985; Lehr & Thomae, 1987; Schaie, 1989*b*; Svanborg, 1985; Thomae, 1976, 1983). In the following, we use the term 'patterns of aging' (Lawton, 1989; Thomae, 1979) to refer to the multi-dimensionality and multi-directionality of the aging process, and to the fact that there is large inter-individual variability in the onset, rate, and direction of age changes.

Inter-individual differences in patterns of aging can be described in terms of differences in person–environment transactions (Lawton, 1989), person–situation interactions (Lerner, 1978; Magnusson, 1988; Magnusson & Endler, 1977; Thomae, 1988), or as the result of processes of social differentiation due for instance to gender, social class, or ethnicity (Dannefer, 1987; Featherman, 1983; Sørensen, Weinert & Sherrod, 1986). The notion of transaction or interaction refers to the fact that aging individuals continuously adapt to situational opportunities and demands that require physical, cognitive, and personality-related competence. At the same time, they also modify certain aspects of the environment by virtue of this competence. While this is true for all phases of the life-span (Lerner, 1978), the specific challenge of aging lies in the fact that the age-correlated power of biological and environmental influences wanes with age and that non-normative factors and individualized pathways become relatively more prominent. That this is so has evolutionary as well as ontogenetic reasons (Baltes & Baltes, 1992). From an evolutionary point of view, aging is a post-reproductive phenomenon and therefore less subject to genetic selection. From an ontogenetic point of view, there is a less developed (less standardized and optimized) culture of old age than is true for earlier periods of the life-span.

To examine a broad spectrum of aging patterns, longitudinal aging studies need to represent a great variety of different genetic and environmental conditions. In contrast to this proposition, most real-time longitudinal studies on aging tend to over-represent healthy individuals with middle or high socio-economic status and middle or high educational background. We do not know to what degree findings from these studies are generalizable to individuals who are living under less favourable or in diverse social conditions (e.g. race, ethnicity, etc).

The bias towards overrepresenting the well educated and the wealthy makes it difficult to evaluate the effects of adverse environmental conditions on the course of aging. It appears that restricted environments are often associated with a relatively high prevalence of pathology, and may lead to a reduction of inter-individual variability because skills and abilities are not activated. Still, individuals seem to be able to maintain subjective feelings of well-being under such conditions unless their physical and emotional resources are depleted (Kruse, 1992). Future longitudinal research on aging needs to undertake a special effort to encompass a broad range of environmental conditions. In particular, the drawing of truly representative samples and the oversampling of certain groups at risk for pathology may be necessary to allow for the systematic comparison of individual and environmental conditions over time. In this case as well, the use of single-subject, microgenetic, and simulation methods holds much promise. By such methods it is possible to specify and intensify particular constellations and reach beyond current reality. Lindenberger, Kliegl, and

Baltes (in press) demonstrated, for instance, how an expertise- and life-history guided selection of subjects (finding a small number of older persons with favourable dispositions for and practice in mental imagination) in combination with intensive memory training (based on strategies of mental imagination) produces new insights into the aging of memory.

INTER-INDIVIDUAL VARIABILITY

In the previous section, we suggested already that one of the major findings of gerontological research is the magnitude of inter-individual differences in functional status among elderly individuals. In contrast to initial assumptions about the uniformity of the aging process (Cowdry, 1939), there are 80-year olds who appear like 60-year olds and vice versa. This substantial inter-individual variability is found both for psychological and behavioural (Lehr & Thomae, 1987; Maddox, 1987; Nesselroade, 1990; Schaie, 1979; Svanborg, 1985) as well as for biomedical indicators (Costa & Andres, 1986; Rowe & Kahn, 1987). The demonstration of such variability, is based on longitudinal and cohort-sequential studies (e.g. Schaie, 1983, 1988, 1990*b*).

While the existence of a wide range of inter-individual variability in old age is an indisputed fact, the relative importance of possible causes for age-related changes in variability is less clear (cf. Holland & Rabbitt, 1991; Schaie et al., in press). Does inter-individual variability in old age reflect, for the most part, the existence of life-long individual differences that are relatively unaffected by aging-related processes? In this case, the basic picture would be one of continuity and stability, and inter-individual differences in intra-individual change, if they were present, would only work in the direction of enhancing already existing differences without altering the rank order of individuals. In the field of personality research, Costa and McCrae (1988) are strong proponents of this view.

However, the transition to late adulthood may also be accompanied by changes in the magnitude and/or stability of individual differences. Some factors may lead to an increase in inter-individual variability. For instance, individuals may differ in the onset and the rate of aging-related decrements in the efficiency of cognitive processing (Schaie, 1989*a*). In addition, differences in life-styles, past work experience, and genetic dispositions may exert a cumulative effect on individual differences in attitudes and behaviour (cf. Baltes, P. B. & Nesselroade, 1978). As a consequence, some, but not all individuals may evince growth in select areas of functioning such as self-related behaviour (Brandtstädter & Baltes-Götz, 1990), wisdom-related knowledge (Baltes, P. B. & Smith, 1990), or professional expertise (Hoyer, 1985). Similarly, health decline will not affect all individuals at the same age and to the same extent.

On the other hand, inter-individual variability may decrease again as individuals approach the very end of their life-time, at least if we assume that the proximity to one's 'natural' death is associated with a lawful decline of bodily functions (i.e. the 'terminal decline' hypothesis; cf. Riegel & Riegel, 1972). Thus, proximity to death, rather than advanced age per se, may reduce phenotypical diversity.

At present, the prediction of inter-individual differences in the onset and magnitude of late-life changes is hampered by a lack of knowledge about relevant antecedent conditions. Without a rather extensive set of a priori assumptions – which may have been obtained on the basis of results from previous longitudinal studies – cross-sectional studies are silent with respect to the mechanisms explaining the existence of functional variability within and across age-groups or cohorts. Therefore, a coalition between real-time, micro-genetic, and simulation methods of longitudinal research is needed to adequately describe and explain the ensemble of causal mechanisms that determine the magnitude of inter-individual variability during the last third of the life span.

Nesselroade (1990), for instance, has shown that a major share of inter-individual variability is due to short-term fluctuations in functioning. He was able to make this case by intensive short-term observations and measurements of personality functioning over several months. Maciel, Heckhausen and Baltes (1992) argued that, to understand longitudinal stability of personality traits (Costa & McCrae, 1988), it is necessary to study the internal comparison standards that people use when responding in self-report questionnaires. Moreover, microgenetic studies provide insights into changes in variability under conditions that have a low likelihood of occurrence in present-day societies. For instance, they can provide optimal environmental conditions with respect to the acquisition of specific cognitive skills in order to test propositions about inter-individual variability in upper limits of functioning (i.e. developmental reserve capacity; Kliegl & Baltes, 1987a, 1987b). Finally, simulation approaches allow for the theory-guided mathematical modelling of age-related changes in inter-individual variability (see Baltes, P. B. & Nesselroade, 1978, for an example).

First example: interindividual variability in late-life cognitive functioning

Both the results of cohort-sequential and real-time longitudinal studies suggest that variability in cognitive functioning increases, rather than decreases, during the transition from middle age to late adulthood (Cunningham & Birren, 1980; Hertzog & Schaie, 1986, 1988). In other words, growing into old age appears to be a source of inter-individual differences in cognitive functioning.

Data from the Seattle Cohort-Sequential Longitudinal Study may serve as an illustration. First, this study revealed major cohort effects in level and direction of psychological functioning (Schaie, 1979, 1983). Such cohort effects suggest that the level and form of cognitive aging functions are much influenced by experience.

Secondly, the Seattle Study informs us – especially because of its multiple-cohort design – about cohort-generalizable age trends. In a comprehensive re-analysis of this data set, Hertzog and Schaie (1986, 1988; see also Schaie, 1989*a*) reported that most individuals between the age of 55 and 70 made a transition from a stability to a decline pattern in general intelligence as measured by sub-tests of the Thurstone Primary Mental Abilities (PMA; Thurstone & Thurstone, 1949). Thus, beyond age 60 or so decline in cognitive functioning was relatively normative, but individuals differed in the age of onset of this decline. Despite the concomitant increase in inter-individual variability with age, individual differences in general intelligence were highly stable, with correlations between adjacent 7-year intervals in the 90s. In other words, the amount of crossover of individual aging trajectories was small when measured against the variability of the sample.

These results seem to suggest that decline in cognitive functioning is quite normative, that the stability of inter-individual differences is quite high, and that the magnitude of inter-individual differences in cognitive functioning increases, rather than decreases in late adulthood. However, a few notes of caution are in order. First, one has to keep in mind that even stabilities in the nineties allow for sizeable inter-individual differences in intra-individual change. Fig. 8.1, taken from the same data set, illustrates this claim. By constucting confidence bands of 2.5 SEM (standard errors of measurement) around individual data points, Schaie (1988, 1990*b*) reported the proportion of individuals evincing a pattern of gain, stability, or loss in intelligence test scores as they traversed the age-span from 60 to 80. Clearly, not all individuals underwent decline, and a substantial minority increased their test scores according to this criterion.

Second, as Hertzog & Schaie (1986; see also Cooney, Schaie & Willis, 1988) pointed out themselves, longitudinal aging samples are generally influenced by a substantial degree of experimental mortality (attrition). It is very likely that individuals suffering a major loss in functional capacity due to severe illness or terminal decline dropped out of the longitudinal sample. Thus, the degree of stability in inter-individual differences observed in the survivors probably is an over-estimation of the stability in the population. As argued in more detail above, careful analyses of sample representativeness, sample selectivity, and longitudinal attrition (Baltes, P. B. et al., 1977) are needed to estimate the magnitude of this effect (cf. Gruenberg, 1986).

Finally, we cannot exclude the possibility that inter-individual variability in cognitive functioning decreases in very old individuals because the data set is restricted, as is true for most studies, to the young–old segment of the elderly population; only few subjects in the sample are above 80 years of age. In young–old populations, the continued existence of high inter-individual variability may be due to the fact that individuals still differ considerably in their closeness to death. Inter-individual variability may be less pronounced when the focus is on old–old rather than young–old individuals, or when courses of aging are plotted backward from death rather than forward from birth (cf. Kleemeier, 1962).

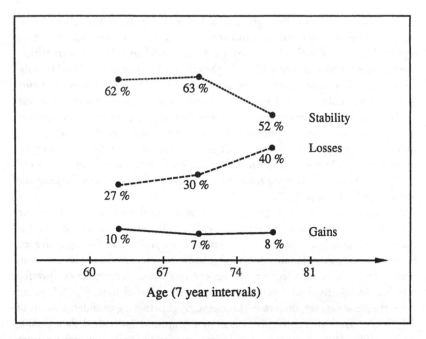

Fig. 8.1.   Percentage of individuals showing stability, losses, or gains in intelligence. (Reanalysed and based on Schaie, 1988, 1990b.)

For this reason, future longitudinal research on aging should be expanded into very old age. Given the high mortality rate in the very old population, this may require deviations from canonical longitudinal methodology. For instance, it may be useful to adjust the time period between adjacent measurement points as a function of age-graded mortality risks, or to closely follow a relatively small member of very old subjects over time (cf. Jones & Nesselroade, 1990). Moreover, death records should be used whenever possible to reorganize existing as well as new data sets in terms of distance from death.

Real-time longitudinal (especially cohort-sequential) research on cognitive aging, then, has provided us with important information on inter-individual variability. This information, however, is largely descriptive. Cognitive training studies, in combination with real-time studies (Schaie & Willis, 1986; Willis, 1991) or as separate research programmes (Baltes, P. B. & Lindenberger, 1988; Baltes, B. B. & Willis, 1982; Kliegl, 1992; Kliegl & Baltes, 1987a,b; Willis, 1987) have supplemented this descriptive information. To what degree are the age functions observed modifiable? To what degree is it possible to produce major changes in rank order by exposing different individuals to differing learning conditions? To what extent can the biologically based decline of cognitive aging be overcome, reversed, or slowed down?

These are the kinds of questions that require the enrichment of real-time longitudinal data with microgenetic and developmental simulation work. We know from training studies in the cognitive domain that a few sessions of instruction and training elevate the performance level of healthy older adults up to two standard deviations above their untrained peers (Baltes & Lindenberger, 1988; Kliegl, Smith & Baltes, 1989). Such results underscore the relevance of environmental conditions in the production of different aging outcomes, and shed new light on the interpretation of variability estimates based on data from real-time longitudinal studies. Furthermore, based on intensive memory training studies (Baltes, P. B. & Kliegl, 1992), we now know that there are definite limits that cannot be overcome, although real-time longitudinal intervention work (necessarily of less intensity) such as that by Schaie and Willis (1986) suggested otherwise. And, to give a final example, we now know through cognitive training research of the microgenetic kind that some subgroups of the elderly (such as persons identified as at risk for Alzheimer dementia) benefit much less from training or may not benefit at all (Baltes, M. M., Kühl & Sowarka, in press). Again, based on simple real-time longitudinal assessment, this information would not be available and real-time age trends would be misinterpreted.

Second example: trait- vs. process-oriented approaches to late-life personality

A central theme of life-span research on personality is the question to what extent inter-individual differences in personality and self-related behaviour are affected by aging (Asendorpf & Weinert, 1990; Bengtson, Reedy & Gordon, 1985; Block, 1981; Brim & Kagan, 1980; Costa & McCrae, 1988; Field & Millsap, 1991; Filipp & Klauer, 1986; Magnusson, 1990; Magnusson & Endler, 1977; Munnichs et al., 1985; Shanan, 1991; Thomae, 1988). Two different views on the issue can be set apart. Trait-oriented approaches (Costa & McCrae, 1988) tend to emphasize continuity of inter-individual differences in personality dimensions, whereas process-oriented approaches (Filipp & Klauer, 1986; Magnusson, 1990) emphasize transformations in coping styles, self-related behaviours, and belief systems as a function of age-graded changes in situational demands. In the following, using longitudinal evidence, we will elaborate on this difference and suggest possible directions for future research.

Based on the assumption of a partly pre-programmed personality structure evolving early in life, many trait theorists posit that inter-individual differences in personality are stable throughout the entire adult life-span, including old age. The results of several real-time longitudinal studies, such as the Baltimore Study (Costa, McCrae & Arenberg, 1983; Costa & McCrae, 1988) and the Normative Aging Study (Costa et al., 1987; Spiro, et al., 1990), seem to support this view. For instance, Costa and McCrae (1988) reported stable pattern of inter-individual differences and sample means in the 'Big Five' (Digman, 1989) personality dimensions over a six-year period.

A recent cohort-sequential study (Schaie, Dutta & Willis, 1991) on the level of functioning focusing on the trait of flexibility versus rigidity is equally consistent with the idea of a basic continuity in personality traits during adulthood. The authors found that the negative correlation between age and flexibility commonly observed in cross-sectional research is probably due, for the most part, to cohort effects. After accounting for cohort effects in their data, the authors still observed a decrease in flexibility after about age 60. However, this decrease was smaller than the corresponding difference between young and old adults in cross-sectional comparisons. The authors argue that the cohort effect may reflect a secular trend due to historical changes on a third variable such as education. Given that flexibility predicts the ability to profit from experience, these data provide an empirical basis for the optimistic assumption that future cohorts of elderly individuals will be increasingly able to maintain and develop their intellectual, self-related, and social potential.

On the other hand, proponents of a more process-oriented view on personality and develoment (Magnusson, 1990; Magnusson & Endler, 1977; Pervin, 1985; Thomae, 1988) argue that certain personality characteristics and self-related behaviours (e.g. coping styles, control beliefs) vary as a function of situational demands. As a consequence, age-graded changes in these aspects of personality are expected to the extent that there is an age-graded change in the demand characteristics of the environment. Such changes would not necessarily lead to a reorganization of personality as it has evolved during the life-course; rather, the consequences would be more or less domain-specific (cf. Lazarus & Folkman, 1984; Lehr, 1991; Maas & Kuypers, 1974; Mussen, 1985; Olbrich, 1985; Shanan, 1991; Thomae, 1988). For instance, the time perspective may change in very old age to the extent that individuals are being confronted with the fact that their life-time is limited (Kastenbaum, 1985; Kruse, 1987; Munnichs, 1966; Thomae, 1981, 1988), but this change will not always lead to changes in other aspects of the self.

Application of microgenetic and simulation methodologies can be expected to bridge the gap between trait- and process-oriented approaches. For example, variations in instructional set has shown that quite different age trajectories result when subjects are asked to describe themselves in the present with or without juxtaposition to the past or when they are asked to characterize the aging of others (Ahammer & Baltes, 1972; Harris, 1975; Heckhausen & Krüger, 1991). Thus, it is likely that the data-gathering scheme employed by Costa, McCrae, and others, where individuals are asked to fill out questionnaires about their present state of mind, is not optimally suited to reveal aging-related changes in personality and the self. There is increasing evidence that irrespective of 'objective' functioning, individuals may continuously adjust their frame of reference such that age changes in personality are compensated by a corresponding change in expectations (cf. Bäckman & Dixon, in press; Maciel et al. (1992). For example, when younger and older adults are asked to describe their health or to characterize their level of satisfaction, fewer age changes result (Baltes, P. B., 1991). It is likely, however, that such lack of age differences or age changes is due to the fact that older adults evaluate their level of functioning in comparison with other older adults and not with their own past. These compensatory shifts in reference groups (Schulz, Heckhausen & Locher, 1991) may become evident if individuals are explicitly asked to review their lives, or to compare the present situation with their recent or remote past (Fooken, 1985; Kruse, 1992; Lehr, 1980; Maas & Kuypers, 1974; Thomae, 1968, 1988). For instance, in addition to asking individuals to answer items from personality questionnaires as it is normally done (e.g. with an implicit but unspecified point of reference), individuals could be asked to answer these items in the way they think they would have answered them a certain time ago (e.g. Ryff & Baltes, 1976; Woodruff & Birren, 1972). They could also be asked whether they have noticed any changes in self-related thoughts and feelings during the last few years, and, if so, in which domains, in what direction, and to what extent.

Real-time longitudinal studies employing these 'pseudo-longitudinal' data gathering techniques such as the Bonn Longitudinal Study and the Berkeley Study have provided a more differentiated picture of continuity and transformation than proponents of the psychometric trait-oriented view who, for the most part, have used standard self-report instruments. The Bonn Longitudinal Study, for instance, conducted extensive interviews to explore individuals' subjective construction of their past, present, and future (Lehr & Thomae, 1987; Schmitz-Scherzer & Thomae, 1983; Thomae, 1976, 1983). At the first of eight measurement occasions ($N = 222$), interviews regarding the past covered the entire biography. Explorations at later measurement occasions concentrated on biographical events and personal experiences which had occurred in-between the preceding and the concurrent measurement point. The Bonn analyses also were not restricted by an extant set of situation-invariant personality traits, but emphasized constructs such as life styles which were more open to developmental transformations.

In recent analyses of these data (Fisseni, 1985; Fooken, 1985; Olbrich, 1985; Thomae, 1988), it was found that individuals experience both continuity and change in different domains of personality, the life situation, and the environment. Changes were experienced primarily regarding the life situation (e.g. as an increase or, sometimes, a decrease in health problems), and with respect to social or physical aspects of the environment (e.g. as changes in the intensity of contacts to relatives, friends, and acquaintances, or as a change in residence from an independent living situation to an institution or the children's home). With respect to personality, basic belief systems and value orientations showed a high degree of stability and continuity, whereas coping styles were more likely to change. For instance, some individuals increased their ability to accept health-related constraints, and to appreciate the positive side of their current life situation. In sum, the results of the study were consistent with the hypothesis that behaviour-oriented aspects of the self are more likely to undergo change than basic personality characteristics.

Results from the Berkeley Study, another real-time longitudinal study investigating personality development from the fourth to the eighth decade of life (Maas & Kuypers, 1974; Mussen, 1985), also focused on the concept of life style. Again, large inter-individual differences in the continuity of life styles were revealed. In particular, life-styles of men exhibited a greater amount of continuity than life-styles of women. The authors argue that the women in the sample were more affected by changes in the family cycle than men. For instance, they were more likely than men to remodel their future time perspectives and life-styles after children had left the house of the parents.

The issue of subjectively experienced continuity and change was also at the center of a recent cross-sectional study (Kruse, 1992). The study was designed to complement the Bonn Longitudinal Study, and comprised 480 participants aged 67 to 103 years. To examine subjectively experienced changes in personality characteristics, individuals were asked to describe the continuities and discontinuities of their own aging process. Thus, the study is a good example for the use of the 'pseudo-longitudinal' method described above in that individuals were explicitly asked to compare the present with the past.

Self-reports indicated that individuals experienced both gains and losses as they were growing into old and very old age. Personality development was primarily characterized by gains. For instance, individuals said that they were increasingly capable of perceiving the possibilities and limitations of their behavioural resources. Moreover, they felt that the increasing constraints on their future time perspective had made them more capable of selecting a set of goals and plans judged to be both important and attainable in the near future (e.g. in the coming weeks or months). Losses were conceived primarily in terms of functional capacity. Examples include increasing sensory and motor impairments, an increase in chronic pain, and the increasing dependence upon health services and caregivers.

INVESTIGATIONS INTO LIMITS OF FUNCTIONING (PLASTICITY)

The systematic exploration of the range (plasticity) of behavioural functioning is another main theme of aging research. Changes in plasticity are increasingly seen as the hallmark of aging (Baltes, P. B., 1987; Lerner, 1984). Plasticity or within-person adaptiveness refers to the fact that individuals perform in different ways and at different levels under varying experiential conditions. In particular, the notion of plasticity points to the latent potential of individuals, to what they could do if conditions were optimal. Kliegl and Baltes (1987) proposed three facets or tiers of functioning which further specify conditions for the assessment of plasticity: 1) baseline capacity indicates what a person can do without intervention or special treatment. 2) baseline reserve capacity denotes an individual's performance when, at one point in time, all available external and internal resources are activated to optimize performance. 3) developmental reserve capacity refers to the kind and level of performance an individual can achieve if continued exposure to an optimal environment has extended the initially available amount of reserve capacity.

It follows from these definitions that age-related changes in plasticity are generally difficult to study by means of real-time longitudinal designs. This is even true if they involve some form of intervention because interventions (if used as an experimental manipulation in real-time longitudinal research) do not approximate the range and intensity necessary to explore the limits of plasticity. Under naturalistic circumstances, individuals do not activate their reserves unless they are forced to do so because of extremely challenging life-events or life-styles. Moreover, standardized assessment procedures as used in large-scale studies are often not appropriate to estimate an individual's possible range of performance. For instance, the administration of a standardized IQ test once per year does not provide an optimal context for the activation of cognitive resources.

To approximate limits (or peaks) of functioning, it is necessary to enlist many hours of practice and often years of guided tutoring (Ericsson, 1990; Ericsson & Smith, 1991). Microgenetic intervention studies and developmental situation studies are designed to approximate peak performances in the laboratory. Here, the focus is on inter-individual differences in short-term – 'microgenetic' – intra-individual change and on maximum possible performance. It is hypothesized that the obtained change function contains important and formerly hidden information about the functional status of an individual. This information may be used not only to estimate the possible range of developmental trajectories available to a given individual but also to understand the matrix of individual differences in aging existing in a given population.

Age differences in plasticity have been studied foremost in the domain of cognitive development, with microgenetic intervention studies demonstrating both the continued existence of cognitive plasticity in old age as well as sizeable age-related reductions in developmental reserve capacity (first research example, below). However, we believe that the notion of plasticity may also lead to a better understanding of the stability and maintained integrity as well as the possible breakdown of personality in old age. For instance, numerous studies have found that the self in old age continues to be a resilient system of coping despite the fact that major losses such as bereavement, chronic illness, and the death of close friends accumulate. Thus, it appears that the plasticity of coping processes is maintained or even refined throughout the entire adult life-span (second research example, below).

First example: old-age cognitive plasticity and its limits

The interest in old-age cognitive plasticity is guided by three main propositions. The first proposition states that descriptive aging research provides but a snapshot of a person's or cohort's location in a population of performance distributions. Because in such descriptive real-time aging research we do not know the life-history of performance conditions that are at the foundation of each person's life circumstances nor their differences between individuals, it is difficult to compare persons as to their basic potential. The second proposition states that there is, especially in old age, reserve capacity which can be activated. This proposition originated in the 1970s (Baltes, P. B., 1973; Labouvie-Vief, 1977), and was originally meant to counteract the focus on decline that was historically dominant in gerontological research. The third proposition states that a loss in plasticity may be a hallmark of aging (Baltes, P. B., 1987; Coper, Jänicke & Schulz 1986; Shock, 1977). As to cognitive aging, these propositions have been applied primarily to the study of experience losses in the strength and range of cognitive potential, especially of 'fluid' intelligence or the 'mechanics' of the mind (Baltes, P. B., Dittmann-Kohli & Dixon, 1984; Cattell, 1971; Horn, 1982; Kliegl, 1992; Salthouse, 1991). Extensive and age-comparative intervention studies (e.g. up to 100 training sessions distributed over 1–2 years) have been conducted to explore the range of and age differences in cognitive plasticity.

Microgenetic intervention studies suggest that all three propositions are basically true, at least with respect to healthy individuals up to their 70s or early 80s. Fig. 8.2, taken from Baltes, P. B. and Kliegl (1992), both exemplifies and resolves this paradox. Subjects in this study participated in 38 experimental sessions distributed over about one year and were trained in the Method of Loci, a mnemonic technique for the ordered recall of word lists (Bower, 1970; Yesavage & Rose, 1984; Kliegl, Smith & Baltes, 1989). In the Method of Loci, subjects overlearn a set of locations or loci in an invariant order. After acquisition of this cognitive routing map, to-be-learned items are sequentially associated with each of the locations of the map by means of a mental image. To recall the items, subjects 'visit' each location, try to remember the mental image, and retrieve the target item.

First, this research shows that simple one-time observations are not sufficient to index a person's level of capacity. Secondly, the research demonstrates that most elderly persons are quite able to learn the Method of Loci, and by using it to perform outside the usual range of performance when recalling lists of words or digits (Baltes, P. B. & Kliegl, 1992; Kliegl et al., 1989). This is illustrated by the large training gains of older adults depicted in Fig. 8.2. The finding of substantive improvement over time is clearly consistent with the proposition that developmental reserve capacity is preserved in old age, and supports earlier findings from other domains of fluid intelligence (for a summary, see Baltes & Lindenberger, 1988).

On the other hand, the data displayed in Fig. 8.2 also support the third proposition of an aging-associated reduction in developmental reserve capacity. Even after very extensive training, old adults were not able to reach the level of performance reached by young adults after very few training sessions. Thus, although older adults were clearly capable of acquiring the Method of Loci and performing outside the range of typical recall performance, they showed sizeable performance deficits when compared to young adults and tested for

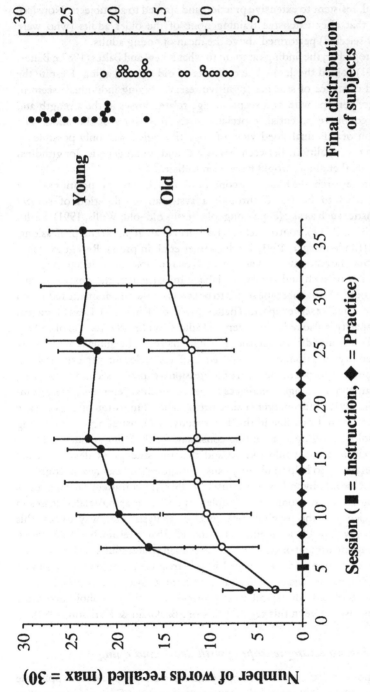

Fig. 8.2. Performance by young and old adults in serial recall of lists of words as a function of mnemonic training (left panel). The bars indicate standard deviations. In the right panel, individual scores are given for the last assessment sessions (36/37). (Taken from Baltes & Kliegl, 1992.)

limits of developmental reserve capacity. This negative age difference was substantial, resistent to extensive practice, and applied to all subjects. Note (see Fig. 8.2) that after extensive training none of the older adults (who were positively selected) performed above the mean of young adults.

Taken together, the findings amount to what Kliegl and Baltes (1987a; Baltes, P. B., 1991) coined the Janus-like character of old age and aging. Despite the continued existence of sizeable cognitive reserves, aging individuals seem to experience, perhaps with no exception, age-related losses in the strength and range of cognitive potential, especially in the mechanics of the mind. The articulation of this dual-sided view of cognitive aging was only possible by developing a coalition between real-time and microgenetic longitudinal research. Neither alone, would have been sufficient.

In future research, the boundary conditions of each of the propositions about plasticity need to be tested through a systematic exploration of subject characteristics such as age (e.g. young–old versus old–old; Willis, 1991), health status (Schaie, 1990b), control beliefs (Lachman et al. in press) and professional expertise (Lindenberger, 1991; Lindenberger et al. in press). Recent evidence suggests that the amount of developmental reserve capacity in old age may vary as a function of such and similar variables. In particular, the onset of senile dementia of the Alzheimer type seems to be associated with a dramatic reduction of developmental reserve capacity (Baltes, M. M. et al. in press). Developmental reserve capacity is also reduced in very old adults (Willis, 1991) and in old adults with cardiovascular disease (Schaie, 1990b). Finally, in the domain of imagery-based memory functioning, the existence of task-relevant pre-experimental knowledge and practice in the form of professional expertise seems to attenuate, rather than eliminate, age differences in developmental reserve capacity (Lindenberger, 1991; Lindenberger et al. in press). That elimination of negative age differences was not possible in this latter study, demonstrating the increasing role of biological aging as a limiting constraint for the aging mind.

In conclusion, we would like to add that the strategy of developmental simulation may also help to identify causes of age-related changes in cognitive plasticity. One may hypothesize, for instance, that effortful attentional processes are among the most prominent variables representing aging-related losses in brain efficiency at the psychological level of analysis. One way to test this hypothesis would be to identify treatments that presumably lead to an analoguous impairment of attentional processes in young adults. The prediction would be that young adults exposed in this treatment would show a similar pattern of cognitive deficits as old adults. A recent study comparing the memory performance of old adults and young sleep-deprived or alcohol-intoxicated subjects is instructive in this regard (Nilsson, Bäckman & Karlsson, 1989).

Second example: coping with death and dying

The notions of plasticity and developmental reserve capacity are also applicable to what Jaspers (1965) termed the boundary situations ('Grenzsituationen') of human existence. Situations of this kind may arise as a consequence of severe chronic illness, confrontation with one's own death and dying, and the death of close persons. The frequency of exposure to such events increases in old age, and some individuals may be confronted with them for the first time. Thus, the likelihood of experiencing a 'boundary situation' is probably higher in late than in early or middle adulthood.

In the following, we proceed from the assumption that there is a structural resemblance between testing-the-limits situations in cognitive intervention and the boundary situations of human existence. In both cases, individuals are confronted with a challenge that strongly deviates from what they normally experience in everyday life. In the case of cognitive intervention, the challenge is mainly on the cognitive plane; in the case of a boundary situation, the challenge concerns central aspects of personality and the self and its adaptive capacity (Brandtstädter & Baltes-Götz, 1990; Brim, 1988, 1992; Filipp & Klauer, 1986; Kruse, 1987; Taylor & Brown, 1988).

An empirical examination of coping with boundary situations in the context of typical large-scale real-time longitudinal studies is difficult because these studies generally have a fixed schedule of measurement and do not preselect for the occurrence of boundary conditions (see, however, Wortman & Silver, 1990). Boundary situations may, or may not, occur between one measurement occasion and the next, and they may already date back for quite some time when the next measurement occasion takes place. Thus, although real-time longitudinal studies provide a differentiated picture of general individual differences in coping styles (Busse & Maddox, 1986; Costa & McCrae, 1988; Costa, McCrae & Arenberg, 1983; Lehr & Thomae, 1987; Mussen, 1985; Palmore et al., 1985; Schmitz-Scherzer & Thomae, 1983), they are not very informative if the goal is to better understand inter-individual differences in coping with boundary situations as well as the microgenesis of that process. Replicated single-subject designs with repeated measurements (for a review, see Jones & Nesselroade, 1990) are more appropriate in this case because both the beginning of measurement and the spacing of measurement intervals can be adopted to each individual and their matrix and flow of life events.

A recent study on death and dying (Kruse, 1987; cf. Kruse, 1991) may serve to illustrate the potential of this approach for a better understanding of individual differences in coping with death and dying as the ultimate boundary situation of human existence. Fifty-five elderly patients with an infaust diagnosis were closely followed by general practitioners and psychologists from the time of their release from hospital until their death. The investigation covered 6 to 24 months, depending upon how long individuals survived. The goal of the study was to examine intra-individual changes in confronting one's death and dying, and to elaborate forms of medical and psychological intervention that would facilitate the acceptance of one's death.

Two results are noteworthy. First, it appeared that patients were seeking out for persons and situations that closely matched their appraisal of and their feelings towards the situation. Thus they made efforts at structuring situations and interactions such that the likelihood of maintaining a sense of subjective continuity was maximized. For instance, patients who were not willing or able to realize impending death refrained from interactions with persons who, according to their judgment, were likely to engage them into conversations about death-related issues. Moreover, these individuals were eager to demonstrate their preserved physical competence.

Secondly, in some individuals, the opportunity to share fears and sorrows with a confidant led to a pronounced improvement in subjective well-being. Initially, these individuals were deeply depressed and resigned; later on, they were able to consciously face – and finally accept – death. The possibility to engage in an intensive exchange was fundamentally new for these patients, given that they had not yet experienced something similar within or outside their families. The unique character of the interaction may have promoted behavioural and experiential development.

On the one hand, the findings of this study support earlier results showing that individual differences among elderly individuals in coping with stressful life events are influenced by personality characteristics and prior experiences with similar situations (Costa & McCrae, 1987; Lazarus & Folkman, 1984; Lehr, 1982; Maas & Kuypers, 1974; Shanan, 1991; Thomae, 1988). The findings, furthermore, demonstrate the usefulness of person-oriented, repeated single-subject designs for the investigation of coping with boundary conditions of human existence. On the other hand, because of a lack of microgenetic and interventive work, we are not yet in a position to specify the constituent processes or the range of individual adaptiveness to boundary situations of human existence. At the same time, this research (Kruse, 1987, 1991), because of its sensitive topic reminds us that we have to consider carefully the ethical implications involved whenever we move from descriptive real-time to experimental longitudinal work.

NORMAL VERSUS PATHOLOGICAL AGING

In essence, the distinction between normality and pathology in aging research is based on the assumption that growing old is not synomymous with becoming sick. Definitions of normal aging vary somewhat depending upon whether a more normative or a more descriptive (i.e. statistical) usage of the term is preferred (cf. Gerok & Brandtstädter, 1992; Fozard, Metter & Bryant, 1990). We prefer a more normative view by defining normal aging as growing old without a manifest illness, be it physical or mental. Pathological aging, on the other hand, refers to aging with clear signs of physical or mental pathology.

The heuristic function of this distinction is to urge researchers to identify those environmental, behavioural, and predisposing systems of influence which predict the incidence of both pathology and health in old age. Thus, the goal is not to classify the universe of aging patterns into two exclusive categories, but to theoretically dissociate two time-related processes in order to better understand the reasons and conditions of their co-occurrence in the real world.

The main goals of longitudinal research on normal and pathological aging are prevention, early diagnosis and prediction of pathology, and rehabilitation. Again, the achievement of these goals requires the combinatorial use of various kinds of longitudinal methodology. Good examples for prevention are studies on cardiovascular disease. By now, several large investigations with random assignment of individuals to treatment and control groups have been carried out on this issue. An important result was that prevention was more effective in reducing morbidity than mortality (Fries, 1990). Studies on early diagnosis focus on the investigation of antecedent conditions of pathology in old age, and on the detection of early disease symptoms (Erlenmeyer-Kimling & Miller, 1986). Finally, longitudinal studies on rehabilitation are concerned with efforts at remediating already existing pathology. In order to explore the possible use of rehabilitative efforts, it is useful, however, to test the effectiveness of interventions in intensive single-subject studies and to offer constellations of treatments not available in reality as it exists today. Note again that this strategy of expanding and re-arranging conditions is at the foundation of microgenetic longitudinal work.

First example: early diagnosis of dementia

Perhaps the most typical example of a chronic disease associated with old age is senile dementia. The incidence rate for senile dementia of the Alzheimer type, for instance, is estimated to be about 5% by age 70, 15% by age 80, and 30% by age 90 (Häfner, 1986; Sørensen et al., 1986; Evans et al., 1989). At the behavioural level, the onset of Alzheimer's disease is marked by a global deterioration of cognitive functioning. Generally, 'fluid' abilities such as reasoning ability, orientation, and episodic memory are affected earlier in the course of the disease than 'crystallized' abilities such as verbal knowledge.

Currently, research efforts are directed toward identifying behavioural and neurophysiological signs of the disease as early and as reliably as possible (Christensen, Hadzi-Pavlovic & Jacomb, 1991). Longitudinal data are an indispensable part in this enterprise because they provide information on events and conditions that predict the incidence of dementia at later measurement occasions (Khatchaturian, 1985; Miller, 1986).

A re-analysis of data from the Aging Twins Study (LaRue & Jarvik, 1987) may serve to illustrate the problems faced by prospective real-time longitudinal studies on the early diagnosis of dementia. The authors examined 64 aging twins. Thirty-six of them were judged to be free of dementia on the basis of a careful mental status examination. A main result was that individuals who were judged to be demented at a mean age of 85 years had achieved lower scores on tests of cognitive functioning 20 years prior to the diagnosis. Moreover, they experienced greater declines in vocabulary and short-term memory over this time period than those surviving to a comparable age without dementia. Thus, the results of this study seem to indicate that individuals who develop dementia in old age experience subtle cognitive declines many years before cognitive impairment becomes clinically evident.

Unfortunately, the interpretation of these data is not without problems. First, we know little about the ways in which sample attrition has influenced the results (Gruenberg, 1986). The original sample comprised 268, rather than 64 individuals. It is possible that individuals with certain types of dementia had a higher chance to drop out of the sample than healthy individuals or individuals with other types of dementia.

Another problem is the wide spacing as well as the small number of measurement occasions. Real-time longitudinal studies of this kind provide only restricted information about inter-individual differences in intra-individual change trajectories. Given the magnitude of inter-individual differences in the level of cognitive functioning present among elderly individuals (Schaie, 1988, 1990b), information on inter-individual differences in intra-individual change may yield a better separation of premorbid and cognitively intact populations (Labouvie, 1986). Thus, the onset of dementia may be better identifiable through measures of change than through measures of status.

Given the methodological and practical problems associated with real-time longitudinal studies on the early diagnosis of dementia, it is worthwhile to explore the potential of microgenetic longitudinal designs. With respect to the issue of dementia, there are theoretical reasons to believe that the microgenetic approach is especially promising. One guiding hypothesis, for instance, is that individuals at risk for dementia profit less from cognitive training than healthy older adults because their learning potential (developmental reserve capacity) is greatly reduced. Thus, it is a lower level of functioning in standard psycho-metric tests rather than the absence of training gains in the course of a few experimental sessions which is expected to predict a future pathology-related cognitive decline in real life.

A recent study (Baltes, M. M. et al., in press) supports this idea. Fifty-six healthy individuals and 25 individuals at risk for dementia were randomly assigned to either a training or a control group. The at-risk diagnosis was based on a standardized psychiatric interview that did not contain a cognitive assessment battery. Individuals in the two training groups received a series of five one-hour training sessions in a test of figural relations, a component of fluid intelligence.

The relevant data are shown in Fig. 8.3. Stepwise hierarchical regressions demonstrated that only healthy elderly profited from training, and that only post-training scores predicted the psychiatric at-risk diagnosis. Albeit prelimi-nary and in need of replication, this study indicates that microgenetic studies with a focus on differential reserve capacity may prove helpful in offering a new window on the 'real-time', longitudinal emergence of dementia.

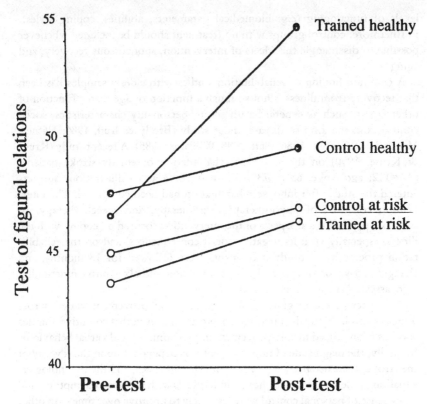

Fig. 8.3.   Microgenetic intervention work on the early diagnosis of dementia (M. M. Baltes, Kühl, & Sowarka, in press). Changes in mean scores from pre- to post-test demonstrate significantly greater plasticity in the healthy trained group compared to the two control groups and the trained at-risk group. Differences in pre-test scores are not significant.

Second example: rehabilitation of pathology in old age

In addition to the identification of precursors and early manifestations of pathology, another task of longitudinal studies on normal versus pathological aging is to explore the degree to which pathological processes can be remediated or attenuated through intervention (Brody & Ruff, 1986; Häfner, 1986; Platt, 1988; Williams, 1985). These rehabilitation studies are microgenetic in nature because they focus on intra-individual change patterns as a consequence of prolonged treatment such as physical exercise, therapy, and drugs.

   Rehabilitation studies have to cover a time period that is sufficiently long to determine the temporal extension (i.e. maintenance) of intervention effects and their possible interaction with age. The number of measurement occasions should be high enough to identify intraindividual change functions, and the scope of the variables under consideration large enough to encompass different levels of functioning (e.g. biomedical parameters, abilities, coping styles). Furthermore, control groups with no treatment should be included whenever possible to disentangle the effects of intervention, spontaneous recovery, and aging.

A common finding of rehabilitation studies with elderly samples has been that recovery from illness is not so much a function of age than a function of other factors such as general health status, personality characteristics, social context, and the kind of disease under study (Brody & Ruff, 1986; Häfner, Moschel & Sartorius, 1986; Platt, 1988; Williams, 1985). A recent study (Kruse & Kruse, 1990) on the ambulant rehabilitation of elderly stroke patients ($N = 112$; age range: 65 to 78 years) may serve as an illustration. Subjects entered the study after inhouse-rehabilitation had been completed. The intervention consisted of physiotherapy, ergotherapy, and speech therapy. In addition, psychological aspects of the intervention focused on coping with the illness, especially with its negative social consequences, and on the rehabilitation process itself. Study participants were followed for 18 months, and changes in psychomotor as well as verbal and non-verbal cognitive functioning were assessed at four measurement occasions.

As expected, the magnitude of performance improvement varied across domains and individuals. First, improvement in non-verbal cognitive abilities was less pronounced than improvement in psychomotor and verbal behaviour. Secondly, the magnitude of improvement was dependent upon the severity of the stroke, the existence and severity of other illnesses, and the psychological situation of the subjects. Specifically, individuals with depressive symptoms and a low sense of personal control were less likely to improve over time than other subjects. Definitely, this study illustrates that non-interventive 'real-time' longitudinal work is insufficient when the task is to identify optimal environmental conditions for rehabilitation. By definition rehabilitation research extends beyond existing realities.

MODELS AND CONCEPTIONS OF SUCCESSFUL AGING

Our final major theme of recent gerontological work is efforts at formulating and testing models of successful aging (Baltes & Baltes, 1990; Gerok & Brandtstädter, 1992; Rowe & Kahn, 1987). This effort encompasses at least three objectives: 1) the specification of relevant outcome variables (what are indicators of successful aging?), 2) the identification of risk and protective factors (which antecedent conditions are related to which desired or undesired outcomes?), and 3) the delineation of processes which are at the foundation of antecedent–consequent linkages (what are the underlying 'basic' mechanisms, behaviourally and societally, which generate the product?). Real-time and microgenetic longitudinal studies, in concert, are relevant for each of these questions and their inter-relationships.

Table 8.1 offers a glimpse at the factors and processes studied in work on

Table 8.1. *Successful aging: examples of positive outcome variables*

Objective role		Subjective role
Length of life	Mental health	Life satisfaction
Biological health	Autonomy	Optimism
Functional health	Social productivity	Personal control
Reserve capacity/adaptivity	Social integration	Self efficacy/agency
. mental		
. physical		
. social		
. economic		

Note:
Because of differences (variations) in personal and cultural traditions and values, no absolute definition of successful aging is possible (Baltes and Baltes, 1990).

successful aging. Depending upon one's view of the system 'human species' and one's preferences for what is significant in civilization and peoples' lifes, different emphases result (Baltes & Baltes, 1990). Some researchers argue for the foremost importance of subjective indicators of the quality of life: 'Add life to years and not only years to life' is their primary motto. Others focus primarily on objective criteria such as length of life or its counterpart, mortality (including aspects of morbidity). Here is not the place to discuss the intellectual dynamics involved in the treatment of these issues. Rather, our focus is on demonstrating the omnipresence of longitudinal research and its use as a generic term rather than as being identical with real-time follow-up studies of single cohorts.

First example: life expectancy and morbidity of old age in the future

A good illustration of the importance of cohort-sequential longitudinal studies is the question of psychological or physical vitality (and its polar counterpoints, that is, morbidity and mortality) in old age. Which factors regulate psychological and physical vitality? How much potential for further improvement is there? Are today's older citizens more or less healthy than those of former generations? What are the prospects in health and well-being for the future of old age? Does the 'greying' of society lead to a healthier or more ailing state of old age? These are issues that take the centre-stage in current gerontology (e.g. M. Baltes, 1989; Baltes, P. B. & Mittelstraß, 1992; Bromley, 1988; Fries, 1990), and their treatment requires the skilful application of the full gamut of longitudinal methods.

Fries (1990), for instance, defines successful aging from a medical or public health point of view, as consisting of 'optimizing life expectancy while at the same time minimizing physical, psychological, and social morbidity' (p. 35). In addition, Fries (1980, 1990) has offered his own 'optimistic' view on the future of old age and the possibility that future generations might increasingly age successfully; that is, live longer and with a smaller and smaller time-span of manifest morbidity. Two components are central to Fries line of argument. First, he argues that there is a definite and biologically based limit to our life-span (say about 85–90 years on average). Second, Fries maintains that within that fixed span of life, it is possible through healthier life-styles and improved medical treatments to delay the frailties of old age until very old age. In short, morbidity in future old age might be increasingly 'compressed' into smaller and smaller time spans before death.

For research endeavours, the Fries model implies an ontogenetic 'longitudinal' and a historical 'cohort-comparative' perspective and prediction. If his compression of morbidity model is correct, the onset of infirmity (morbidity) in more recent and especially future cohorts (generations) would occur later and later in old age; and in addition, the life-time available for healthy aging would increase more than the average life expectancy. The model, furthermore, implies that compression of morbidity should be evident only if the lifetime of individuals has reached an age sufficiently close to their biological maximum (Fries, Greene, & Levine, 1989).

In current gerontology, this optimistic view of Fries on the future of old age is juxtaposed by more pessimistic views (e.g. Krämer, 1992; Schneider & Brody, 1983; Schneider & Guralnik, 1990; Verbrugge, 1984). According to these pessimistic views, just the opposite is true for future aging cohorts. When populations, on average, live longer and longer, the likelihood increases for old age to become an increasingly sick state of life. And indeed, such a pessimistic view also has its empirical and theoretical foundations. Consider just the following two perspectives. In modern times, more and more biologically 'vulnerable' or 'weak' persons receive enough medical and social support to reach old age. In other words, the demographic 'greying' of society is actually correlated with a decrease of the magnitude of 'positive selection' during ontogenesis. In addition, there may be an added effect of life-prolonging efforts of medical technology during the very last phase of life. In short, the argument of the pessimist view of the future of old age goes: the older a population, the larger the proportion of biologically 'weak' and 'sick' individuals; and this, in addition to the illnesses which are characteristics of old age in the first place.

The evaluation of such opposing views requires longitudinal work: real-time, cohort-comparative, and interventive (Fries, 1989, 1990). For instance, to estimate the power and causal direction of risk factors (such as smoking, hypertension, obesity, or physical inactivity), it is necessary to observe longitudinally individuals as they age, who differ in these characteristics, and who have changed status in the risk factors involved (see also, Rutter, 1988a). Secondly, to understand and estimate the role of historical change and its connection with ontogenetic processes, it is imperative to conduct cohort-comparative longitudinal work, that is, to follow the longitudinal development of several generations.

The need for real-time, cohort-comparative, and interventive longitudinal work applies to each of the components of Fries' model. One component is the assumption of a biologically fixed maximum life-span. This assumption evolved and is continuously tested by comparing age-specific life expectancies in successful cohorts, such as life expectancies of 70-year-olds in 1900 vs. 1950. Fries' conclusion in this regard is that there has been very little cohort or historical increase in life expectancy for the very old of each generation. Such a plateauing of life expectancy for the very old suggests to Fries that his assumption of a biologically fixed life-span is a reasonable one.

The second major assumption of Fries' compression of morbidity model is that older persons of the same age become healthier and healthier. Such a finding is part of the Goteborg Longitudinal Study which reports increased health for the average 70-year-olds across recent cohorts (Svanborg, 1985). Fries (1990) summarizes major American work which equally attests to a decrease in age-specific incidence of chronic disease. House et al. (1990) add another variation. In addition to cohort comparisons, they include variations of socio-economic status. This added comparison elucidates an important factor of social differentiation. By this addition, House et al. (1990) were able to show that the compression of morbidity model (more healthier than sick life-time associated with living longer) seems to be true for the upper, but not for the lower end of the socio-economic stratum.

The discourse surrounding the debate about the compression of morbidity model also makes explicit the importance of interventive and microgenetic longitudinal work. There is an increasingly large body of data aimed at examining the role of factors aimed at reducing risk or improving protection or 'reserve capacity' as we call it in our own work on the aging mind (Baltes, P. B. & Lindenberger, 1988; Kliegl & Baltes, 1987a, b). Bortz (1991), for instance, summarizes extant intervention work on the role of physical activity on morbidity and mortality, Fries (1990) offers a synopsis on the effect of medical interventions aimed at studying the effect of changes in health habits including the use of seat belts, and Masoro (1991), in his recent Kleemeier Award address at the Annual Meetings of the Gerontological Society of America (in press), demonstrates how longitudinal data on the effect of nutrition on longevity were elucidated by long-term and short-term animal research, in which the mechanisms and components involved were made more explicit through simulations of different life-histories (see Denenberg et al. (1968) for an early line of work on the experimental simulation of life-histories).

The corpus of data on morbidity and mortality and the future of an aging society is too extensive to be summarized here. The issue is further complicated by the fact that morbidity and mortality are not as highly correlated as one might assume (Fries, 1990). We also do not want to take a particular position on the nature of the evidence. The point here is to show the importance of viewing longitudinal methodology as a generic term with many faces. If the goal is to empirically evaluate the tenability of the compression of morbidity model, it is imperative to carry out cohort-sequential and experimental-interventive work.

Second example: psychological mechanisms of good (successful) aging

The same general perspective applies to the psychological study of aging well (Baltes & Baltes, 1990; Featherman, Smith, & Peterson, 1990). To illustrate, we focus on the role of certain processes of life management which individuals use to regulate their aging, behaviourally and experientially (e.g., Baltes, M. M. & Carstensen, 1991: Brandtstädter & Baltes-Götz, 1990, and this volume; Brim, 1992; Schulz et al., 1991).

One meta-model of successful aging is that of 'selective optimization with compensation' (Baltes & Baltes, 1990). This model is a meta-model in the sense that its basic components (selection, optimization, compensation) identify general, quasi-universal characteristics of successful aging. A central feature of life-span development is the management of a shifting balance between gains and losses. During adulthood, with increasing age, the balance shifts towards a less positive ratio until, in old age, losses begin to outweigh gains, at least in our subjective pattern of expectations about the life course (Baltes, P. B., 1987; Heckhausen, Dixon & Baltes, 1989).

To achieve the management of this life-span developmental task, Baltes and Baltes (1990) posit that individuals, as they age, 'select' (passively or actively) domains for continued achievement and withdrawal, and they attempt to 'optimize' their functioning in the areas selected. In addition, they search for, and practise, 'compensation' when their levels of potential or skill fall below required levels. The model of selective optimization with compensation, then, proceeds from the assumption that, despite much individual variation, there is a fixed framework for the course of life: a reduction in reserve capacity implies less and less potential for positive change (gains). Continued plasticity (Lerner, 1984) permits, however, optimization and compensation aimed at maximizing gains in select areas and minimizing losses in others.

How this generic task of the management of a shifting balance between gains and losses is realized, depends, of course, upon the specific personal and environmental conditions. The model is generic (universal), its implementation, however is person and culture-specific. Table 8.2 offers three examples (music, running, and golf) using personal histories and observations offered by three persons who have focused on different domains as targets of selective optimization with compensation.

What about longitudinal research on the process selective optimization with compensation? The example used for illustration is the role of expectations and management strategies which operate when selection, optimization, and compensation take place, passively or actively. Among the central putative mechanisms of personal management of a shifting ratio between gains and losses are changes in goals and goal transformations (Brim, 1992) as well as changes in styles or forms of action control and coping (Baltes & Baltes, 1986; Brandtstädter & Baltes-Götz, 1990, this volume). We are also interested in learning

Table 8.2. *Selective optimization with compensation: everyday examples*

Source	Selection	Optimization	Compensation
Concert pianist (Rubinstein)	Fewer pieces	More practice	More contrasts in speed of play
Long-distance runner	Easier courses Fewer competing activities	More practice New strategies (e.g. diet)	New and varied shoewear Prevention of injuries (e.g. warm-up)
Senior golfer (Morehouse)	Fewer and shorter courses Time of day	More sensori-motor training Shift practice from driving range to green and short play	Change in club selection (e.g. higher woods, longer shafts) Change stance to calibrate for loss of balance

whether these processes of management of a shifting ratio of gains and losses are effective in the sense that they protect the aging person from a loss of self-esteem.

The significance of descriptive real-time longitudinal work on these topics has become paramount. First, longitudinal research has shown that older individuals, indeed, do not show the widely held expectation of a major loss in self-esteem and sense of control (Bengtson et al., 1985; Lachman, 1986). Older persons, by and large, report levels of well-being, self-esteem, and personal control that are comparable to levels reported by younger adults. Such an outcome, because the 'objective' state of older individuals is expected to be less positive (Baltes & Baltes, 1990), may be considered a surprise and needs explanation. Here, longitudinal research on styles of life management and coping becomes relevant, and there is a dearth of relevant work. As Brandt-städter and his colleagues (Brandtstädter & Baltes-Götz, 1990) have demon-strated, however, older adults exhibit coping strategies that focus increasingly on accommodative rather than assimilative goal definitions and goal realiza-tions. With age, we become more inclined to adjust to new levels of what is possible in principle: certain goals are ignored, other goals are lowered, still other goals are transformed, and goals are stretched in time (Brim, 1992).

Such real-time longitudinal work needs expansion, however, and there is beginning to be evidence about how descriptive longitudinal work can be combined with microgenetic simulation of the developmental processes involved. One example is consideration of processes of self-referent thought in the management of gains and losses, and of our expectations about our futures changing with age (Baltes, M. M. & Carstensen, 1991; Schulz et al., 1991; Cross & Markus, 1991). Markus and her colleagues, for instance, have focused on the role of possible selves and how the choice of one's self-focus can be used in maintaining self-esteem and giving new direction to life.

Of particular significance as an exemplary case of microgenetic longitudinal work on the nature of coping in old age is the short-term, but highly intensive, observational work conducted by Baltes, M. M. and her colleagues in nursing homes and private residences (Baltes, M. M., 1988; Baltes, M. M. & Wahl, 1991; Baltes, Wahl & Reichert, 1991; Wahl, in press). When older adults show increasing passivity in mind and behaviour, the traditional view was that this is a function of lack of autonomy, dependency, or learned helplessness. By observing in detail, over weeks and months, the specific nature of interpersonal transactions between elderly persons and their social partners surrounding dependency-events and by combining such descriptive observational work with interventive strategies, Margret Baltes and her colleagues demonstrated that the traditional 'longitudinal' picture of the aging process needs re-interpretation. First, they showed that there is more plasticity in the age-associated evolution of dependency than would be expected from real-time longitudinal research. Secondly, they could demonstrate that not all of dependency is dysfunctional. When older adults show dependent behaviour, this is often not due to a lack of competence. Rather, dependent behaviour in the elderly can be associated with positive outcomes such as a sense of control over the social environment and the production of social contact. Through microgenetic longitudinal work, then, it was possible to elucidate with more clarity the multi-dimensional and multi-functional nature of dependency and its modifiability (plasticity). Achieving this level of insight would have been impossible with real-time longitudinal work alone.

OUTLOOK

The foregoing research illustrations from the study of human aging converge on the same general conclusion: real-time longitudinal studies, of course, are an essential part of research on human aging. They are a required part of developmental scholarship. But, despite their complexity, especially in implementation and quality control (Magnusson & Bergman, 1990), simple real-time studies are not enough. To understand antecedent–consequent relationships in ontogenesis, their degrees of magnitude, their causal directions, the nature of the underlying mechanisms, and the intricate relationship between ontogenesis and social change, its is necessary to rely on a broad spectrum of well-coordinated longitudinal designs: descriptive and interventive, single cohort and cohort-comparative, real-time and simulated-time.

As a concluding observation, we reiterate another argument why we firmly believe that research in human aging needs to treat 'real-time' longitudinal research in a perspective which includes a cautionary stance about its final power as a measure of what is true and possible in human development. Of all the periods of the life-span, old age is the newest in terms of the history of civilization. In one important sense, old age is 'young', that is, it does not have the benefit of a long and carefully refined cultural history of human care and tradition as would be true for childhood or adolescence. Were we to attend, therefore, predominantly to findings from real-time longitudinal studies of extant cohorts, we would continuously reify the cultural past, we would omit other outcomes that are possible in principle (Baltes, P. B. & Mittelstraß, 1992). The future of old age, therefore, is also critically dependent on what researchers can create and simulate in their laboratories and not only on what culture has accomplished thus far. Let us revisit the example of cognitive aging as an example. Real-time longitudinal work suggested that the reality of the aging mind was decline, at least after the sixth decade of life. It was, however, short-term and interventive 'microgenetic' work which helped us understand not only the nature of the processes involved, but especially the conditions for continued plasticity.

Aging and old age, then, are not fully fixed biological and cultural realities. They are in flux. It is also for this reason that we argue for an expanded conception of longitudinal methodology. The final power of real-time longitudinal methodology hinges on its creative combination with other kinds of longitudinal designs that permit us to look more closely at the constituent processes and to look beyond.

REFERENCES

Ahammer, I. M. & Baltes, P. B. (1972). Objective vs. perceived age differences in personality: how do adolescents, adults, and older people view themselves and each other? *Journal of Gerontology*, **27**, 46–51.

Aitken, A. C. (1934). Note on selection from a multivariate normal distribution. *Proceedings of the Edinburgh Mathematical Society*, **4**, 106–10.

Asendorph, J. B. & Weinert, F. E. (1990). Stability of patterns and patterns of stability in personality development. In D. Magnuson & L. R. Bergman (eds.), *Data quality in longitudinal research*, pp. 181–197. New York: Cambridge University Press.

Bäckman, L. & Dixon, R. A. (in press). Psychological compensation: a theoretical framework. *Psychological Bulletin*.

Baltes, P. B. (1968). Longitudinal and cross-sectional sequences in the study of age and generation effects. *Human Development*, **11**, 145–71.

Baltes, P. B. (1973). Strategies for psychological intervention in old age. *Gerontologist*, **13**, 4–6.

Baltes, P. B. (1987). Theoretical propositions of life-span developmental psychology: on the dynamics between growth and decline. *Developmental Psychology*, **23**, 611–26.

Baltes, M. M. (1988). The etiology and maintenance of dependency in the elderly: three phases of operant research. *Behavior Therapy*, **19**, 301–19.

Baltes, M. M. (ed.). (1989). *Erfolgreiches Altern. Bedingungen und Variationen*. Bern: Huber.

Baltes, P. B. (1991). The many faces of human ageing: toward a psychological culture of old age. *Psychological Medicine*, **21**, 837–54.

Baltes, M. M. & Baltes, P. B. (eds.) (1986). *The psychology of control and aging*. Hillsdale: NJ: Erlbaum.

Baltes, P. B. & Baltes, M. M. (1990). Psychological perspectives on successful aging: the model of selective optimization with compensation. In P. B. Baltes and M. M. Baltes (eds.), *Successful aging: Perspectives from the behavioral sciences*, pp. 1–34. New York: Cambridge University Press.

Baltes, P. B. & Baltes, M. M. (1992). Gerontologie: Begriff, Herausforderung und Brennpunkte. In P. B. Baltes & J. Mittelstraß (eds.), *Zukunft des Alterns und gesellschaftliche Entwicklung*, pp. 1–34. (Special Report of Committee on Aging and Societal Development of the Academy of Sciences and Technology in Berlin). Berlin: de Gruyter.

Baltes, M. M. & Carstensen, L. (1991). Possible selves and their fertility in the process of successful aging: a commentary on Cross and Markus. *Human Development*, 34, 256–60.

Baltes, P. B. & Goulet, L. R. (1971). Exploration of developmental variables by manipulation and simulation of age differences in behaviour. *Human Development*, 14, 149–70.

Baltes, P. B. & Kliegl, R. (1992). Further testing of limits of cognitive plasticity: negative age differences in a mnemonic skill are robust. *Developmental Psychology*, 28, 121–5.

Baltes, P. B. & Lindenberger, U. (1988). On the range of cognitive plasticity in old age as a function of experience: 15 years of intervention research. *Behavior Therapy*, 19, 283–300.

Baltes, P. B. & Mittelstraß, J. (eds.). (1992). *Zukunft des Alterns und gesellschaftliche Entwicklung*. (Special Report of Committee on Aging and Societal Development of the Academy of Sciences and Technology in Berlin). Berlin: de Gruyter.

Baltes, P. B. & Nesselroade, J. R. (1978). Multivariate antecedents of structural change in development: a simulation of cumulative environmental patterns. *Multivariate Behavioral Research*, 13, 127–52.

Baltes, P. B. & Nesselroade, J. R. (1979). History and rationale of longitudinal research. In P. B. Baltes & J. R. Nesselroade (eds.), *Longitudinal research in the study of behavior and development*, pp. 1–29.

Baltes, P. B. & Smith, J. (1990). The psychology of wisdom and its ontogenesis. In R. J. Sternberg (ed.), *Wisdom: its nature, origins, and development*, pp. 87–120. Cambridge University Press: New York.

Baltes, M. M. & Wahl, H.-W. (1991). The behavioural system of dependency in the elderly: Interaction with the social environment. In M. Ory, R. P. Abeles, & P. D. Lipman (eds.), *Aging, health, and behavior*. Beverly Hills, CA: Sage.

Baltes, P. B. & Willis, S. L. (1982). Plasticity and enhancement of intellectual functioning in old age. In F. I. M. Craik, & E. E. Trehub (eds.), *Aging and cognitive processes*. New York: Plenum Press.

Baltes, P. B., Cornelius, S. W. & Nesselroade, J. R. (1979). Cohort effects in developmental psychology. In J. R. Nesselroade & P. B. Baltes (eds.), *Longitudinal research in the study of behavioral development*, pp. 61–87. New York: Academic Press.

Baltes, P. B., Dittmann-Kohli, F. & Dixon, R. A. (1984). New perspectives on the development of intelligence in adulthood: toward a dual-process conception and a model of selective optimization with compensation. In P. B. Baltes & O. G. Brim, Jr. (eds.), *Life-span development and behavior*, vol. 6, pp. 33–76. Academic Press: New York.

Baltes, M. M., Kühl, K.-P. & Sowarka, D. (in press). Testing the limits of cognitive reserve capacity: a promising strategy for early diagnosis of dementia?

Baltes, P. B., Reese, H. W. & Nesselroade, J. R. (1977). *Life-span developmental psychology: an introduction to research methods*. Monterey, CA: Brooks Cole (reprinted 1988 – Hillsdale, NJ: Erlbaum).

Baltes, M. M., Wahl, H. W. & Reichert, M. (1991). Successful aging in institutions? *Annual Review of Gerontology and Geriatrics*.

Bengtson, V. L., Reedy, M. N. & Gordon, C. (1985). Aging and self-conceptions:

personality processes and social contexts. In J. E. Birren & K. W. Schaie (eds.), *Handbook of the psychology of aging*, 2nd edn., pp. 544–593. New York: Van Nostrand Reinhold.

Birren, J. E. (1988). A contribution to the theory of the psychology of aging: as a counterpart of development. In J. E. Birren & V. L. Bengston (eds.), *Emergent theories of aging*, pp. 153–176. New York: Springer.

Block, J. (1981). Some enduring and consequential structures of personality. In A. I. Rabin (ed.), *Further explorations in personality*, pp. 27–43. New York: Wiley.

Blossfeld, H.-P., Hamerle, A. & Mayer, K. U. (1989). *Event history analysis: Statistical theory and application in the social sciences.* Hillsdale, NJ: Erlbaum.

Bortz, W. M. (1991). *Living short and dying long.* New York: Bantam.

Bower, G. H. (1970). Analysis of a mnemonic device. *American Scientist*, **58**, 496–510.

Brandtstädter, J. & Baltes-Götz, B. (1990). Personal control over development and quality of life perspectives in adulthood. In P. B. Baltes & M. M. Baltes (eds.), *Successful aging: perspectives from the behavioral sciences*, pp. 197–224, Cambridge University Press: New York.

Brim, G. (1988). Losing and winning. *Psychology Today*, **9**, 48–52.

Brim, G. (1992). *Ambition: How we manage success and failure throughout our lives.* New York: Basic Books.

Brim, O. G., Jr. & Kagan, J. (1980). Constancy and change: a view of the issues. In O. G. Brim, Jr. & J. Kagan (eds.), *Constancy and change in human development*, pp. 1–25. Cambridge, MA: Harvard University Press.

Brody, S. J. & Ruff, G. E. (eds.) (1986). *Aging and rehabilitation.* New York: Human Sciences Press.

Bromley, D. B. (1988). Approaching the limits. *Social Behaviour*, **3**, 71–84.

Busse, E. W. & Maddox, G. L. (eds.) (1985). *The Duke longitudinal study of normal aging 1955–1980.* New York: Springer.

Busse, E. W. & Maddox, G. L. (eds.) (1986). *The Duke longitudinal studies of normal aging in 1955–1980.* New York: Springer.

Cattell, R. B. (1971). *Abilities: their structure, growth, and action.* Houghton Mifflin: Boston.

Christensen, H., Hadzi-Pavlovic, D. & Jacomb, P. (1991). The psychometric differentiation of dementia from normal aging: a metaanalysis. *Psychological Assessment: A Journal of Consulting and Clinical Psychology*, **3**, 147–55.

Collins, L. M. & Horn, J. L. (eds.) (1991). *Best methods for the analysis of change. Recent advances, unanswered questions, future directions.* Washington, DC: American Psychological Association.

Cooney, T. M., Schaie, K. W. & Willis, S. K. (1988). The relationships between prior functioning on cognitive and personality dimensions and subject attrition in longitudinal research. *Journals of Gerontology: Psychological Sciences*, **43**, 12–17.

Coper, H., Jänicke, B. & Schulze, G. (1986). Biopsychological research on adaptivity across the life span of animals. In P. B. Baltes, D. L. Featherman, & R. M. Lerner (eds.), *Life-span development and behavior*, vol. 7, pp. 207–232. Hillsdale: NJ: Erlbaum.

Costa, P. T., Jr & Andres, R. (1986). Patterns of age changes. In I. Rossman (ed.), *Clinical Geriatrics*, pp. 23–30. Lippincott: New York.

Costa, P. T., Jr. & McCrae, R. R. (1987). Neuroticism. somatic complaints, and disease: is the bark worse than the bite? *Journal of Personality*, **55**, 299–316.

Costa, P. T. Jr. & McCrae, R. R. (1988). Personality in adulthood: a six-year longitudinal study of self-reports and spouse ratings on the NEO Personality Inventory. *Journal of*

Personality and Social Psychology, **54**, 853–63.

Costa, P. T. Jr., McCrae, R. R. & Arenberg, D. (1983). Recent longitudinal research on personality and aging. In K. W. Schaie (ed.), *Longitudinal studies of adult psychological development*, pp. 103–121. New York: Guilford.

Costa, P. T. Jr., Zonderman, A. B., McCrae, R. R., Cornoni-Huntley, J., Locke, B. Z. & Barbano, H. E. (1987). Longitudinal analyses of psychological well-being in a national sample: stability of mean-levels. *Journal of Gerontology*, **42**, 50–5.

Cowdry, E. V. (ed.). (1939). *Problems of ageing. Biological and Medical Aspects*. Williams and Wilkins: Baltimore.

Cross, S., & Markus, H. (1991). Possible selves across the life-span. *Human Development*, **34**, 230–55.

Cunningham, W. R. & Birren, J. E. (1980). Age changes in the factor structure of intellectual abilities in adulthood and old age. *Educational and Psychological Measurement*, **40**, 271–90.

Dannefer, D. (1987). The Matthew effect and the life course: aging as intracohort differentiation. *Sociological Forum*, **2**, 211–36.

Denenberg, V. H., Karas, G. G., Rosenberg, F. M. & Schell, S. F. (1968). Programming life histories: an experimental design and initial results. *Developmental Psychobiology*, **1**, 3–9.

Digman, J. M. (1989). Five robust trait dimensions: development, stability, and utility. *Journal of Personality*, **57**, 195–214.

Dinkel, R. H. (1992). Demographische Alterung: ein Überblick unter besonderer Berücksichtigung der Mortalitätsentwicklungen. In P. B. Baltes & J. Mittelstraß (Hrsg.), *Zukunft des Alterns und gesellschaftliche Entwicklung*, pp. 62–94. (Special Report of Committee on Aging and Societal Development of the Academy of Sciences and Technology in Berln). Berlin: de Gruyter.

Elder, G. H. (1986). The life course and social change. In G. H. Elder Families and lives: developments in life course studies. *Journal of Family History*.

Ericsson, K. A. (1990). Peak performance and age: an examination of peak performance in sports. In P. B. Baltes & M. M. Baltes (eds.), *Successful aging: perspectives from the behavioral sciences*, pp. 164–195. New York: Cambridge University Press.

Ericsson, K. A. & Smith, J. (1991). *Toward a general theory of expertise*. New York: Cambridge University Press.

Erlenmeyer-Kimling, L. & Miller, N. E. (eds.) (1986). *Life-span research on the prediction of psychopathology*. Hillsdale, NJ: Lawrence Erlbaum.

Evans, D. A., Funkenstein, H., Albert, M. S., Scherr, P. A., Cook, N. R., Chown, M. J., Hebert, L. E., Hennekens, C. H. & Taylor, J. O. (1989). Prevalence of Alzheimer's disease in a community population of older persons – higher than previously reported. *Journal of the American Medical Association*, **262**, 2551–6.

Featherman, D. L. (1983). The life-span perspective in social science research. In P. B. Baltes & O. G. Brim, Jr. (eds.), *Life-span development and behavior*, vol. 5, pp. 1–59. New York: Academic Press.

Featherman, D. L., Smith J. & Peterson, J. G. (1990). Successful aging in a 'post-retired' society. In P. B. Baltes & M. M. Baltes (eds.), *Successful aging: Perspectives from the behavioral sciences*, pp. 50–93. Cambridge University Press: New York.

Field, D. & Millsap, R. E. (1991). Personality in advanced old age: continuity of change? *Journal of Gerontology*, **46**, 299–308.

Filipp, S.-H. & Klauer, T. (1986). Conceptions of self over the life span: reflections on the dialectics of change. In P. B. Baltes & M. M. Baltes (eds.), *The psychology of control and aging*, pp. 167–205. Erlbaum: Hillsdale, NJ.

Fisseni, H. J. (1985). Perceived unchangeability of life and some biographical correlates. In J. M. A. Munnichs, P. Mussen, E. Olbrich, P. G. Coleman (eds.), *Life-span and change in a gerontological perspective*, pp. 103–131. New York: Academic Press.

Fooken, I. (1985). Old and female: psychosocial concomitants of the aging process in a group of older women. In J. M. A. Munnichs, P. Mussen, E. Olbrich, & P. G. Coleman (eds.), *Life-span and change in a gerontological perspective*, pp. 77–101. New York: Academic Press.

Fozard, J. L., Metter, E. J. & Bryant, L. J. (1990). Next steps in describing aging and disease in longitudinal studies. *Journal of Gerontology: Psychological Sciences*, **45**, 116–27.

Fries, J. F. (1980). Aging, natural death, and the compression of morbidity. *New England Journal of Medicine*, **303**, 130–5.

Fries, J. F. (1989). The compression of morbidity: near or far? *The Milbank Memorial Quarterly*, **67**, 208–32.

Fries, J. F. (1990). Medical perspectives upon successful aging. In P. B. Baltes & M. M. Baltes (eds.), *Successful aging: perspectives from the behavioral sciences*, pp. 35–49. New York: Cambridge University Press.

Fries, J. F., Green, L. W. & Levine, S. (1989). Health promotion and the compression of morbidity. *The Lancet*, **3**, 481–3.

Gerok, W. & Brandtstädter, J. (1992). Normales, krankhaftes und optimales Altern: Variationen und Modifikationsspielräume. In P. B. Baltes & J. Mittelstraß (Hrsg.), *Zukunft des Alterns und gesellschaftliche Entwicklung*, pp. 356–385. (Special Report of Committee on Aging and Societal Development of the Academy of Sciences and Technology in Berlin). Berlin: de Gruyter.

Gollob, H. F. & Reichardt, C. S. (1991). Interpreting and estimating indirect effects assuming time lags really matter. In L. M. Collins & J. L. Horn (eds.), *Best methods for the analysis of change. Recent advances, unanswered questions, future directions*, pp. 243–259. Washington, DC: American Psychological Association.

Gruenberg, E. M. (1986). Discussion: two views of time. In L. Erlenmeyer-Kimling & N. E. Miller (eds.), *Life-span research on the prediction of psychopathology*, pp. 287–293. Hillsdale, NJ: Lawrence Erlbaum.

Häfner, J. (1986). *Psychologische Gesundheit im Alter*. Stuttgart: Fischer.

Häfner, J., Moschel, G. & Sartorius, N. (eds.) (1986). *Mental health in the elderly*. New York: Springer.

Harris, L. (1975). *The myth and reality of aging in America*. Washington, DC: National Council on the Aging.

Heckhausen, J. & Krüger, J. (1991). *Developmental expectations for the self and most other people: age-grading in three functions of social comparison*. Manuscript under review. Max Planck Institute for Human Development and Education, Berlin, FRG.

Heckhausen, J., Dixon, R. A. & Baltes, P. B. (1989). Gains and losses in development throughout adulthood as perceived by different adult age groups. *Developmental Psychology*, **25**, 109–21.

Hertzog, C. & Schaie, K. W. (1986). Stability and change in adult intelligence: 1. Analysis of longitudinal covariance structures. *Psychology and Aging*, **1**, 159–71.

Hertzog, C. & Schaie, K. W. (1988). Stability and change in adult intelligence: 2. Simultaneous analysis of longitudinal means and covariance structures. *Psychology and Aging*, **3**, 122–30.

Holland, C. A. & Rabbitt, P. (1991). Social and psychological gerontology: The course and causes of cognitive change with advancing age. *Reviews in Clinical Gerontology*, 1, 81–96.

Horn, J. L. (1982). The theory of fluid and crystallized intelligence in relation to concepts of cognitive psychology and aging in adulthood. In F. I. M. Craik & S. E. Trehub (eds.), *Aging and cognitive processes*, pp. 847–870. New York: Plenum Press.

House, J. S., Kessler, R. C., Herzog, A. R., Mero, R. P., Kinney, A. M. & Breslow, M. J. (1990). Age, socioeconomic status, and health. *The Milbank Quarterly*, 68, 383–411.

Hoyer, W. J. (1985). Aging and the development of expert cognition. In T. M. Schlechter & M. P. Toglia (eds.), *New directions in cognitive science*, pp. 69–87. Norwood, NJ: Ablex.

Hoyer, W. J., & Hannon, D. J. (in press). Individual differences in visual-cognitive aging: toward a formal model. In D. Detterman (ed.), *Current topics in human intelligence*.

Jaspers, K. (1965). *Philosophie*. Heidelberg: Springer.

Jones, K. (1991). The application of time series methods to moderate span longitudinal data. In L. M. Collins & J. L. Horn (eds.), *Best methods for the analysis of change. Recent advances, unanswered questions, future directions*, pp. 75–87. Washington, DC: American Psychological Association.

Jones, C. J. & Nesselroade, J. R. (1990). Multivariate, replicated, single-subject, repeated measures designs and P-technique factor analysis: a review of intraindividual change studies. *Experimental Aging Research*, 16, 171–83.

Kastenbaum, R. (1985). Dying and death: a life-span approach. In J. E. Birren & K. W. Schaie (eds.), *Handbook of psychology and aging*, pp. 619–646. New York: Van Nostrand Reinhold.

Khatchaturian, Z. S. (1985). Progress of research on Alzheimer's disease. Research opportunities for behavioral scientists. *American Psychology*, 40, 1251–5.

Kleemeier, R. W. (1962). Intellectual change in the senium. *Proceedings of the Social Statistics Section of the American Statistical Association*, 290–5.

Kliegl, R. (1992). *Gedächtnis für Gedankenbilder: Altersunterschiede in Entwicklungskapazität und kognitiven Mechanismen*. Max-Planck-Institut für Bildungsforschung, Berlin, FRG.

Kliegl, R. & Baltes, P. B. (1987a). Das Janusgesicht des Alters: Über Washstum und Abbau in Intelligenz und Gedächtnis. In E. H. Graul, S. Pütter & D. Lowe (eds.), *Medicenale XVII*, pp. 1–22. Iserlohn: Medice.

Kliegl, R. & Baltes, P. B. (1987b). Theory-guilded analysis of development and aging mechanisms through testing-the-limits and research on expertise. In C. Schooler & K. W. Schaie (eds.), *Cognitive Functioning and Social Structure over the Life Course*, pp. 95–119. Norwood, NJ: Ablex.

Kliegl, R. & Lindenberger, U. (1988). *Age-related susceptibility to intrusion errors in cued recall.* Paper presented at the Second Cognitive Aging Conference, Atlanta, USA.

Kliegl, R., Smith, J. & Baltes, P. B. (1989). Testing-the-limits and the study of adult age differences in cognitive plasticity of a mnemonic skill. *Developmental Psychology*, 25, 247–56.

Krämer, W. (1992). Altern und Gesundheitswesen: Probleme und Lösungen aus der Sicht der Gesundheitsökonomie. In P. B. Baltes & J. Mittelstraß (eds.), *Zukunft des Alterns und gesellschaftliche Entwicklung*, pp. 563–580. (Special Report of Committee on Aging and Societal Development of the Academy of Sciences and Technology in Berlin.) Berlin: de Gruyter.

Kruse, A. (1987). Competence in old age: Coping with chronic disease, dying, and death.

Comprehensive Gerontology, **C1**, 1–11.

Kruse, A. (1990). Potential im Alter. *Zeitschrift für Gerontologie*, **23**, 205–15.

Kruse, A. (1991). Caregivers coping with chronic disease, dying and death of an aged family member. *Reviews in Clinical Gerontology*, **1**, 411–15.

Kruse, A. (1992). *Kompetenz im Alter in ihren Bezügen zur objektiven und subjektiven Lebenssituation.* Darmstadt: Steinkopff.

Kruse, A. & Kruse, W. (1990). Ambulante Rehabilitation älterer Patienten. *Zeitschrift für Allgemeinmedizin*, **26**, 677–86.

Labouvie, E. W. (1980). The measurement of individual differences in intraindividual changes. *Psychological Bulletin*, **88**, 54–9.

Labouvie, E. W. (1986). Methodological issues in the prediction of psychopathology: A life-span perspective. In L. Erlenmeyer-Kimling & N. E. Miller (eds.), *Life-span research on the prediction of psychopathology*, pp. 137–156. Hillsdale, NJ: Lawrence Erlbaum.

Labouvie-Vief, G. (1977). Adult cognitive development: in search of alternative interpretations. *Merrill-Palmer Quarterly*, **23**, 227–63.

Lachman, M. E. (1986). Personal control in later life: stability, change, and cognitive correlates. In M. M. Baltes & P. B. Baltes (eds.), *The Psychology of Control and Aging*, pp. 207–236. Erlbaum: Hillsdale, NJ.

Lachman, M. E., Weaver, S. L., Bandura, M., Elliott, E. & Lewkowicz, C. J. (in press). Improving memory and control beliefs through cognitive restructuring and self-generated strategies. *Journal of Gerontology: Psychological Sciences*.

LaRue, A. & Jarvik, L. F. (1987). Cognitive function and prediction of dementia in old age. *International Journal of Aging and Human Development*, **25**, 79–89.

Lawley, D. N. (1943–44). A note on Karl Pearson's selection formulae. *Proceedings of the Royal Society of Edinburgh*, **62**, 28–30.

Lawton, N. P. (1989). Environmental proactivity in older people. In V. L. Bengtson & K. W. Schaie (eds.), *The course of later life*, pp. 15–24. New York: Springer.

Lazarus, R. S. & Folkman, S. (1984). *Stress, appraisal, and coping.* New York: Springer.

Lehr, U. (1980). Die Bedeutung der Lebenslaufpsychologie für die Gerontologie. *Aktuelle Gerontologie*, **10**, 257–69.

Lehr, U. (1982). Social-psychological correlates of longevity. In C. Eisdorfer (ed.), *Annual Review of Gerontology & Geriatrics*, vol. 3, pp. 102–147. New York: Springer.

Lehr, U. (1991). *Psychologie des Alterns.* Heidelberg: Quelle & Meyer.

Lehr, U. & Thomae, J. (eds.) (1987). *Formen seelischen Alterns.* (Patterns of psychological aging). Stuttgart: Enke.

Lerner, R. M. (1978). Nature, nurture, and dynamic interactionism. *Human Development*, **21**, 1–20.

Lerner, R. M. (1984). *On the nature of human plasticity.* New York: Cambridge University Press.

Lindenberger, U. (1991). *Aging, professional expertise, and cognitive plasticity.* Stuttgart: Klett–Cotta.

Lindenberger, U., Kliegl, R. & Baltes, P. B. (in press). Professional expertise does not eliminate negative age differences in imagery-based memory performance during adulthood. *Psychology and Aging*.

Maas, H. & Kuypers, J. (1974). *From thirty to seventy: a forty-year longitudinal study of adult life styles and personality.* San Francisco: Jossey-Bass.

McArdle, J. J. & Hamagami, F. (1991). Modeling incomplete longitudinal and cross-sectional data using latent growth structural models. In L. M. Collins & J. L. Horn (eds.), *Best methods for the analysis of change. Recent advances, unanswered questions, future directions*, pp. 276–298. Washington, DC: American Psychological Association.

McArdle, J. J., Hamagami, F., Elias, M. F. & Robbins, M. A. (1991). Structural modeling of mixed longitudinal and cross-sectional data.

McClelland, J. L. (1989). Parallel distributed processing: Implications for cognition and development. In R. G. M. Morris (ed.), *Parallel distributed processing: implications for psychology and neurobiology*, pp. 8–45. Oxford: Clarendon Press.

Maciel, A. G., Heckhausen, J. & Baltes, P. B. (1992). A life-span perspective on the interface between personality and intelligence. In R. J. Sternberg & P. Ruzgis (eds.), *Intelligence and Personality*. New York: Cambridge University Press.

Maddox, G. L. (1987). Aging differently. *Gerontologist*, 27, 557–64.

Magnusson, D. (1988). *Individual development from an interactional perspective: A longitudinal study*. Hillsdale, NJ: Lawrence Erlbaum.

Magnusson, D. (1990). Personality research – challenges for the future. *European Journal of Personality*, 4, 1–18.

Magnusson, D. & Bergman, L. R. (1990). *Data quality in longitudinal research*. New York: Cambridge University Press.

Magnusson, D. & Endler, N. S. (1977). Present status and future aspects. In D. Magnusson & N. S. Endler (eds.), *Personality at the crossroads; Current issues in interactional psychology*, pp. 1–17. Hillsdale, NJ: Lawrence Erlbaum.

Manton, K. G. & Woodbury, M. A. (1983). A mathematical model of the physiological dynamics of aging and correlated mortality selection: II. application to Duke Longitudinal Study. *Journal of Gerontology*, 38, 406–13.

Masoro, E. J. (1991). Kleemeier Award Lecture. *44th Annual Scientific Meeting of the Gerontological Society of America* 1991.

Mayer, K. U. (1990). Lebensverläufe und sozialer Wande. *Kölner Zeitschrift für Soziologie und Sozialpsychologie, Sonderheft*, 31, 7–21.

Miller, N. E. (1986). The prediction of psychopathology across the life span: The value of longitudinal research. In L. Erlenmeyer-Kimling & N. E. Miller (eds.), *Life-span research on the prediction of psychopathology*, pp. 1–15. Hillsdale, NJ: Lawrence Erlbaum.

Munnichs, J. M. A. (1966). *Old age and finitude*. Basel: Karger.

Munnichs, J. M. A., Mussen, P., Olbrich, E., & Coleman, P. G. (eds.) (1985). *Life-span and change in a gerontological perspective*. New York: Academic Press.

Mussen, P. (1985). Early adult antecedents of life satisfaction at age 70. In J. M. A. Munnichs, P. Mussen, E. Olbrich & P. G. Coleman (eds.), *Life-span and change in a gerontological perspective*, pp. 45–61. New York: Academic Press.

Muthén, B. O. (1991). Analysis of longitudinal data using latent variable models with varying parameters. In L. M. Collins & J. L. Horn (eds.), *Best methods for the analysis of change. Recent advances, unanswered questions, future directions*, pp. 1–24. Washington, DC: American Psychological Association.

Nesselroade, J. R. (1990). Adult personality development: Issues in addressing constance and change. In A. E. Rabe, R. A. Zucker, R. A. Emmons & S. Frank (eds.), *Studying Persons and Lives*, pp. 41–85. New York: Springer.

Nesselroade, J. R. (1991). Interindividual differences in intraindividual change. In L. M. Collins & J. L. Horn (eds.), *Best methods for the analysis of change. Recent advances, unanswered questions, future directions*, pp. 92–105. Washington, DC: American Psychological Association.

Nesselroade, J. R. & Reese, H. W. (1973). *Life-span developmental psychology: methodological issues.* New York: Academic Press.

Nilsson, L.-G., Bäckman, L. & Karlsson, T. (1989). Priming and cued recall in elderly, alcohol intoxicated, and sleep deprived subjects: a case of functionally similar memory deficits. *Psychological Medicine,* 19, 423–33.

Olbrich, E. (1985). Coping and development in the later years. In J. M. A. Munnichs, P. Mussen, E. Olbrich & P. G. Coleman (eds.), *Life-span and change in a gerontological perspective,* pp. 133–155. New York: Academic Press.

Palmore, E., Busse, E. W., Maddox, G. L., Nowlin, J. B. & Siegler, I. C. (1985). *Normal aging III.* Durham, NC: Duke University Press.

Pervin, L. A. (1985). Personality: Current controversies, issues, and direction. *Annual Review of Psychology,* 36, 85–114.

Platt, D. (1988). *Experimental gerontology.* New York: Springer.

Powell, D. A., Furchtgott, E., Henderson, M., Prescott, L., Mitchell, A., Hartis, P., Valentine, J. D. & Milligan, W. L. (1990). Some determinants of attrition in prospective studies on aging. *Experimental Aging Research,* 16, 17–24.

Putz, F. & Schwarz, K. (eds.) (1984). *Neuere Aspekte·der Sterblichkeitsentwicklung.* Wiesbaden.

Riegel, K. F. & Riegel, R. M. (1972). Development, drop, and death. *Developmental Psychology,* 6, 306–19.

Rovine, M. J. & Delaney, M. (1990). Missing data estimation in developmental research. In A. von Eye (ed.), *Statistical Methods in Longitudinal Research,* 1, pp. 35–79. New York: Academic Press.

Rowe, J. W. & Kahn, R. L. (1987). Human aging: usual and successful. *Science,* 237, 143–9.

Rubin, D. B. (1991). Comments on chapters 16 and 17. In L. M. Collins & J. L. Horn (eds.), *Best methods for the analysis of change. Recent advances, unanswered questions, future directions,* pp. 305–309. Washington, DC: American Psychological Association.

Rudinger, G. & Wood, P. K. (1990). N's, times and number of variables in longitudinal research. In D. Magnusson & L. R. Bergman (eds.), *Data Quality in Longitudinal Research,* pp. 157–180. New York: Cambridge University Press.

Rutter, M. (ed.) (1988a). *Studies of psychosocial risk: the power of longitudinal data.* New York: Cambridge University Press.

Rutter, M. (1988b). *Longitudinal data in the study of causal processes: some uses and some pitfalls.* In M. Rutter (ed.), *Studies of psychosocial risk: The power of longitudinal data,* pp. 1–28. New York: Cambridge University Press.

Ryff, C. & Baltes, P. B. (1976). Value transition and adult development in women: the instrumentality-terminality sequence hypothesis. *Developmental Psychology,* 12, 567–8.

Salthouse, T. A. (1991). *Theoretical perspectives on cognitive aging.* Hillsdale, NJ: Erlbaum.

Schaie, K. W. (1965). A general model for the study of developmental problems. *Psychological Bulletin,* 64, 92–107.

Schaie, K. W. (1979). The primary mental abilities in adulthood: an exploration in the development of psychometric intelligence. In P. B. Baltes & O. G. Brim, Jr. (eds.), *Life-span development and behavior,* (vol. 3, pp. 67–115). New York: Academic Press.

Schaie, K. W. (1983). The Seattle Longitudinal Study: a 21-year exploration of psychometric intelligence in adulthood. In K. W. Schaie (ed.), *Longitudinal studies of adult psychological development,* pp. 64–135. New York: Guilford.

Schaie, K. W. (1988). Variability in cognitive function in the elderly: Implications for societal participation. In A. D. Woodhead, M. A. Bender & R. C. Leonard (eds.), *Phenotypic Variation in Populations*, pp. 191–211. New York: Plenum Press.

Schaie, K. W. (1989a). The hazards of cognitive aging. *Gerontologist*, **29**, 484–93.

Schaie, K. W. (1989b). Individual differences in rate of cognitive change in adulthood. In V. L. Bengtson & K. W. Schaie (eds.), *The course of later life*, pp. 65–85. New York: Springer.

Schaie, K. W. (1990a). Late life potential and cohort differences in mental abilities. In M. Perlmutter (ed.), *Late life potential*. Washington, DC: Gerontological Society of America. New York: Cambridge University Press.

Schaie, K. W. (1990b). The optimization of cognitive functioning in old age: Predictions based on cohort-sequential and longitudinal data. In P. B. Baltes & M. M. Baltes (eds.), *Successful Aging: Perspectives from the behavioral sciences*, pp. 94–116. New York: Cambridge University Press.

Schaie, K. W., Dutta, R. & Willis, S. L. (1991). Relationship between rigidity-flexibility and cognitive abilities in adulthood. *Psychology and Aging*, **6**, 371–83.

Schaie, K. W. et al. (in press). The role of genetics in adult intellectual development [Tentative title]. *Nebraska Symposium on Motivation*, **39**.

Schaie, K. W. & Willis, S. L. (1986). Can adult intellectual decline be reversed? *Developmental Psychology*, **22**, 223–32.

Schmitz-Scherzer, R. & Thomae, H. (1983). Constancy and change of behavior in old age: findings from the Bonn Longitudinal Study on Aging. In K. W. Schaie (ed.), *Longitudinal studies of adult psychological development*, pp. 191–221. New York: Guilford.

Schneider, E. L. & Brody, J. A. (1983). Aging, natural death, and the compression of morbidity: another view. *New England Journal of Medicine*, **309**, 854–6.

Schneider, E. L. & Guralnik, J. M. (1990). The aging of America: impact on health costs. *Journal of the American Medical Association*, **263**, 2335–40.

Schulz, R., Heckhausen, J. & Locher, J. L. (1991). Adult development, control, and adaptive functioning. *Journal of Social Issues*, **47**, 177–96.

Shanan, J. (1991). Who and how: Some unanswered questions in adult development. *Journal of Gerontology*, **46**, 309–16.

Shock, N. W. (1977). System integration. In C. E. Finch and L. Hayflick (eds.), *Handbook of the biology of aging*, pp. 639–665. New York: Van Nostrand Reinhold.

Siegler, I. C. & Botwinick, J. (1979). A long term longitudinal study of intellectual ability of older adults: the matter of selective subject attrition. *Journal of Gerontology*, **34**, 242–5.

Siegler, R. S. (1988). Strategy choice and the development of multiplication skill. *Journal of Experimental Psychology: General*, **117**, 258–75.

Siegler, R. S. & Crowley, K. (1991). The microgenetic method. *American Psychologist*, **46**, 606–20.

Sjostrom, K. P. & Pollack, R. H. (1971). The effect of simulated receptor aging on two types of visual illusions. *Psychonomic Science*, **23**, 147–8.

Sørensen, A. B., Weinert, F. E. & Sherrod, L. (eds.) (1986). *Human development and the life course: multidisciplinary perspectives*. Hillsdale, NJ: Erlbaum.

Spiro, A., Aldwin, C. M., Levenson, M. R. & Bosse, R. (1990). Longitudinal findings from the Normative Aging Study: II. Do emotionality and extraversion predict symptom change? *Journal of Gerontology*, **45**, 136–44.

Svanborg, A. (1985). Biomedical and environmental influences on aging. In R. N. Butler & H. P. Gleason (eds.), *Productive aging: enhancing vitality in later life*, pp. 31–52. New York: Springer.

Taylor, S. E. & Brown, J. D. (1988). Illusion and well-being: a social psychological perspective on mental health. *Psychological Bulletin*, **103**, 193–210.

Thomae, H. (1968). *Das Individuum und seine Welt: eine Persönlichekeitstheorie*. Göttingen: Hogrefe.

Thomae, H. (1976). *Patterns of aging: findings from the Bonn Longitudinal Study of Aging: contributions to human development*, **3**. Basel: Karger.

Thomae, H. (1979). The concept of development and life-span development psychology. In P. B. Baltes & O. G. Brim (eds.), *Life-span Development and Behavior*, **2**, New York: Academic Press.

Thomae, H. (1981). Expected unchangeability of life stress in old age: a contribution to a cognitive theory of aging. *Human Development*, **24**, 229–39.

Thomae, H. (1983). *Alternsstile und Alternsschicksale*. Bern: Huber.

Thomae, H. (1988). *Das Individuum and seine Welt: eine persönlichkeits Theorie*. Göttingen: Hogrefe.

Thurstone, L. L. & Thurstone, T. G. (1949). *Examiners manual, SRA Primary Mental Abilities* (Form 11.17). Chicago: Science Research Associates.

Verbrugge, L. (1984). Longer life but worsening health? Trends in health and mortality of middle-aged and older persons. *The Milbank Quarterly*, **62**, 475–519.

Wahl (in press). Forschung über Altersheime [Tentative title]. *Psychologische Rundschau*.

Werner, H. (1948). *Comparative psychology of mental development*. New York: International Universities Press.

Williams, T. F. (ed.) (1985). *Rehabilitation in the Aging*. New York: Raven Press.

Willis, S. L. (1987). Cognitive training and everyday competence. In K. W. Schaie (ed.), *Annual Review of Gerontology and Geriatrics*, **7**, pp. 159–188. New York: Springer.

Willis, S. L. (1991). Age/cohort differences in cognitive training. *Paper presented at the 44th Annual Meeting of the Gerontological Society of America* (GSA), November 22–26, San Francisco.

Wohlwill, J. F. (1970). The age variable in psychological research. *Psychological Review*, **77**, 49–64.

Woodruff, D. & Birren, J. E. (1972). Age changes and cohort differences in personality. *Developmental Psychology*, **6**, 252–9.

Wortman, C. B. & Silver, R. C. (1990). Successful mastery of bereavement and widowhood: a life-course perspective. In P. B. Baltes & M. M. Baltes (eds.), *Successful aging: perspectives from the behavioral sciences*, **8**, pp. 225–264. New York: Cambridge University Press.

Yesavage, J. A. & Rose, T. L. (1984). Semantic elaboration and the method of loci: a new trip for older learners. *Experimental Aging Research*, **10**, 155–9.

9   Development, aging, and control: empirical and theoretical issues

JOCHEN BRANDTSTÄDTER

During the last two or three decades, growing resources have been invested in large-scale research projects on adult development and aging (for overviews, see Deeg, 1989; Migdal, Abeles & Sherrod, 1981; Schaie, 1983; Thomae, 1987). This research has documented the broad range and variability of developmental patterns in middle and later adulthood, but it still gives only a fragmentary picture of the underlying dynamics of developmental change in middle and later adulthood. Recent claims emphasizing modifyability, contextual specifity, lack of connectivity and discontinuity of development (cf. Gergen, 1980; Brim & Kagan, 1980) may be seen not only as propositions about the fundamental nature of development but also as symptoms of theoretical perplexity. It is true that simplistic notions of stability and ordered change in adult development are largely discredited by the bulk of evidence. Nevertheless, we should be aware that difficulties in finding order and coherence may result from theoretical deficiencies rather than reflect a fundamental feature of development itself.

Related to these points, it has to be noted that, even with the most refined longitudinal or sequential designs we do not capture developmental laws, but, at best, regularities in need of theoretical explanation. Developmental researchers should not be content with simply documenting patterns of continuity and change, but inquire more deeply into the regulative processes and generative mechanisms on historical, social, personal as well as physical or biological levels that bring about, maintain, or forestall continuity and change across the life span (cf. Baltes, 1987; Dannefer & Perlmutter, 1990).

In the following, I will focus more closely on a theoretical perspective which in my view holds much promise for future research on adult development and aging. I am referring to a theoretical point of view which conceives of development as a personal and social construction, as a process which is actively controlled and shaped within personal and social contexts of action. In fact, many regularities of development critically depend on actions or interventions. As an example, losses in intellectual and physical functioning are often seen as inevitable implications of the aging process, but it is obvious that this presumably normal or necessary developmental sequence critically depends on our potentials for corrective and preventive intervention, which are, in principle, open to change. This type of argument can be extended to many areas of development and aging. Neither the social nor even the biological constraints of development over the life-span are to be considered a priori as fixed or unalterable. Rather, forms and patterns of development and aging that emerge in a given cultural and historical context largely depend on the resources of control that are available on social and personal levels, as well as on prevailing normative constructions of successful development and aging. Even the genetic regulation and canalization of development cannot be adequately understood without considering the selective and constructive activities by which individuals shape their developmental niche (cf. Lewontin, 1982; Scarr & McCartney, 1983; see also Scarr, this volume).

To prevent possible misunderstandings: I do not want to propose an action perspective on human development as a new paradigmatic stance. First, this perspective is not entirely novel: elements of an action perspective are already present in the seminal contributions of Charlotte Bühler (1933), and can be found even much earlier in the philosophical writings of Johann Nikolaus Tetens (1777) concerning the 'perfectibility' of human development (for more detailed historical considerations, see also Höhn, 1958; Brandtstädter, 1990). Secondly, I feel no need to add a further item to the menagerie of (organismic, humanistic, dialectical, contextualistic, transactional, aleatoric, etc.) 'paradigms' that have been promulgated, sometimes with programmatic fervour, as guiding schemes of developmental research. In my view, any comprehensive analysis of development and aging encompasses different explanatory stances: (a) a personal or intentional stance which focuses on development-related cognitions, values and actions, and which focuses on the self-reflective processes that regulate and maintain development over the life-span; (b) a sub-personal stance, which focuses on the physical, physiological and biological aspects of development and aging; and (c) a transpersonal stance, centring on social and cultural constraints of development that cannot simply be subsumed under personal-intentional or physical schemes of explanation. These explanatory stances are neither exchangeable nor reducible to each other; each generates its own questions and problem solutions (cf. Brandtstädter, 1990). From this point of view, attempts to oppose these different stances or to proclaim one of them as the only useful or legitimate 'paradigm' for research on development and aging, seem bootless. The merits of a given paradigm or explanatory stance should be judged not on an a priori base, but with regard to the yield of research programmes and theories that are generated within a specific paradigmatic framework.

In the following, I shall try to illustrate my claims concerning the heuristic value of an action perspective on development and aging by some selected research examples. I shall first elaborate on the concept of development-related action. I will then give a brief description of our own research and discuss some selected findings, paying special attention to issues of perceived control over personal development and implications for optimal development and successful aging. Finally, I will address some methodological implications and challenges for future research.

PERSONAL CONTROL OVER DEVELOPMENT: SOME PRELIMINARY EXPLICATIONS

From an action perspective on development, the adult person is not simply seen as the passive subject of age-related change, but as an active, purposeful agent who shapes and tries to optimize his or her own developmental prospects (cf. Brandtstädter, 1986, 1990; Lerner & Busch-Rossnagel, 1981; Magnusson, 1990). Correspondingly, development over the life-span is conceived as a sequence of changes which from a personal point of view involves gains and losses in different domains of functioning (cf. Baltes, 1987; Heckhausen, Dixon & Baltes, 1989), and which continually induces, and is in turn modified by, personal efforts to keep this balance positive (which may be more or less successful). Fig. 9.1 portrays some basic features of this process.

The basic propositions sketched in Fig. 9.1 may be summarized as follows. It is assumed that the adult individual continuously constructs cognitive representations of his or her past and future development over the life-span. These cognitive representations are knowledge based, i.e. they are mediated by general and self-referential beliefs about development over the life-span (which may, of course, be influenced to a greater or lesser degree by prevailing stereotyped beliefs about development and aging). The cognitive representations form the basis for the individual's evaluation of personal developmental prospects, which at the same time depends on the developmental goals, aspirations, and identity projects the individual is committed to. The evaluative appraisal of developmental prospects comprises a wide range of emotional reactions. Individuals may look back on their personal development with pride, satisfaction, gratitude, but also with shame, anger, or disgust; considering future developmental prospects, they may feel hopeful, calm, confident, but also uneasy, discouraged, or worried. Generally, such emotional evaluations are linked with, or give rise to, specific action tendencies. Most important, negative evaluations of personal developmental prospects, such as the expectation of developmental losses in later phases of life, should induce corrective or preventive actions that aim at altering the anticipated course of development. At this stage, generalized or specific control beliefs related to personal development become important as moderating variables. Thus, self-corrective tendencies should be less expressed when the person harbours self-beliefs of low efficacy with regard to personal development or considers developmental changes as largely preordained (see also Bandura, 1989).

The central tenet of an action perspective on development, then, is that adult development and aging cannot be adequately understood without regard to the self-reflective and self-regulative loops that link developmental changes to the individual's construction of personal development over the life span, which is also open to change. This should not be read to imply that individuals are the sole or omnipotent producers of their development. Such an assumption would give a seriously biased portrayal of human development. Like any other human

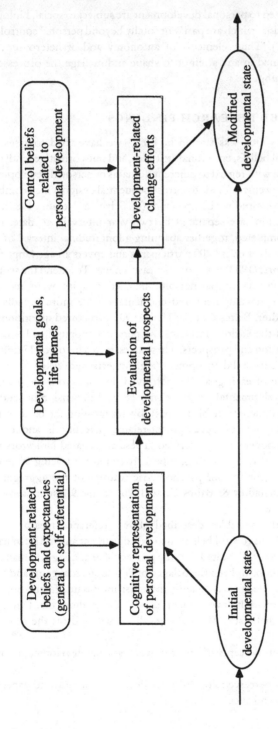

Fig. 9.1. Development-related action: cognitive, evaluative and executive processes.

activity, actions related to personal development are subject to social, biological and physical constraints which are partly or totally beyond personal control (see Brandtstädter, 1990). Thus, elements of autonomy and of heteronomy are inseparably intertwined in any attempt to shape and manage the processes of development and aging.

SELECTED RESEARCH FINDINGS

In a larger project which was started in 1983,[1] we have tried to assess the expectations, control beliefs, emotional attitudes, and self-corrective tendencies that individuals have with regard to different domains of personal development. The sampling strategy corresponds to a cross-sequential design which combines cross-sectional and longitudinal comparisons (cf. Schaie & Herzog, 1982). The longitudinal replications are separated by two-year intervals; to date, three waves have been completed, together spanning a longitudinal interval of four years. Our panel involves over 1200 participants and covers an age range from 30 to 60 years at the first (1983) occasion of measurement. To extend the scope of investigation to contexts of partnership, married couples were recruited (aspects of marital codevelopment and coorientation are more broadly discussed in Brandtstädter, Baltes-Götz & Heil, 1990). Structured questionnaires were used to assess the various facets of the person's appraisal of his or her developmental situation and prospects. These assessments involved 17 different goal dimensions of personal development (e.g. subjects were asked to rate the personal importance of each goal, the perceived distance from the goal, the extent to which developmental progress on each goal dimension depends on personal effort or on uncontrollable factors). By aggregating the basic ratings, various global indicators of development-related perceptions and control beliefs and action tendencies were derived. These aggregated indicators were found to be highly reliable and, thus, especially suited for tracing systematic longitudinal change (for further psychometric features of the aggregational variables, see Brandtstädter & Baltes-Götz, 1990). Table 9.1 summarizes the assessment procedure.

In addition to the variables described above, reference measures were included for generalized control beliefs, marital adjustment and life satisfaction.

As Brim (1989) recently pointed out, the process of arranging and managing our lives and life designs to keep the balance of developmental gains and losses favourable over the life-span is 'one of the most important, fascinating, and overlooked aspects of adult development (p. 50)'. The findings that I am going to discuss bear on that issue. More specifically, I will address the following questions:

1 How do self-percepts of control over personal development change with age?
2 How does perceived control over development relate to aspects of well-being and successful aging?

Table 9.1. *Assessment of development-related attitudes and beliefs: developmental goals, basic ratings, and aggregated indicators of personal development*

Developmental goals	Goal-related ratings	Aggregated indicators
Health, physical well-being	(for each goal g):	Subjective developmental deficit $\left(\sum_{g} d_g\, pi_g\right)$
Emotional stability		
Wisdom, mature understanding of life	importance of g (pi_g)	
Self-esteem	perceived distance from g (d_g)	Autonomous control over development $\left(\sum_{g} ar_g\, pi_g\right)$
Social recognition	extent to which attainment of g depends on own behaviour (ar_g)	
Occupational efficiency		Heteronomous control over development $\left(\sum_{g} br_g\, pi_g\right)$
Assertiveness, self-assurance	extent to which attainment of g depends on conditions beyond personal control (br_g)	
Harmonious partnership		Subjective developmental reserve $\left(\sum_{g} dr_g\, pi_g\right)$
Empathy	subjective reserve potential for attainment of g (dr_g)	
Personal independence		Anticipated developmental gain $\left(\sum_{g} er_g\, pi_g\right)$
Family security	expected change toward or away from g (er_g)	
Prosperity, comfortable standard of living		Perceived marital support $\left(\sum_{g} sp_g\, pi_g\right)$
Intellectual efficiency	extent to which attainment of g is seen as supported by the spouse (sp_g)	
Self-development		
Physical fitness		
Satisfying friendship		
Commitment to ideals		

3 How does the subjective balance of developmental gains and losses change with age, and what strategies are used to keep this balance positive?

I will not attempt to give ultimate answers to these questions, but rather, my objective is to pinpoint some important concerns for future research. Nevertheless, the cross-sequential findings that we have gathered so far in many respects challenge some widespread and entrenched beliefs about adult development and aging. Above all, they put into question a common stereotype according to which the later phases of life are generally characterized by growing despondency, depression and dissatisfaction. The general picture that emerges from our findings rather points to a considerable resilience of the aging person to the adversities and losses related to the aging process, a resilience that is perhaps primarily due to a self-protective adjustment of goals and developmental options, rather than on the use of self-deceptive defences.

Development-related control beliefs

According to widespread opinion, the aging person experiences a general decline in perceived control over his or her life and personal development (e.g. Seligman, 1975). The assumption of age-related deficits in perceived control also seems to be shared by many theorists in the field of development and aging (see Rodin, Timko & Harris, 1985). Accumulated evidence from cross-sectional and longitudinal investigations, however, is inconclusive with respect to the question of how control beliefs change with age (for reviews, see Krampen, 1987; Lachman, 1986; Rodin, 1986). This inconsistency may stem partly from the fact that many studies in this field have adopted a unidimensional–bipolar (internal vs. external) concept of perceived control. Our findings do not easily fit with such a simple conception.

As shown in Table 9.1 above, two indicators of perceived control over development were considered in our study. Participants had to rate their self-percepts of control with respect to 17 different goal dimensions; by aggregating over goals, a global indicator of autonomous control over development (CDA) was formed. Furthermore, participants rated the impact of uncontrollable factors on personal development with respect to each goal dimension. Aggregation of these ratings yielded a global indicator of heteronomous control over development (CDH).[2] These indicators have some variance in common with traditional measures of generalized control beliefs; the relationships are moderate, but significant and conceptually consistent (for details, see Brandtstädter & Baltes-Götz, 1990). Individual differences in autonomous control are impressively stable; over a four-year longitudinal interval, the autocorrelation is .52. In comparison, inter-individual differences in heteronomous control seem to fluctuate more strongly; the four-year stability for this indicator is .37.

Regarding the cross-sequential patterns, let us first consider the findings for

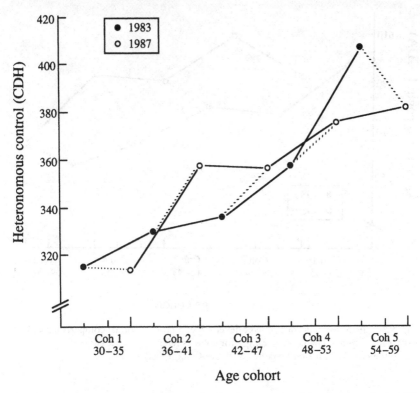

Fig. 9.2. Heteronomous control over development: cross-sectional comparisons and 4-year longitudinal change (age ranges for cohorts refer to first occasion of measurement). (From Brandtstädter & Baltes-Götz, 1990.)

heteronomous control over development. Fig. 9.2 gives the cross-sectional gradients for the 1983 and 1987 occasions, as well as the longitudinal changes within the four-year interval (indicated by hatched lines).

Both the longitudinal and the cross-sectional findings indicate that in middle and later adulthood – at least up to the early 60s – personal development is increasingly seen as affected by influences outside personal control. The cross-sectional as well as the longitudinal effects are highly significant (there were no interactions with gender). The age-related increase in heteronomous control most probably reflects the cumulation of uncontrollable events and losses in the later phases of life (cf. also Folkman et al., 1987). These findings so far seem to be in good agreement with allegations of an age-related loss in perceived control.

The results for the index variable of autonomous control over development, however, introduce another twist. Cross-sectional effects for this indicator fall short of significance, and longitudinal comparisons even indicate a significant increase in self-attributed influence on personal developmental prospects (Fig.

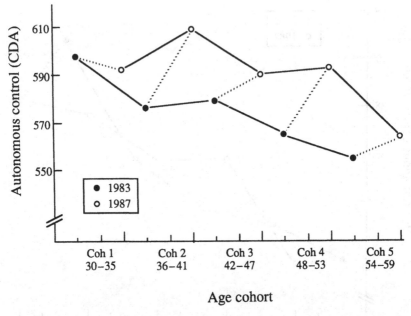

Fig. 9.3.   Autonomous control over development: cross-sectional comparisons and 4-year longitudinal change (age ranges for cohorts refer to first occasion of measurement). (From Brandtstädter & Baltes-Götz, 1990.)

9.3). In interpreting these data, one should note that age-related longitudinal changes may be partly confounded with effects related to repeated testing. In the overall picture, however, our findings do not support the assumption of a general age-related loss in perceived control over personal development.

As one may extrapolate from these findings, the indicators of autonomous control and of heteronomous control should not be considered as opposite poles of an underlying one-dimensional construct. Statistically, these indicators constitute nearly orthogonal features of perceived control. Thus, one cannot exclude that individuals who see their development as strongly influenced by factors outside personal control may nevertheless feel that they can play an active role in optimizing their development and aging. Such a pattern of beliefs hardly fits a unidimensional (internal vs. external) conception of control, but it is not self-contradictory. Our findings indicate that with advancing age, the dependence of development on controllable factors as well as on aleatoric influences beyond control is increasingly recognized. Presumably, the experience of a growing vulnerability of life processes and of diminishing reserve capacities brings to attention not only the heteronomous constraints of development, but as well the importance of active efforts for optimizing personal developmental prospects.

PERCEIVED CONTROL OVER DEVELOPMENT AND
EVALUATION OF PERSONAL DEVELOPMENTAL
PROSPECTS

According to theoretical notions of control and self-efficacy, self-percepts of control should have a broad range of beneficial effects on personal development (cf. Baltes & Baltes, 1986; Bandura, 1981; Heil & Krampen, 1989; Rodin, 1987). Almost by definition, people having a strong sense of control over personal development should be less vulnerable to feelings of helplessness and depression; in coping with adversities, they should be more persistent and expend more problem-focused effort. Believing that one has control over aversive and threatening events also reduces the emotional strain associated with these events; there is ample evidence that positive action–outcome expectancies may buffer the pathogenetic impact of situational stress (cf. Bandura, 1989; Peterson & Seligman, 1987; Holahan, Holahan & Belk, 1984). By contrast, people who entertain doubts in their efficacy to achieve the goals to which they are committed should have difficulties in finding sense and meaning in their lives. From a conceptual point of view, a belief that one cannot become the person that one wants to be, or cannot live up to one's own aspirations, is certainly a central ingredient of depression.

Our findings are largely consistent with these propositions. Thus, autonomous Control generally goes with features of successful development and well-being such as high life satisfaction and dyadic adjustment, while heteronomous control shows an opposite pattern of relationships (cf. Brandtstädter, 1991). As part of the assessment procedure, participants in our panel study also described their feelings with regard to past and future personal development on selected adjective scales. The canonical analysis shown in Table 9.2 addresses these emotional implications. The first and strongest canonical correlation links a combination of high autonomous and low heteronomous control over development to a pattern of self-ascribed emotional states characterized by retrospective emotions such as pride and gratitude and future-related emotions such as hope and confidence. Interestingly, the cognitive–emotional syndrome linking self-percepts of control to an optimistic, zestful outlook on personal development also emerges when we consider differential longitudinal change within the four-year interval.

A note of caution should be added with regard to issues of causal priority. Changes in emotional states are often deemed to causally depend on changes in control beliefs (cf. Peterson & Seligman, 1984). In our study, the cross-lagged panel correlations between the various measures of perceived control and personal well-being taken at the different occasions yielded were virtually identical, thus giving no evidence of a simple antecedent-consequent type of causal ordering. There are, of course, different possible reasons for such an outcome (cf. Kenny, 1979; Rogosa, 1988). In the present case, it seems most

Table 9.2. *Self-percepts of control over development and development-related emotions: results of canonical correlation analysis (T1: first wave, 1983; T3 — T1: change scores 1987–1983)*

Variables	Canonical factors (T1)		Canonical factors (T3–T1)	
Set A				
(Self-percepts of control)	*A1*	*A2*	*A'1*	*A'2*
Autonomous control	.89	.45	.60	.80
Heteronomous control	−.30	.95	.87	−.50
Set B				
(Self-ascribed emotions or feelings)	*B1*	*B2*	*B'1*	*B'2*
Pride	.54	.37	.45	.39
Exhaustion	−.51	.60	.38	−.45
Depression	−.56	.56	.26	−.60
Indifference	−.55	.17	.09	−.53
Gratitude	.47	.15	−.33	.54
Hope	.66	.13	.03	.70
Discouragement	−.67	.50	.47	−.43
Fear	−.46	.54	.60	−.18
Confidence	.67	−.10	−.19	.43
Venturesomeness	.79	.26	.15	.51
Canonical correlations	.45***	.29***	.21***	.19**

Note:
N(T1): 1111, N(T3 − T1): 674. Listwise deletion of missing data.
***$p < .001$, **$p < .01$.

plausible to assume that the variables of perceived control and subjective well-being do not fit into a simple antecedent–consequent scheme, but form a complex nonrecursive system involving reciprocal influences. This would be in line with experimental evidence indicating that depression is not only induced by, but also generates or primes mood-congruent cognitions (cf. Blaney, 1986; Bower, 1981).

Age-related changes in perceived quality of life

In our study, the individual's appraisal of personal developmental prospects was assessed in different ways. From the subjects' ratings of perceived distance from developmental goals, a general indicator of subjective developmental deficit was derived (see above, Table 9.1). Fig. 9.4 gives the cross-sequential findings for this developmental parameter.

The picture of findings is rather consistent in this case. Cross-sectional and longitudinal effects are both highly significant, indicating that over the age-

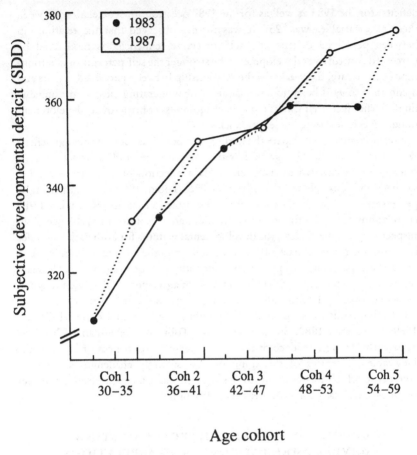

Fig. 9.4. Subjective developmental deficit: cross-sectional comparisons and 4-year longitudinal change (age ranges for cohorts refer to first occasion of measurement).

range considered, individuals experience a growing distance from personally valued goals and a gradual worsening of the balance between developmental gains and losses (see also Heckhausen et al., 1989).

Let me briefly digress to a further observation that bears on the functional linkage between self-corrective action and the perception of developmental deficits. In addition to the various assessments considered so far, we also asked our participants to rate the degree of intended self-corrective change for a broad range of behavioural domains. From these ratings which involved 48 different behavioural facets, a sum index of self-corrective tendency was formed as a global measure of the subject's inclination to alter habitualized ways of living. As should be expected from an action-theory point of view, self-corrective tendencies were found to significantly increase with perceived developmental deficits (for the 1983 as well as for the 1987 occasion, the correlation between these two variables was .23). It was further observed that the relationship between perceived deficits and self-corrective tendencies is moderated by perceived control over development: the stronger the self-percepts of heteronomous control are, the weaker is the relationship between perceived deficits and inclination toward behavioural change. This moderating effect is presumably due to the fact that beliefs of heteronomous control over development undermine action-outcome expectancies.

It is instructive to compare the findings for perceived developmental deficits with cross-sequential changes in a traditional measure of life satisfaction. As a reference measure, we used in our study a selection of items from the life satisfaction index (Neugarten, Havighurst & Tobin, 1961). Not surprisingly, perceived developmental deficits and life satisfaction are inversely related (the correlations are $-.35$ for the 1983 occasion, and $-.36$ for the 1987 occasion, respectively). Nevertheless, the developmental patterns for both variables differ in important respects. Apart from a slight drop in the age range from 30 to 35 years, the cross-sequential picture gives no indication of an age-related decrease in life satisfaction (Fig. 9.5). This finding is in agreement with a wide range of cross-sectional and longitudinal investigations indicating that reported life satisfaction tends to be stable through middle and later adulthood (cf. Blazer, 1989; Newmann, 1989; Stock et al., 1983; Tobin & Lieberman, 1976). The apparently strong resilience of the elderly against experiences of loss and the inevitable adversities of the aging process strongly challenges a common stereotype which relates aging to despondency and fatalistic resignation, but obviously also calls for a theoretical explanation.

BEYOND PERSONAL CONTROL: ADJUSTING DEVELOPMENTAL GOALS AND ASPIRATIONS TO SITUATIONAL CONSTRAINTS

The findings that I have presented so far confront us with a puzzling question: how do the elderly manage to maintain a generally positive outlook on development, even though they face morbidity, death, impairment, and losses in many domains of life and personal development? Lazarus and Golden (1981) have advanced the proposition that the elderly cope with problems of old age partly by denying, avoiding or misconstruing its implications. Obviously, one might object to this view that the aging person should have some expertise of what aging means and implies personally.

I would propose a somewhat different account that does not primarily centre on functional self-deceptions, but rather on self-protective changes in goals and preferences. This approach was suggested by the following observations. For nearly all developmental goals presented to our participants, rated personal importance of a goal was inversely related to the perceived distance from that

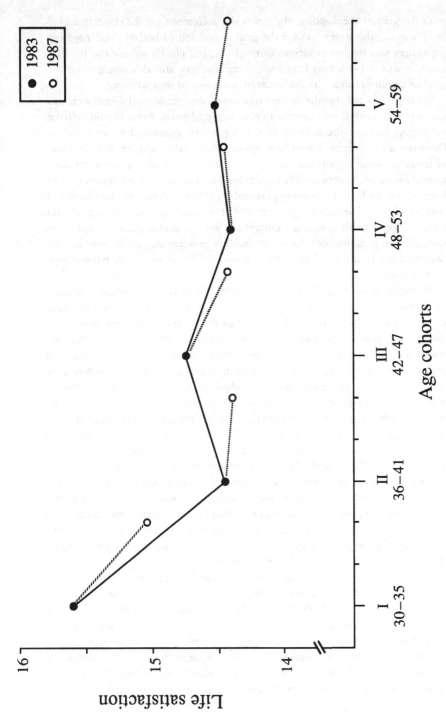

Fig. 9.5. Life satisfaction: cross-sectional comparisons and 4-year longitudinal change (age ranges for cohorts refer to first occasion of measurement). (From Brandtstädter, 1991.)

goal: the greater the distance, the lower the preference for the respective goal (with a noticeable exception for the goal dimension of health). This negative regression was low to moderate throughout, but clearly significant; furthermore, it was stable across longitudinal replications, and also emerged on the level of intraindividual change between occasions of measurement.

We hypothesized that the inverse relation of importance and distance ratings might partly result from a process of preference adaptation that should help the individual to keep the balance of developmental gains and losses positive. Developmental deficits should be tolerated more easily when they involve areas of lesser personal importance, and the aversive emotional impact of developmental losses might conceivably be alleviated by a compensatory devaluation of barren goals or by downgrading personal aspirations. A testable implication is that the observed negative regression of distance on importance ratings should tend to disappear when we select individuals with an unfavourable or depressive outlook on personal development. Such a moderating effect was in fact observed for 15 out of 17 goal dimensions (see Brandtstädter & Baltes-Götz, 1990, for details).

To account for these findings, we had to adjust our theoretical approach. Obviously, individuals can cope with losses and deficits in two basically different ways. On the one hand, perceived discrepancies between factual and desired developmental outcomes may induce active attempts to alter or transform the situation so that it fits more closely with personal preferences and aspirations. This is the aspect to which notions of control and self-efficacy usually refer. On the other hand, individuals may also adjust their system of preferences and aspirations to situational constraints in a way that alleviates the negative emotional impact of initially aversive events. I have denoted these distinct, but nevertheless complementary modes of coping as assimilative and accommodative, respectively. Accommodative readjustments of goals, aspirations and beliefs should become predominant to the extent that active-assimilative attempts to solve the problem turn out as unavailing. From this point of view, feelings of helplessness and depression do not appear as the terminal outcome of perceived loss of control over personally relevant areas of life, but rather as functional phenomena that precede, and may enhance, the rearrangement of personal goals and developmental options (see also Klinger, 1975). In certain respects, this theoretical framework converges with the distinctions of problem-focused vs. emotion-focused coping (Lazarus & Launier, 1978; Moos & Billings, 1982) and of primary vs. secondary control (Rothbaum, Weisz & Snyder, 1982). It is important, however, to note that accommodative changes in the system of personal preferences are to a large extent not intentional; we cannot change our beliefs and commitments merely because it seems advantageous to do so, even if such changes may eventually be enhanced by self-management techniques (cf. Karoly & Kanfer, 1982). Accordingly, it would not seem appropriate to subsume accommodative processes

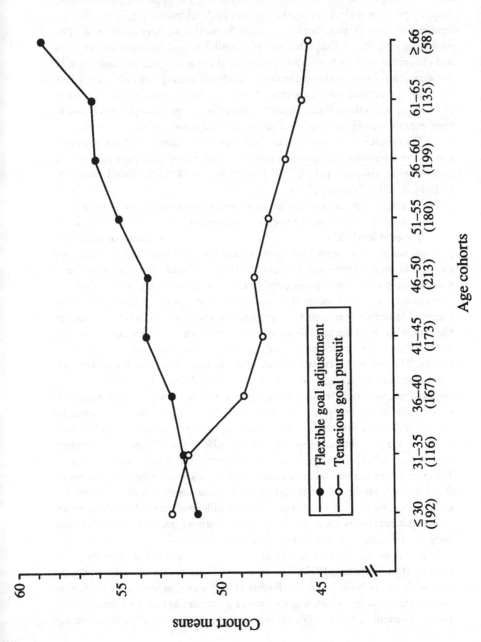

Fig. 9.6. Tenacious goal pursuit and flexible goal adjustment: cross-sectional comparisons. (From Brandtstädter, 1991.)

under a sweeping notion of personal control (for a broader discussion, see Brandtstädter & Renner, 1992).

The dual-process model of assimilative and accommodative modes of coping seems to offer a conceptual scheme for resolving the apparent paradox that, despite a progressively deteriorating balance of developmental gains and losses, reported life satisfaction does not generally decline in later adulthood. The model suggests that the experience of irreversible losses, uncontrollable events and chronic strains in later adulthood should enhance gradual dominance of accommodative over active-assimilative modes of coping with advancing age. Such an age-related shift in styles of coping might conceivably enhance a comforting outlook on life even under limited developmental prospects and to keep experiences of loss and decline within emotionally manageable proportions. These assumptions, of course, challenge earlier generalizations from age-comparative research, according to which '... older people ... cope in much the same way as younger people' (McCrae, 1982, p. 459; cf. also Lazarus & DeLongis, 1983; Aldwin, 1991).

To investigate the hypothesis of an assimilative-to-accommodative shift in modes of coping, we designed a questionnaire to assess these different modes on a dispositional level. The instrument comprises two scales, denoted as flexible goal adjustment and tenacious goal pursuit (or flexibility and tenacity, for short). The tenacity scale taps a tendency to cling to barren commitments and to tenaciously pursue one's goals even in the face of obstacles. This reflects an assimilative mode of coping. The items comprised in the flexibility scale, by contrast, indicate a readiness to disengage from barren commitments, to adapt aspiration levels to the feasible range and to find positive meaning in aversive events. These are obviously central features of an accommodative mode of coping. The two scales are statistically nearly independent, which indicates that the constructs of tenacity and flexibility tap different, but not necessarily opposed, dispositional features of coping competence. Despite their independence, both scales are positively related to various measures of successful development and well-being (for details of construction and psychometric qualities, see also Brandtstädter & Renner, 1990). Apart from these findings, several lines of evidence speak for the conceptual validity of these constructs. For example, evidence from moderation analyses shows that flexibility alleviates the negative impact of perceived developmental deficits and losses on life satisfaction (Renner, 1990). Results from an independent study with coronary disease patients further indicate that patients scoring high in flexibility have less difficulty revising their life-style (Scherler, 1989).[3]

Fig. 9.6 shows first cross-sectional age comparisons for flexibility and tenacity (Brandtstädter, 1991). The data come from our panel study, where the new scales were introduced on the last (1987) wave, as well as from further independent studies which together cover a broader age range than our main panel. As predicted, the scales exhibit clearly opposite regressions on the age variable; the linear correlations with age are .23 and − .23 for flexibility and tenacity, respectively, the difference being highly significant. Considering the independence of these variables and their convergent relation with variables of well-being and successful development, the opposite regressions on the age variable are particularly intriguing.

Again, we should be aware of the possible different sources of variance in cross-sectional data sets. Comparison of the 1987 data with results from a large independent sample obtained in early 1991 did not reveal any history-graded effects on the variables of flexibility and tenacity. While the theoretical arguments that I have advanced strongly favour an interpretation in terms of ontogenetic or age-graded change, we will have to wait for the results of longitudinal replications to rule out alternative interpretations with greater confidence.

SOME METHODOLOGICAL AFTERTHOUGHTS

To conclude, let me briefly outline some methodological desiderata for future research on adult development and aging.

There is no need to reiterate the well-known merits of longitudinal and sequential approaches here in detail. Obviously, it would be impossible to model intra-individual change and inter-individual differences in intra-individual change without longitudinal information. The search for coherence and continuity in developmental data, as well as any causal analysis, necessarily requires longitudinal observations. Long-range developmental outcomes, as well as incompatibilities within sequentially ordered systems of developmental tasks, become visible only from a diachronic perspective that extends over broader segments of an individual's developmental history; thus, issues of optimal development and successful aging can be successfully treated only within a longitudinal approach. The data presented here demonstrate once again the interpretive advantages of combining cross-sectional and longitudinal comparisons within a sequential strategy (cf. Schaie & Hertzog, 1982).

To inquire more thoroughly the generative mechanisms of development and aging, however, we should be prepared to go beyond the basic scheme of systematizing observations by age, cohort, and occasions of measurement. Developmental researchers usually agree that the age variable has no explanatory power in and of itself. The same reservation holds for the categories of cohort and occasions. Formally, these variables do not qualify as nomological predicates that could figure in theoretical propositions (cf. Stegmüller, 1969). Issues of design should be related to, but cannot replace, theoretical propositions; to analyse the mechanisms that produce certain longitudinal and sequential patterns, we have to extend the context of observation. It should be broad and explicit enough to yield insights not only as to the how, but also as to the why of age-related developmental change. Sequential strategies can capture and eventually disentangle the effects of factors correlated with the categories of age, birth cohort, and occasion of measurement, but they do not by themselves identify these factors.

Extending in this way the context of measurement may enhance a more systematic and comprehensive understanding of the processes of development and aging. We certainly cannot hope to gain such an understanding by focusing on single constructs or on the trajectories of isolated variables which only represent, as it were, fragments of the aging person (cf. Kenyon, 1988; Weinert, 1992). A rich, multi-variate observational basis is not a methodological cure-all, of course. Theoretical order can emerge only to the extent that the different measurements and observations can be meaningfully connected.

In our research efforts, we have adopted an action-theory framework as an organizing scheme, assuming that development-related goals, emotions, control beliefs and action tendencies constitute functionally inter-related facets within the process of personal control over development. To elaborate this theoretical framework, we will have to combine our cross-sequential approach with other strategies of investigation. As already mentioned, for example, we attempt to trace experimentally the microprocesses involved in accommodative adjustments of goals and aspirations. We expect that this complementary research will enhance a deeper understanding of age-comparative findings. This brings me to a final point. Future developmental research on adult development and aging, in my view, should freely adopt what might be called a post-modern methodological stance: a posture which in an opportunistic manner combines longitudinal observations with experimental process research, biographical analyses, case studies, simulation techniques, and other strategies of investigation that may help to illuminate the dynamics of development over the life-span.

NOTES

1. This project is funded by the German Research Foundation (DFG). The author is grateful to Bernhard Baltes-Götz, Werner Greve, Friedrich E. Heil, Günter Krampen, Gerolf Renner, and Dirk Wentura, who assisted in various phases of this research.

2. In the aggregation formulas, the inclusion of importance ratings (pi_g) as weighting factors reflects the assumption that an individual's general sense of control over personal development should be affected to a greater extent by self-percepts of control on developmental dimensions of higher personal relevance. An interesting implication is that strategic changes in the individual's system of preferences and priorities may help to maintain a sense of power and control even in face of a factual decrease in control potentials. I will return to this point in a later section.

3. In ongoing experimental work, we are investigating the assumption that differences in flexible goal adjustment are related to the availability and production of cognitions

that lend positive instrumental and semantic meaning to an initially aversive situation. This line of investigation draws on the priming and retrieval paradigms used in the experimental analysis of semantic memory.

REFERENCES

Aldwin, C. M. (1991). Does age affect the stress and coping process? Implications of age differences in perceived control. *Journal of Gerontology: Psychological Sciences*, **46** (4), 174–80.

Baltes, P. B. (1987). Theoretical propositions of life-span developmental psychology: on the dynamics between growth and decline. *Developmental Psychology*, **23**, 611–26.

Baltes, M. M. & Baltes, P. B. (eds.) (1986). *The psychology of aging and control*. Hillsdale, NJ: Erlbaum.

Bandura, A. (1981). Self-referent thought: a developmental analysis of self-efficacy. In J. H. Flavell & L. Ross (eds.), *Social cognitive development. Frontiers and possible futures*, pp. 200–239. Cambridge: Cambridge University Press.

Bandura, A. (1989). Perceived self-efficacy in the exercise of personal agency. *The Psychologist: Bulletin of the British Psychological Society*, **10**, 411–24.

Blaney, P. H. (1986). Affect and memory: a review. *Psychological Bulletin*, **99**, 229–46.

Blazer, D. (1989). Depression in late life: an update. *Annual Review of Gerontology & Geriatrics*, **9**, 197–215.

Bower, G. (1981). Mood and memory. *American Psychologist*, **36**, 129–48.

Brandtstädter, J. (1986). Personal and social control over development: some implications of an action perspective in life-span developmental psychology. In P. B. Baltes & O. G. Brim Jr. (eds.), *Life-span development and behavior*, vol. 6, pp. 1–32. New York: Academic Press.

Brandtstädter, J. (1990). Development as a personal and social construction. In K. Gergen & G. Semin (eds.), *Everyday understanding. Social and scientific implications*, pp. 83–107. London: Sage.

Brandtstädter, J. (1991). Personal control over development: Some developmental implications of self-efficacy. In R. Schwarzer (ed.), *Social cognitive mediators of action: the role of expectancies* (in prep.).

Brandtstädter, J. & Baltes-Götz, B. (1990). Personal control over development and quality of life perspectives in adulthood. In P. B. Baltes & M. M. Baltes (eds.), *Successful aging. Perspectives from the behavioral sciences*, pp. 197–224. New York: Cambridge University Press.

Brandtstädter, J. & Renner, G. (1990). Tenacious goal pursuit and flexible goal adjustment: explication and age-related analysis of assimilative and accommodative strategies of coping. *Psychology and Aging*, **5**, 58–67.

Brandtstädter, J. & Renner, G. (1992). Coping with discrepancies between aspirations and achievements in adult development: a dual-process model. In L. Montada, S.-H. Filipp & M. R. Lerner (eds.), *Life crises and experiences of loss in adulthood*, pp.301–319. Hillsdale, NJ: Erlbaum.

Brandtstädter, J., Baltes-Götz, B. & Heil, F. E. (1990). Entwicklung in Partnerschaften: Analysen zur Partnerschaftsqualität bei Ehepaaren im mittleren Erwachsenenalter. *Zeitschrift für Entwicklungspsychologie und Pädagogische Psychologie*, **22**, 183–206.

Brim, O. G. (1989). Losing and winning. *Psychology Today*, **22**, 48–52.

Brim, O. G. Jr. & Kagan, J. (1980). Constancy and change: A view of the issues. In O. G. Brim Jr. & J. Kagan (eds.), *Constancy and change in human development*, pp. 1–25. Cambridge, MA: Harvard University Press.

Bühler, C. (1933). *Der menschliche Lebenslauf als psychologisches Problem*. Leipzig: Hirzel.

Dannefer, D. & Perlmutter, M. (1990). Development as a multidimensional process: individual and social constituents. *Human Development*, **33**, 108–37.

Deeg, D. J. H. (1989). *Experiences from longitudinal studies of aging*. Nijmegen: NIG Trendstudies, Nr. 3.

Folkman, S., Lazarus, R. S., Pimley, S. & Novacek, J. (1987). Age differences in stress and coping processes. *Psychology and Aging*, **2**, 171–84.

Gergen, K. J. (1980). The emerging crisis in life-span developmental theory. In P. B. Baltes & O. G. Brim Jr. (eds.), *Life-span development and behavior*, vol. 3, pp. 31–63. New York: Academic Press.

Heckhausen, J., Dixon, R. A. & Baltes, P. B. (1989). Gains and losses in development throughout adulthood as perceived by different adult age groups. *Developmental Psychology*, **25**, 109–21.

Heil, F. E. & Krampen, G. (1989). Action theoretical approaches to the development of control orientations in the aged. In P. S. Fry (ed.), *Psychological perspectives of helplessness and control in the elderly*, pp. 99–118. North-Holland: Elsevier.

Höhn, E. (1958). Entwicklung als aktive Gestaltung. In H. Thomae (ed.), *Entwicklungspsychologie*, pp. 312–325. Göttingen: Hogrefe (= Handbuch der Psychologie in 12 Bänden, Bd. 3).

Holahan, C. K., Holahan, C. J. & Belk, S. (1984). Adjustment in aging: The roles of life stress, hassles, and self-efficacy. *Health Psychology*, **3**, 315–28.

Karoly, P. & Kanfer, F. H. (eds.) (1982). *The psychology of self-management. From theory to practice*. New York: Plenum.

Kenny, D. A. (1979). *Correlation and causality*. New York: Wiley.

Kenyon, G. M. (1988). Basic assumptions in theories of human aging. In J. E. Birren & V. L. Bengtson (eds.), *Emergent theories of aging*, pp. 3–18. New York: Springer.

Klinger, E. (1975). Consequences of commitment to and disengagement from incentives. *Psychological Review*, **82**, 1–25.

Krampen, G. (1987). Entwicklung von Kontrollüberzeugungen: Thesen zu Forschungsstand und Perspektiven. *Zeitschrift für Entwicklungspsychologie und Pädagogische Psychologie*, **19**, 195–227.

Lachman, M. E. (1986). Locus of control in aging research. *Journal of Psychology and Aging*, **1**, 34–40.

Lazarus, R. S. & DeLongis, A. (1983). Psychological stress and coping in aging. *American Psychologist*, **38**, 245–54.

Lazarus, R. S. & Golden, G. Y. (1981). The function of denial in stress, coping, and aging. In J. L. McGaugh & S. B. Kiesler (eds.), *Aging. Biology and behavior*, pp. 283–307. New York: Academic Press.

Lazarus, R. S. & Launier, R. (1978). Stress-related transactions between person and environment. In L. A. Pervin & M. Lewis (eds.), *Perspectives in interactional psychology*, pp. 287–327. New York: Plenum Press.

Lerner, R. M. & Busch-Rossnagel, N. A. (eds.) (1981). *Individuals as producers of their development*. New York: Academic Press.

Lewontin, R. C. (1982). Organism and environment. In H. C. Plotkin (ed.), *Learning, development and culture*, pp. 151–170. Chichester: Wiley.

McCrae, R. R. (1982). Age differences in the use of coping mechanisms. *Journal of Gerontology*, **37**, 454–60.

Magnusson, D. (1990). Personality development from an interactional perspective. In L. A. Pervin (ed.), *Handbook of personality: theory and research*, pp. 193–222. New York: Guilford Press.

Migdal, S., Abeles, R. & Sherrod, L. (1981). *An inventory of longitudinal studies of middle and old age*. New York: Social Science Research Council.

Moos, R. H. & Billings, A. G. (1982). Conceptualizing and measuring coping resources and processes. In L. Goldberger & S. Breznitz (eds.), *Handbook of stress: Theoretical and clinical aspects*, pp. 212–230. New York: Free Press.

Neugarten, B. L., Havighurst, R. J. & Tobin, S. S. (1961). The measurement of life satisfaction. *Journal of Gerontology*, **16**, 134–43.

Newmann, J. P. (1989). Aging and depression. *Psychology and Aging*, **4**, 150–65.

Peterson, C. & Seligman, M. E. P. (1984). Causal explanations as a risk factor for depression: theory and evidence. *Psychological Review*, **91**, 347–74.

Peterson, C. & Seligman, M. E. P. (1987). Explanatory style and illness. *Journal of Personality*, **55**, 237–65.

Renner, G. (1990). *Flexible Zielanpassung und hartnäckige Zielverfolgung: zur Aufrechterhaltung der subjektiven Lebensqualität in Entwicklungskrisen*. Unpublished doctoral dissertation. University of Trier, Trier.

Rodin, J. (1986). Health, control and aging. In M. M. Baltes & P. B. Baltes (eds.), *The psychology of control and aging*, pp. 139–165. Hillsdale, NJ: Erlbaum.

Rodin, J. (1987). Personal control through the life course. In R. P. Abeles (ed.), *Life-span perspective and social psychology*, pp. 103–119. Hillsdale, NJ: Erlbaum.

Rodin, J., Timko, C. & Harris, S. (1985). The construct of control: biological and psychosocial correlates. *Annual Review of Gerontology and Geriatrics*, **5**, 3–55.

Rogosa, D. (1988). Myths about longitudinal research. In K. W. Schaie, R. T. Campbell, W. Meredith & S. L. Rawlings (eds.), *Methodological issues in aging research*, pp. 171–209. New York: Springer.

Rothbaum, F., Weisz, J. R. & Snyder, S. S. (1982). Changing the world and changing the self. A two-process model of perceived control. *Journal of Personality and Social Psychology*, **42**, 5–37.

Scarr, S. & McCartney, K. (1983). How people make their own environments. A theory of genotype–environment effects. *Child Development*, **54**, 424–35.

Schaie, K. W. (ed.) (1983). *Longitudinal studies of adult psychological development*. New York: Guilford Press.

Schaie, K. W. & Hertzog, C. (1982). Longitudinal methods. In B. B. Wolman (ed.), *Handbook of developmental psychology*, pp. 91–115. Englewood Cliffs: Prentice-Hall.

Scherler, J. (1989). *Entwicklungserleben bei Patienten mit koronaren Herzkrankheiten*. Unpublished master's thesis. University of Trier, Trier.

Seligman, M. E. P. (1975). *Helplessness: on depression, development and death*. San Francisco: Freeman.

Stegmüller, W. (1969). *Wissenschaftliche Erklärung und Begründung* (= Probleme und Resultate der Wissenschaftstheorie und Analytischen Philosophie, Bd. 1). Berlin: Springer.

Stock, W. A., Okun, M. A., Haring, M. J. & Wilter, R. A. (1983). Age and subjective well-being: a meta-analysis. In R. J. Light (ed.), *Evaluation studies: Review annual*, vol. 8, pp. 279–302. Beverly Hills, CA: Sage.

Tetens, J. (1777). *Philosophische Versuche über die menschliche Natur und ihre Entwickelung.* Leipzig: M. G. Weidmanns Erben und Reich.

Thomae, H. (1987). Gerontologische Längsschnittstudien. Ziele – Möglichkeiten – Grenzen. In U. Lehr & H. Thomae (eds.), *Formen seelischen Alterns*, pp. 1–6. Stuttgart: Enke.

Tobin, S. & Lieberman, M. (1976). *Last home for the aged.* San Francisco: Jossey-Bass.

Weinert, F. E. (1992). Altern in psychologischer Perspektive. In P. B. Baltes & J. Mittelstrass (eds.), *Zukunft des Alterns und gesellschaftliche Entwicklung*, pp. 180–203. Berlin: de Gruyter.

10 Some methodological issues in longitudinal research: looking ahead

LARS R. BERGMAN

THE NEED FOR A LONGITUDINAL APPROACH

Longitudinal studies are vital for studying individual development and cannot normally for this purpose be replaced by other kinds of studies. This has been asserted many times (see Chapter 1 in this volume; Magnusson, 1988; Mednick, Harway & Finello, 1984). The main reason for using a longitudinal approach is really common-sense: If you want to understand how an individual develops over time, you have to study the individual over time. All other approaches are more indirect and have to make questionable assumptions for the results to be applicable for statements about individual development. For overviews of longitudinal versus other designs, the reader is referred to Baltes (1968) and Baltes and Nesselroade (1979).

The above should not be interpreted to mean that a longitudinal study always is necessary when development or change is to be studied. For instance, within epidemiology, a case-control study can be faster, cheaper, and more efficient than a longitudinal study for the (preliminary) study of the aetiology of a certain decease.

THE RESEARCH PROCESS

The research process can be described as having the following components:
1 The process starts from the specific aspect of reality that is at the focus of enquiry.
2 By some kind of data collection procedure, the raw data are produced.
3 The raw data are often further processed to give the variable values used in the analyses (transformed, summed to form indices and so on).
4 Statistical analyses are performed.
5 The results are interpreted in relation to the theoretical formulations.
6 Theoretical work (formulating and reformulating theories). The process is, of course, a feed-back system, and what is going on at later stages in the process also influences the design of the activities at earlier stages of the process.

It is often said that a researcher should carefully observe the raw data and be open to new and interesting relationships that may exist (as well as to, e.g. extreme values indicating possible errors). However, when a heavily theory-oriented approach is used, a specific statistical method is usually applied and the results are interpreted in terms of rejecting or retaining the theory that was proposed in advance often without any careful observation and description taking place. The usefulness of the results will then be a hostage to the appropriateness of the theoretical formulations being tested. Within the longitudinal field where highly complex phenomena often form the focus of investigation, current theories are often painfully inadequate and the danger in restricting contacts with reality to the testing of such theories should be obvious. The point that more emphasis should be given to careful description and observation has been made many times, for instance by Cronbach (1975) and by Magnusson (1988). See also Chapter 1 in this volume. In the context of risk research, Bergman (1988a) said that '. . . longitudinal risk data are too precious a commodity to be used mainly for a theoretical one-shot'. (pp. 363, 364). The approach advocated here can perhaps best be described as result-centred according to the terminology of Greenwald et al. (1986).

An obvious reason for the popularity of extensive model building and model testing is the advent of modern powerful computers, making easy what was previously practically impossible. This, of course, paves the ground for methodological breakthroughs. However, some dangers also arise. 1) A researcher may come all the way to interpreting the results without ever having actually examined the raw data, and 2) reruns can easily be performed after successive modifications of statistical models and of data (e.g. of cut-off points) which create risks of overfit or, even worse, of inadvertently adjusting the results after one's expectations. In the old days, a single statistical multivariate analysis was a major undertaking, and usually the researcher invested a great deal of time and theoretical effort in making sure that the appropriate analysis was performed.

A serious problem in longitudinal research can be the fading relevancy of the data. When the time has come to carry out the major analyses that were the focus of the longitudinal programme, the theoretical framework that decided the design of the study, the data to be collected, and the variables to be constructed, may have become obsolete. This problem has been discussed by, for instance, Bergman and Magnusson (1990) and by Janson (1990). Thus, when collecting the data in a longitudinal programme, one must be theoretically broad-minded or even eclectic. The primary raw data should also be retained to permit new codings, etc based on theories that are of interest at the time of the final analyses.

Taking a bird's eye view on the longitudinal research process and the amount of effort spent at the different stages of the process, one is struck by two facts. The first is the enormous amount of time, money, and energy that has to be invested to collect longitudinal data of high quality, and the other is the frequent emphasis, once the data have been collected, on theoretical work and statistical analysis/modelling. In the present author's opinion, both these items deduct from energy spent on constructing good measurements and on refining the measurements before analysis, and deduct from energy spent on obtaining good samples. Some signs of this are found in the dominance of measurement procedures developed in a cross-sectional context that are also used in longitudinal research, and the not unfrequent use of convenience samples that are not adequate for the inferences the longitudinal programme is focused at. These methodological issues will be discussed briefly in the following two sections.

Some of the issues brought up here have been discussed from different perspectives in the two previous methodological volumes in this series (Magnusson & Bergman, 1990; Magnusson et al. 1991) as well as by Magnusson in this volume.

MEASUREMENT IN A LONGITUDINAL CONTEXT

The aim of capturing development by studying individuals over time leads to many complications from a measurement point of view. In this section some central measurement issues in a longitudinal context are discussed.

The measurement of individual change

The measurement of individual change is a vital issue in many scientific studies of processes in the life sciences. For this purpose, longitudinal data are necessary. The study of individual change should be separated from the study of mean change (which sometimes can be performed using cross-sectional samples). Few areas within the behavioural sciences are so complex, so full of misunderstandings and so debated as how to measure change (for overviews, see Bergman, 1972*a*; Burr & Nesselroade, 1990; Harris, 1963).

Consider, for instance, the situation when change is measured as the difference between the time 2 and time 1 score on a variable. The interpretability of this difference is then affected by the following two factors:

1 Is the same quality measured at the two points in time? If this is questionable, the meaning of the change score is also questionable.

2 Making standard test theoretical assumptions, it is easy to show that, for scores within the normal reliability range, the reliability of the change score tends to be low when the correlation between the time 1 and time 2 scores is high.

Often a high correlation is viewed as reassuring in that it may indicate that the same quality is measured at the two points in time but, on the other hand, a high correlation often indicates that the reliability of the change score is low – a sort of a catch 22 situation.

A fair amount of psychometric and statistical work has been devoted to the properties of change scores. For instance, it has been shown that the use of a difference score as one variable in a correlational study tends to lead to interpretational difficulties (Bereiter, 1963). One problem is the often negatively biased correlation of the difference score with the initial score. To counteract this, various base-free measures have been constructed, but these seem to introduce other complications (Werts & Linn, 1970). Also, such simple operations as linear transformations of the involved variables can alter the results obtained (Bergman, 1972*b*). A conclusion reached by many researchers is that change scores should usually be avoided altogether and that one way to study the relationship of change to other variables is to use the post-test measurements directly while controlling for the pre-test measurements (Cronbach and Furby, 1970; Werts & Linn, 1970). However, in recent years, there has been a renewed interest in using change scores (Maxwell & Howard, 1981; Rogosa and Willett, 1985).

It seems reasonable to conclude that many of the problems in change measurement stem from the fact that the variables used in longitudinal studies were originally constructed in cross-sectional settings. It is not surprising that such variables create problems when they are used to extract information about change, a purpose for which they were not constructed. This has been noted long ago (Bereiter, 1963), but surprisingly little has been done about constructing direct measures of change. Microgenetic studies may be an exception (e.g. Kliegl & Baltes, 1987) in which one designs direct measures of process characteristics that are not just measurements based on snapshots of moments in time. Hopefully, such measures can then be taken over by real-time longitudinal studies.

Absolute and relative measurements

The discussion here is restricted to nomothetic measurements. The term 'absolute' may seem strange since all measurements are in some way relative. It is here meant to indicate the opposite end of a continuum which starts with a situation where the score of an individual has meaning only in relation to the other individuals' scores in the group under study (like a z-score or a T-score). The properties required of measurements used in studies of individual change or development are, of course, dependent on the purpose of the study. Frequently the purpose is to study correlations between variables, either directly or by using such correlations as an input in more sophisticated methods of analysis. Since correlation coefficients are invariant to linear transformations and, since the usual experience is that correlations do not change much if monotonic transformations of the involved variables are undertaken, there is some support for a fairly relaxed attitude towards measurement properties of the variables involved in such studies. However, there is often also a relaxed attitude towards the scaling level of the involved variables which, for instance, has been expressed as '. . . the numbers don't know where they came from' (Lord, 1953, p. 751). As long as the distributional properties of the involved variables satisfy the conditions of the statistical methods used, it is considered all right to use them. However, this is a dangerous assumption as has been pointed out by, for instance, Townsend and Ashby (1984), since the interpretation of the figures and summary statistics used in such situations becomes very difficult. The reader is referred to Velleman and Wilkinson (1993).

In certain situations, purely relative scores are not sufficient. There is a growing awareness that raw scores may contain important information that is lost by routine conversion into standardized or normalized scores. One obvious example when absolute measurements have to be used is in studying intellectual growth for the purpose of constructing age-dependent intelligence functions (Thorndike, 1966). Another example is found in an ongoing study of the development of patterns of adjustment problems (Bergman & Magnusson, 1991). In this study, the focus is on the growth of individuals' profiles of adjustment problems, and the prevalence of an adjustment problem must be interpreted both in relation to other problems and in relation to the same problem studied at another age. For this purpose, a strictly relative scaling would not be useful and a multivariate quasi-absolute scaling procedure was developed.

Aggregation level

It is well known that results pertaining to a given level of aggregation of observational units cannot normally be interpreted at a lower level of aggregation. For instance, the correlation between two variables measured for the population of Stockholm at the individual level cannot be inferred from the correlation between the two variables measured with the city block mean as the observational unit. Aggregation can be performed over different kinds of units such as individuals, items, situations, and points in time. Within a longitudinal context, it is common to aggregate items to form a scale, using school classes as observational units, and using a measure from a single point in time to represent all possible measures from the surrounding time period. Without going into this complex area it must here suffice to state that it is important to be aware of the aggregation level one is working at and to be sure that it corresponds to the level at which one wants to make inferences. For reasons of economy of information handling it is sometimes necessary to perform the analyses at a higher level of aggregation than the one at which the inferences are to be made. The burden of proof is then on the researcher to show that the results are interpretable at the desired level. For discussions of the problems of aggregation, the reader is referred to Bakketeig *et al.* (1991) and to Bergman and Magnusson (1990).

The impact of errors of measurement

Sizeable errors of measurement are ubiquitous in all life sciences and their handling is a challenge to longitudinal research methodology. On p. 221, some effects of errors of measurement on the study of change were discussed. Generally speaking, a fair amount of work has been performed in statistical modelling to handle the presence of 'benign' errors of measurement (usually error components that are uncorrelated to other components, non-systematic, etc). For instance, it is a very useful property of linear structural modelling, e.g. LISREL (Jöreskog and Sörbom, 1989), that measurement errors (including correlated errors) can be incorporated in the model. This is not the place for a detailed discussion but a few comments about unsolved problems caused by errors of measurement are in place.

1 Sometimes errors of measurement can be 'malign', for instance, if they are correlated to each other, and especially if they are correlated to the true scores. Examples of such errors that often are neglected are errors introduced by interviewer behaviour and characteristics (Groves, 1989), and errors introduced by recall bias. For the purpose of studying errors, retest or reinterview data can be useful (Andrews, 1984; Bergman, 1988a).

2 A question of basic importance is whether different respondents have the same response function (Saris, 1988) or whether they have different response functions. If the latter is the case, the same observed score can imply a different position on the latent continuum, dependent on which respondent it pertains to. This issue can be compared to that of social desirability (Edwards, 1957). There are ways of minimizing such effects, the effectiveness of which depends on the nature of the variables under study. In some contexts, the usefulness of cognitive laboratories for questionnaire design should be pointed out (Bergman, 1993; Lessler & Sirken, 1985).

SAMPLING IN LONGITUDINAL STUDIES

In longitudinal settings, like in many other settings within the behavioural, social and life sciences, samples of subjects have to be used that are not ideal from a statistical viewpoint.

1 Often non-random samples have to be used, due to practical consider-ations. For instance, to achieve an efficient data collection at a reasonable cost, entire school classes in certain schools, or all children of a specific age and living in a specific area, are selected.

2 Some longitudinal studies require a very intensive and expensive data collection for each subject, which precludes a large sample. Sometimes a sample size of, say, 50 subjects is the practical maximum. Unfortuna-tely, this opens the door to a strong influence of random fluctuations on the results.

Together, these two circumstances imply limitations in the usefulness of methods for estimation based on sampling theory in the analysis of longitudinal data.

The frequent lack of statistical representativeness of the sample must be considered when judging to what extent the results obtained can be generalized – problems that sometimes are more or less ignored by researchers who perform significance tests, etc on non-random samples without discussion or qualifications. It is extremely important that the generalization aspects of results from a non-random longitudinal sample are carefully discussed by the researcher because such considerations can be difficult to formulate for other researchers and are vital for the conclusions (Bergman, 1972*c*).

A special problem in this context is caused by drop-out or sample attrition (Bailar, 1989). Due to cumulative effects, there may be incomplete data for a considerable proportion of the sample and the drop-out can be selective. This is discussed by, for instance, Bergman and Magnusson (1990) and Cox et al. (1977). Fortunately, longitudinal data offer special ways of handling drop-out by using information from other points in time for subjects with incomplete data either directly for estimation of parameters, for imputation or for estimation of the characteristics of the drop-out (Kasprzyk et al., 1989).

The necessity of using small samples in longitudinal research often creates serious problems for the researcher when interpreting the results. Both estimation and significance testing can be problematic (too wide confidence intervals and too low power, respectively). For instance, for a simple random sample of 50 observations a percentage estimate around 50% will result in a 95% confidence interval that is 28%. However, there are ways of improving this situation if careful attention is paid to the sample design. Often it is feasible first to draw a large sample from which 'cheap' information is collected, e.g. by using questionnaires. This large sample is to be characterized by the fact that some of the 'cheap' variables are correlated with the 'expensive' variables being collected from an intensive small sample. A two-phase sampling procedure (double sampling) can then be used for computing estimates leading to substantially decreased mean square errors as compared to a common simple random sampling (Cochran, 1977). For instance, instead of using just the sample mean for the small sample as an estimator of the population mean, a more complex estimator can be used which takes into account the difference in means between the small and the large sample for a suitable 'cheap' variable. For general overviews of sampling considerations in a longitudinal context, the reader is referred to Goldstein (1979) and to Kasprzyk et al. (1989).

It is the present author's opinion that substantial gains in the quality of longitudinal studies can be made by paying close attention to modern sampling techniques both in data analysis and especially in sample design. The attitude within the longitudinal field towards sampling issues appears sometimes to be too relaxed. 'Modellers' (see next section) tend to defend this by pointing out that the model is assumed to hold for everyone and hence is tested also for non-random samples. Without denying that there is something in the argument, it should be obvious that this can be a dangerous position to take – often it is reasonable to assume that a model does not hold for everyone and only

Table 10.1 *Examples of problem classes and statistical methods used to elucidate them*

Class of problem	Statistical method frequently used
What are the relationships between variables measured at different points in time?	Correlational analysis, e.g. path analysis, regression analysis.
Testing/finding a model explaining the relationships between variables measured at different points in time.	Covariance structure modelling, e.g. LISREL.
Modelling/describing development in a single variable measured at many points in time.	Growth curve models and time-series analysis.
The impact of events taking place in continuous time.	Event history analysis.
Modelling/describing growth of categorical phenomena.	Log-linear models, configural frequency analysis, prediction analysis.
Modelling/describing classifications based on profiles of values and how they evolve.	Methods based on latent structure analysis and cluster analysis.

approximates reality. If this is the case, the danger of wasting effort and pursuing the wrong path, using a too rigid model approach, should be apparent.

Some statistical methods in longitudinal research

It is a truism that the statistical method used for elucidating a problem should be suited to that problem. Without any claims of completeness, Table 10.1 lists some classes of problems and the statistical methods frequently used to elucidate them.

Space limitations preclude a discussion of all the statistical methods in longitudinal research that are indicated in Table 10.1 and these are, of course, only a sub-set of the plethora of methods that are in use. The reader is referred to Magnusson, Bergman, Rudinger, and Törestad, (1991) for a discussion of different statistical methods focused on the matching of problems and methods and to von Eye (1990a,b) and Rovine and von Eye (1991) for presentations of a large variety of statistical methods.

There are at least two aspects that are important in the choice of a statistical method for analysing one's longitudinal data, viz. 1) that the information the method provides really answers the problem in hand, and 2) that the method produces trustworthy results. Unfortunately, it is common for methods to be used for which the conditions necessary for a valid interpretation of the results probably are not satisfied. This choice of an unsuitable method may happen for practical reasons (the method used is easily available), for reasons of prestige (the method used is considered sophisticated), or out of sheer ignorance. It is an important inter-disciplinary activity for the European scientific community to continue the methodological training programme started by the European Science Foundation and to assist in establishing clearing houses where methodological knowledge and computer programs can be made available to longitudinal researchers who are not methodological experts.

On pp. 226–31 a mainstream method will be presented for each of two classes of problems, namely finding a model for longitudinal relationships between variables and describing the development of individual profiles. On pp. 231–5, the two approaches will be compared with regard to assumptions and to the matching between problems and methods. The two methods were chosen because a discussion and comparison of them will elucidate important issues in the choice of a statistical method.

Modelling the relationships between variables using a covariance structure model

A standard situation when covariance structure modelling is applied in a longitudinal context can be described as follows. The researcher has a more or less precise theoretical model for the causal relationships between certain variables. He or she has an empirical data set with several indicators measuring each of the variables of interest. The existing knowledge is used for constructing 1) a measurement model specifying how the observed indicators are related to the (unobservable) latent variables of interest, and 2) a model for the causal relationships between the latent variables. The model is then tested on the empirical data set to see whether the model is sufficient for explaining the relationships between the observed variables. A widely used approach for analysing covariance structures is the powerful LISREL system (Jöreskog, 1973, 1979; Jöreskog and Sörbom, 1989). Often, the study is rather descriptive with a fair amount of successive modifications made of the model on the basis of preliminary model fit.

An example of this approach is furnished by a study made by Olsson and Bergman (1977) in which the problem under study was the age differentiation hypothesis postulated by Garrett (1946) as 'Abstract or symbol intelligence changes in its organization as age increases from a fairly unified and general ability to a loosely organized group of abilities or factors' (p. 373). For studying this problem, scores on six ability tests and two achievement tests were available from the age 10 and 13 for 353 boys and 375 girls. It was decided that covariance structure modelling would shed light on this problem by analysing the relationships between the observed variables and the hypothesized latent variables and the relationships among the latent variables. First a measurement model was constructed at each point in time and then the latent variables were connected in a complete model according to theoretical expectations. The model was built for girls and it was successively modified to fit the data but, of course, only in ways that were judged to be theoretically meaningful. In the testing, the fit of successively simpler models were compared to the fit of a more complex model with more free parameters, and the simpler model was preferred if it fitted the data almost as well. The final model for girls, which fitted the data nicely, was then tested on the data set for boys and fitted those data rather well.

The model for girls is summarized in Fig. 10.1 below with circles indicating latent variables and squares indicating observed variables. It is seen from Fig. 10.1 that the factors can be described as developing fairly independently of each other indicating differentiation in this sense. Identical factor structures fitted the data at both ages. The factor correlations were also computed and were often lower at age 13; and the inductive factor and knowledge factor, which were virtually one at age 10, had become clearly differentiated at age 13. Lack of space precludes a more detailed discussion of the results, but it should be obvious that the chosen approach provided substantial information of relevance to the problem at hand. (In its latest version, LISREL also offers the possibility of incorporating in the model means for factors and observed values which could shed additional light on the issue discussed here.)

Describing the development of individual patterns

It is assumed here that information is available at several points in time for a group of individuals. The information from the different points in time can relate to the same variables or to different variables. However, at each point in time, it is considered vital to characterize an individual by his, or her, profile of values at that point in time, and it is the growth of such individual profiles that constitutes the focus of interest. Below, an example of this approach is presented concerning the growth of boys' patterns of intrinsic adjustment problems. It is based on data from the IDA-programme (Magnusson, 1988). For technical details about the sample, variables, and cross-sectional classifications the reader is referred to Bergman and Magnusson (1984a, b); this presentation only gives an outline of the procedures and concentrates on the longitudinal aspects.

The study concerned boys' intrinsic adjustment problems at age 10 and age 13. The longitudinal sample comprised 367 boys. At age 10, the following indicators of problems were used: doesn't like school work, doesn't like school generally, psychosomatic reactions, low self-esteem, and feelings of low peer-status. At age 13 indicators very similar to the four last ones were used as well as a new one: heavy work load. To form the values in each indicator, self-reports were used most frequently, and sometimes information from different sources was combined. A quasi-absolute scaling procedure was used to produce four-point scales for each indicator rendering values considered comparable for the different indicators and for the two ages.

There are several ways of approaching a description of the growth of individual profiles (Bergman & Magnusson, 1991). Here, longisectional cluster

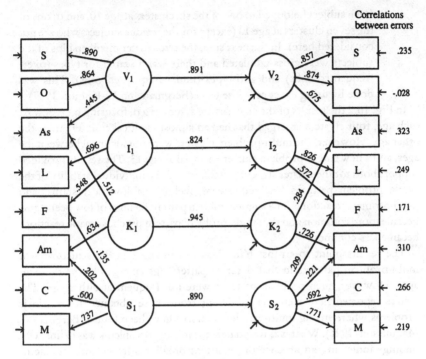

Fig. 10.1. A structural model for describing the relationships of the abilities between ages 10 and 13 for girls. S = Similarities; O = Opposites; As = Achievement in Swedish; L = Letter groups; F = Figure series; Am = Achievement mathematics; C = Cube counting; M = Metal folding; Goodness to fit: x^2 = 76.305 with 74 d.f.; p = .4043; Tucker and Lewis reliability = .999.

analysis was used (Lienert & Bergman, 1985). It is a fairly basic method which is suitable here for illustrative purposes. The analysis was performed in the following way.

1 A cross-sectional classification was performed at each of the two ages. For this purpose, cluster analysis was used (Ward's method provided a start classification for a RELOCATE procedure). Following the RESIDAN rationale (Bergman, 1988*b*), not every child was classified, but a residue of outliers or unique subjects was formed (3% and 4% of the subjects at age 10 and 13, respectively). However, for the present purpose this aspect of the study will not be further commented upon. At age 10, a six-cluster solution was chosen which 'explained' 68% of the error sum of squares, and at age 13 a seven-cluster solution was chosen which 'explained' 70% of the error sum of squares. It was found that the clusters were reasonably tight, and that the members of a cluster could be considered as subjects having similar value profiles.

2 Each subject belonged to one of the six clusters at age 10, and to one of the seven clusters at age 13 (except for the residue subjects who are not considered here). In the next step, the two cluster memberships of the subjects were cross-tabulated and there was a search for types (over-frequented cells) and anti-types (under-frequented cells). This was done by using exact cell-wise tests (Bergman and El-Khouri, 1987).

In Fig. 10.2 the results of the analyses are summarized, focusing on types. At each age, four clusters emerged that had an almost identical counterpart at the other age. However, the multi-problem clusters were not identical between the ages, and a new single-problem cluster emerged at age 13. The results provided support both for the cluster structure stability and the individual stability of the single problem patterns low self-esteem, feelings of low peer status, and psychosomatic reactions. The single-problem pattern feelings of low peer status became more common and the single-problem pattern psychosomatic reactions became less common.

The results point to an instability between the ages in the structuring of multi-problem patterns in that different patternings emerged at the different ages. However, such problem patterns were not frequent at either age. The results reported here were very different from those obtained for extrinsic problems where strong multi-problem patterns have been found (Bergman & Magnusson, 1991). What was found here for intrinsic problems was in line with findings indicating an absence of persistent broad syndromes of intrinsic or emotional problems (e.g. Rutter, 1981; Achenbach & Edelbrock, 1978). The most pronounced developmental streams included children characterized by patterns containing low self-esteem and/or psychosomatic reactions showing patterns of continued problems of these kinds.

The above example concerned the domain of intrinsic problems. If the patterns of intrinsic problems are correlated with patterns of problems taken from the domain of extrinsic problems, some connections are found. For instance, children characterized by problem patterns containing feelings of low peer status are, more frequently than expected by change, also characterized by extrinsic patterns containing poor peer relations and conduct problems (Berg-man & Magnusson 1984a, b). However, the main conclusion is the lack of correspondence between intrinsic and extrinsic patterns – children character-ized by some kind of intrinsic maladjustment syndrome are only slightly more likely to be characterized by a syndrome of extrinsic maladjustment and vice versa. This supports the basic distinction often made between externalizing and internalizing problems (Achenbach & Edelbrock, 1978).

Hopefully, the presented example of a pattern analysis have shown the possibility of this approach in capturing more of the *Gestalt* of the information, and in giving results that are more person-oriented.

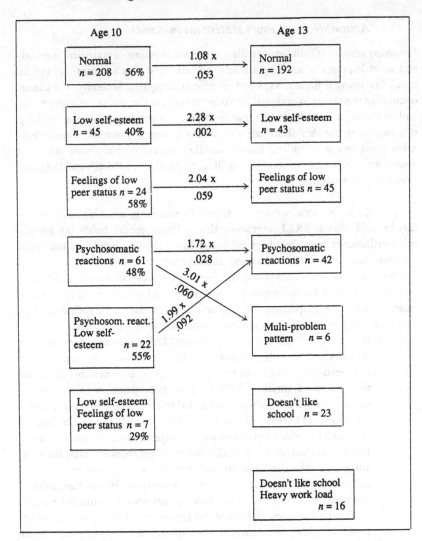

Fig. 10.2.   Longitudinal stream of patterns of boys' intrinsic adjustment problems. $n = 367$. *Note* The figures above and below the arrows indicate the ratio between the observed and expected frequency of a cluster combination and the significance level of the deviance of this ratio from one, respectively. An arrow is drawn only if $p = .10$. The percentages refer to the proportion of subjects in a cluster at age 10 who are found in the normal cluster at age 13.

Assumptions of some statistical methods

For many reasons it is difficult to discuss the assumptions of statistical methods and what happens when they are not fulfilled. First, the assumptions can be invalid in many different ways and to different degrees. Secondly, the consequences of the errors introduced also depend on how the results are interpreted, and on the aspects of the results that are of interest in the specific case. To keep this section reasonably short, we will take as a starting point the assumptions often made in a longitudinal context for the two kinds of methods discussed above, viz. covariance structure modelling, particularly, LISREL and longisectional cluster analysis.

Covariance structure models Generally speaking, and a bit simplified, it can be said that LISREL stipulates that a linear model holds (a) for the relationships between the observed variables on the one hand and the latent variables and the errors of measurement on the other (measurement model) and (b) for the relationships among the latent variables (structural model). A multivariate normal distribution is often assumed as well, and the error terms must have certain properties. We will here concentrate on the following four crucial assumptions that often are made when using this approach.

1 It is assumed that the model (almost) holds for everyone and that, therefore, it is only necessary to have a sufficiently large sample irrespective of whether or not this sample is a random sample from the population of interest. This kind of assumption is often basic in statistical model building and has led to a long controversy between what Groves (1989) call 'modellers' and 'describers'. At the heart of the matter is whether the researcher judges it is reasonable to assume that a (specified) model of reality holds at least approximately for every subject or whether he or she believes instead, for instance, that it is difficult to find even an approximate general model and that different segments of a population can best be described by different models. This issue was discussed already by Lewin (1931). From the describer's point of view, the characteristics of the sample are vital for the conclusions reached, and weighing procedures can be necessary to adjust the estimates.

2 It is assumed that the errors are not correlated to the true values. This assumption does not always hold and can be hard to check (see also p. 223). It is made in most models containing error terms, outside covariance structure modelling as well, and the effects of violations are hard to evaluate since they, among other things, depend on the exact nature of the violations. For instance, in a simple case Bergman and Magnusson (1990) showed that the correlation between a predictor and an outcome can be expected to be inflated if there is a positive

correlation between errors and true scores, i.e. an inversion of the well-known attenuation effect.

3 If the postulated model is correct, all the necessary information is contained in the first- and second-order moments. However, if the model is not true, and interactions and non-linear relationships exist, then these moments would not necessarily contain sufficient information. For instance, it has been pointed out that strong interactions can prevail in a data set where all pairwise correlations are zero (e.g. Bergman, 1988*b*). Obviously, a covariance structure model would then not detect these interactions. This points to an unpleasant property of almost every modelling approach – certain serious deviances from the model cannot be detected, and an inadequate model can fit the data. This is one aspect of the lack of power of many statistical tests against alternative hypotheses that really build on different assumptions. When the researcher tests a model, and specifies a null hypothesis, he or she also must be aware of the fact that only certain alternative hypotheses have the power of falsifying the null hypothesis.

4 It is frequently assumed that the model that is found is in some sense the 'right' one. However, it is possible that different models fit the data equally well and the researcher must be very careful before interpreting the results as supporting his or her theory. This problem is amplified by the frequent use of successive model modifications before arriving at the final model. Information and knowledge outside that provided by the analysis is necessary to achieve a firm basis for theoretical conclusions.

For a further discussion of assumptions, and other aspects in the application of covariance structure models, the reader is referred to Breckler (1990).

In many areas in longitudinal research, highly complex phenomena are studied and experiments are rarely possible. In the present author's opinion, it would seem that, in many cases, there is but a limited basis on which to found realistic, strict models of such phenomena, and that there has first to be a cumulative growth of descriptive knowledge (summarized by micro-theories) before it makes sense to concentrate on a model testing approach. An interactional paradigm in developmental research in which interactions and non-linear relationships are stressed has also become more pronounced during the last decades (Magnusson & Allen, 1983). Together, these items suggest that, in the early stages of many developmental fields, one should worry about the tenability of the above assumptions and not invest too much effort on model building and testing within the covariance structure modelling framework without first undertaking a thorough descriptive groundwork and a check out of the assumptions. A system like LISREL is a wonderful tool but its greatest enemy can be the indiscriminate and over-enthusiastic user.

Longisectional cluster analysis   The assumptions on which person-oriented methods build vary with the specific method. Generally speaking, more assumptions have to be made in model-based approaches like latent structure analysis and log linear analysis, and less assumptions have to be made in more descriptive approaches like cluster analysis or configural frequency analysis. In accordance with the previous discussion about assumptions, the issue of the scale level of the involved variables will not be discussed. Following the rationale in the previous section, the discussion is also restricted to the method previously presented and discussed. Major assumptions in longisectional cluster analysis are as follows.

1 Whether one believes the classification to encompass everyone or whether the existence of a unique set of subjects is recognized. Often it does not seem reasonable to assume that all individuals follow a limited number of developmental patterns, and there are some studies showing that atypical patterns can be a personality attribute and not just an artefact of errors of measurement (Bergman, 1988*b*). Thus, there appear to be good theoretical (Bergman, 1988*b*) and technical (Edelbrock, 1979) reasons, for not classifying everyone.

2 That the chosen similarity or dissimilarity coefficient appropriately reflects the properties of the data set one is interested in. This choice is very basic since different coefficients are sensitive to different properties of the (dis)similarity between two subjects' profiles. For instance, the correlation coefficient is sensitive only to profile form, not level, and squared Euclidean distance is sensitive to both form and level (Cronbach & Gleser, 1953). The researcher must decide which aspects of the correspondence between two profiles are of importance for his or her particular problem. Another related question is whether it is sufficient to consider only pairwise similarity (cf. point 3. above). Generally speaking, this restriction normally poses no severe problems; one reason being that the number of subjects normally is much larger than the number of variables, and the (dis)similarity matrix therefore tends to contain much more information than an ordinary correlation matrix.

3 That the chosen variables give an adequate reflection of the sub-system one wants to study. This choice is crucial since it has been shown that the exchange of even one variable for another in the profile can considerably alter the whole clustering solution (Milligan, 1981). Thus, cluster analysis cannot be used exploratively as easily as factor analysis to bring order and structure into an area where variables afterwards can be eliminated/added/combined. Presumably, misconceptions in this respect lie behind many conflicting and confusing results obtained within the cluster analysis area. The assumption that

the 'right' variables constitute the profile is very basic. Since standard cluster analysis contains no way of handling errors of measurement, and since profiles are sensitive to errors of measurement it also makes sense to use only variables with a high reliability and as few as possible (Bergman & Magnusson, 1983, 1987).

4 Suppose that a classification has been undertaken for a number of subjects, using information in k variables and giving a value profile for each subject. It must then be assumed that the k-dimensional reality can be reasonably well summarized by one categorical variable, i.e. by the clusters. This, of course, is not always the case which explains much of the criticism against typologies in psychology and psychiatry (Anastasi, 1958; Ekman, 1951). However, it should be observed that in a typological approach typically no dimensional data are ever produced – the types are constructed directly, often using more or less subjective ratings. Hence the assumption that the categorical variable gives a valid reflection of a multi-dimensional reality is hard to check. If, on the other hand, e.g. cluster analysis is used on dimensional data to produce a classification, its appropriateness can be checked since the k-dimensional data are available (Bergman & Magnusson, 1987).

5 In longisectional cluster analysis, a cross-tabulation of cluster membership between two points in time follows the cluster analysis made separately at each point in time. It is then assumed that the cluster membership combination contains the necessary information for interpreting pattern development. If this assumption is not tenable, some other approach must be used (for instance, longitudinal cluster analysis). However, it should be noted that, as opposed to the standard situation when studying change using parametric methods, there are no assumptions involved about having measured the same qualities at the different points in time (or having obtained the same clusters at the different points in time).

Conclusion In the above, the obvious importance has been discussed of being aware of the assumptions contained in the methods used, the extent to which they are satisfied in the practical situation, and the importance of the deviations for the interpretations one wants to make. The discussion underlines the importance of keeping an open mind and preferably of using different kinds of analyses on the same data set to provide a binocular view. As well, it underlines the importance of replication and cross-validation to ascertain the validity and generalizability of the results; a recommendation often made but rarely followed (Rutter & Pickles, 1990).

THE APPLICATION OF CHAOS THEORY IN STUDIES
OF INDIVIDUAL DEVELOPMENT

Chaos has been defined as the occurrence of stochastic behaviour in a deterministic system. During the last decade, there has been a great increase in the interest in this area, mainly in physics, meteorology, and mathematics (for overviews, see Gleick, 1987; Crutchfield et al., 1986). It has been shown that simple deterministic models can exhibit chaotic properties under specific conditions, and that systems behaving in a very complicated fashion sometimes can be modelled by a very simple deterministic model. Such examples have been found in biology and epidemiology as well (e.g. Rapp, 1986; Pool, 1989).

Chaos models are sometimes characterized by the following properties:

1 A simple mathematical deterministic model of an iterative kind is assumed, where output values generated by the function are input values in the function for deciding the output values in the next step, and so on.

2 The model is iterated a large number of times to see if the output from the system stabilizes to one or more attractors, e.g. after a few hundred iterations settles down to produce the same output value or output vector of values. Or, if the system instead produces what appears to be a stochastic output; unpredictable and never settling down to a limited number of attractors, i.e. chaos occurs.

3 Chaos usually occurs only for specific parameter values and for such value one can find an extreme sensitivity of the system for differences in the initial values that are fed into the function. For instance, a difference in the fifth decimal place in the starting values can, after only a small number of iterations, produce output that is completely different (the so-called 'butterfly effect' coined by Lorenz, cf. Gleick, 1987). Already in 1903 Poincaré noted this and pointed out that prediction can become impossible in such situations (Poincaré, 1946).

4 Even in chaos there is some kind of order and so-called 'strange attractors' can be found. The emergence of attractors, period doubling, and chaos as parameter values change can be analysed by the new mathematics. For instance, a new mathematical constant called the *feigenvalue* has been found with a value of 4.669 which can be interpreted as the ratio between the scales of successive period doublings (or more generally as the scaling ratio of a large class of one-humped mappings, see, for instance, Stewart, 1989).

To exemplify a very simple function that can exhibit chaotic behaviour the following iterative function is sometimes used:

$$X(t+1) = k(X(t) (1 - X(t))$$

with a starting value between null and one and a k value between one and four. For small k values, the function value, after a number of iterations, settles down to a single attractor value. When k increases, the number of attractor values increases as well and, at about $k = 3.58$, chaos occurs.

The attraction of chaos theory to developmental modelling is obvious. Since this kind of thinking opens up the possibility of understanding complex behaviour by simple models which explain random or stochastic behaviour. For instance, van Eenwyk (1991) has discussed the application of chaos theory to Jungerian psychology, and he has pointed to several aspects of the new mathematics that correspond to Jung's thinking and which provide new concepts and ideas. This extends into developmental issues like symptom formation and recovery from psychotic episodes.

However, some problems with applying chaos theory in the longitudinal field must be noted.

1 The extreme sensitivity to initial values in a chaos situation, and the dependence on parameter values, mean that errors of measurement can pose tricky problems for the study of such systems. On the other hand, periodic aspects and the presence/absence of chaos are, for some kinds of systems, not at all sensitive to the choice of starting values and can refer to broad ranges of parameter values.

2 It is reasonable to claim that human development must be described as an open system in which the individual is in continuous interaction with his or her environment (Magnusson & Allen, 1983). It thus seems doubtful to adopt a mathematical model which depends solely on the starting values of the system and on some fixed parameter values. Except for special applications limited to short time-spans, it would appear that a chaos model must be constructed in a way that at least allows for time-dependent changes in the parameter values.

DISCUSSION

A growing rapprochement between longitudinal researchers and methodological experts will hopefully lead to a decrease in the gap between the methods the experts are interested in developing and working with, and the methods that the longitudinal researchers need for answering their questions. The book by Magnusson et al. (1991) is one example of this. It is my guess that the more general acceptance of the interactional meta-theoretical framework and the growing awareness that the individual fruitfully can be seen as an evolving complex open system will lead to a sharply increased demand for new methods suited for research along these lines. Until now, surprisingly little effort has been spent on developing, for instance, pattern analysis oriented methods, as compared to methods based on linear models. Considering the comparatively low sophistication of many of the methods dealing with individual configurations or structures, a considerable method improvement can be hoped for if large-scale systematic work is undertaken in this field.

The mathematics of non-linear science and chaos is an exciting new tool and, hopefully, young mathematicians will be interested in taking part in multi-disciplinary work creating developmental models based on such concepts. Especially interesting is the search for critical attractors using these techniques which nicely answers to the concept of stable system states or configurations in developmental processes as discussed in Bergman and Magnusson (1991). As pointed out above, there are many issues that have to be resolved before this new tool can be used. Nevertheless, it is a promising avenue of research that is really new and basically different from the methods originating from statistics which are stochastic, not deterministic.

The stochastic approach is in many ways sound and useful, but it is possible to feel some apprehension about the frequent tolerance of large error components as long as they are incorporated in a model that fits the data. The fact remains that modelled error is still error, and error indicates deficiencies in the chosen model in explaining the phenomenon under study. One awaits with interest results of the beginning interaction between non-linear science and statistical science (Berliner, 1992; Chatterjee & Yilmaz, 1992).

As was pointed out in a previous section, viewing the research process as a whole, it can be argued that, comparatively speaking, too much effort is spent on statistical analysis and data collection and too little on measurement issues. One example of this is the dominance in longitudinal research of measures developed in a cross-sectional setting. Hopefully, this will change with growing sophistication. In survey research, there also exists a large body of methods and procedures for improving measures and for measuring error that advantageously can be applied within the longitudinal field. The survey research approach to measurement and error is summarized by Groves (1989), and data quality issues within the longitudinal field are discussed in Magnusson and Bergman (1990).

One important development that can be expected in the application of statistical models in longitudinal research is when researchers in earnest will start asking the question 'who is to be modelled?'. In practice, a model is often applied to all available subjects (perhaps with some extreme outliers removed) and without consideration for the fact that there may be theoretical reasons to expect that the model does not apply to some sub-sets of the sample. It is a challenge to find procedures for excluding subjects believed not to fit the model before the analysis; procedures preferably based on theoretical considerations and not on technical/statistical considerations. Such procedures are discussed within some fields, for instance, within random control trials, decisions about the eligibility of subjects can be theory based. This approach would also strengthen the modeller's position relative to the describer's in that the results would be less sensitive to sample characteristics. Naturally, this line of reasoning is also relevant in a classification setting, and there are some results indicating that the formation of a residue (not classifying everybody) can increase the interpretability of the results (Bergman, 1988).

Hopefully, this chapter has given the reader a flavour of some different approaches that are possible within the longitudinal framework. In spite of the large investments in time, effort, and money, longitudinal research programmes alone can answer many of the most important questions about individual development. Alternatives like cross-sectional designs have serious drawbacks, and microgenetic studies can replace a longitudinal study only in very specific situations. Often more sophisticated designs than a simple longitudinal design are then called for when, for instance, longitudinal and cross-sectional data from many generations are combined in the same study (for a discussion of these issues the reader is referred to Baltes and Nesselroade, 1979). As argued in a previous section, an increasing use of state-of-the-art sampling and estimation techniques can also be expected within the longitudinal field. Such methods can enhance the information value of the small samples which have to be used in many longitudinal studies.

The problems in making causal inferences based on non-experimental data are well known. Although this problem can be alleviated if a longitudinal design is used, it is still so that only a properly conceived randomized trial design can offer reasonable assurance on this point (see, e.g. Sacks, Chalmers & Smith, 1982). It is said with some justification that randomized experiments are usually not possible in an ordinary longitudinal setting for ethical and practical reasons. However, in the present author's opinion, the possibilities for randomized or natural experiments are often not explored sufficiently in a longitudinal study. For instance, ethical considerations are usually no obstacle for giving a treatment to a randomized group that is believed to enhance development in some specific way that is predicted by the researcher's theory. Sometimes events also occur affecting the longitudinal sample, or parts of it, that can be used to perform natural experiments. It is a strength of a longitudinal study that measures before the exposure then are available.

In medicine, especially concerning the acceptance of new drugs, there is a tendency to downgrade findings that are not supported by results from randomized trial studies. Results from case-control studies and non-experimental longitudinal studies tend not to be considered as sufficient evidence.[2] Also within the longitudinal field, in general, it can be a good idea to stress more the inconclusiveness of non-experimental findings and more strongly emphasize some kind of experimental verification of aspects of a developmental theory before it is seriously considered. Realistic kinds of experimental designs will then, in many cases, be natural experiments and other kinds of quasi-experimental designs and not classical randomized experiments.

NOTES

1. The author is grateful to Gunnar Eklund, David Magnusson and Dag Sörbom for highly useful comments on a previous version of this paper.
2. Personal communication with Gunnar Eklund.

REFERENCES

Achenbach, T. & Edelbrock, C. (1978). The classification of child psychopathology: a review and analyses of empirical efforts. *Psychological Bulletin*, **85**, 1275–301.

Anastasi, A. (1958). *Differential psychology*. New York: MacMillan.

Andrews, F. (1984). Construct validity and error components of survey measures: a structural modelling approach, *Public Opinion Quarterly*, **48**, No. 2, pp. 409–22.

Bailar, B. A. (1989). Information needs, surveys and measurement errors. In D. Kasprzyk, G. Duncan, G. Kalton, & M. P. Singh (eds), *Panel surveys*. New York: Wiley.

Bakketeig, L., Magnus, P. & Sundet, J. M. (1991). Differential development of health in a life-span perspective. In D. Magnusson, L. R. Bergman, G. Rudinger & B. Törestad (eds), *Problems and methods in longitudinal research: stability and change*, pp. 95–106. Cambridge: Cambridge University Press.

Baltes, P. B. (1968). Longitudinal and cross-sectional sequences in the study of age and generation effects. *Human Development II*, 145–71.

Baltes, P. B., & Nesselroade, J. R. (1979). History and rationale of longitudinal research. In J. R. Nesselroade & P. B. Baltes (eds), *Longitudinal research in the study of behavior and development*, pp. 1–39. New York: Academic Press.

Bereiter, C. (1963). Some persistent dilemmas in the measurement of change. In C. Harris (ed.), *Problems in measuring change*. pp. 3–20, Madison: University of Wisconsin Press.

Bergman, L. R. (1972c). Inferential aspects of longitudinal data in studying developmental problems. *Human Development*, **15**, 287–93.

Bergman, L. R. (1972a). Change as the dependent variable. *Reports from the Psychological Laboratories*, University of Stockholm, Suppl. 14.

Bergman, L. R. (1972b). Linear transformations and the study of change. *Reports from the Psychological Laboratories*, University of Stockholm, No. 352.

Bergman, L. R. (1988b). You can't classify all of the people all of the time. *Multivariate Behavioral Research*, **23**, 425–41.

Bergman, L. R. (1988a). Modelling reality: some comments. In M. Rutter (ed.), *Studies of psychosocial risk. The power of longitudinal data*, pp. 354–66. Cambridge: Cambridge University Press.

Bergman, L. R. (1993). Pretesting questionnaires at Sweden's statistics measurement, evaluation and development laboratory. *Journal of Official Statistics* (in press).

Bergman, L. R. & El-Khouri, B. (1987). EXACON – a Fortran 77 program for the exact analysis of single cells in a contingency table. *Educational and Psychological Measurement*, **47**, 155–61.

Bergman, L. R. & Magnusson, D. (1983). The development of patterns of maladjustment. *Report from the project Individual Development and Adjustment*, University of Stockholm, No. 50.

Bergman, L. R. & Magnusson, D. (1984a). Patterns of adjustment problems at age 10: an empirical and methodological study. *Reports from the Department of Psychology*, University of Stockholm, No. 615.

Bergman, L. R. & Magnusson, D. (1984b). Patterns of adjustment problems at age 13: an empirical and methodological study. *Reports from the Department of Psychology*, University of Stockholm, No. 620.

Bergman, L. R. & Magnusson, D. (1987). A personal approach to the study of the development of adjustment problems: an empirical example and some research strategical considerations. In D. Magnusson & A. Öhman (eds), *Psychopathology: an interactional perspective*. New York: Academic Press.

Bergman, L. R. & Magnusson, D. (1990). General issues about data quality in longitudinal research. In D. Magnusson & L. R. Bergman (eds), *Data quality in longitudinal research*. Cambridge: Cambridge University Press.

Bergman, L. R. & Magnusson, D. (1991). Stability and change in patterns of extrinsic adjustment problems. In D. Magnusson, L. R. Bergman, G. Rudinger & B. Törestad (eds), *Problems and methods in longitudinal research: stability and change*. Cambridge: Cambridge University Press.

Berliner, L. M. (1992). Statistics, probability and chaos. *Statistical Science*, 7, 69–90.

Breckler, S. J. (1990). Applications of covariance structure modeling in psychology: cause for concern? *Psychological Bulletin*, 107, 260–73.

Burr, J. A. & Nesselroade, J. R. (1990). Change measurement. In A. von Eye (ed.), *Statistical methods in longitudinal research*, vol. 1. San Diego: Academic Press.

Chatterjee, S. & Yilmaz, M. R. (1992). Chaos, fractals and statistics, *Statistical Science*, 7, 49–68.

Cochran, W. G. (1977). *Sampling techniques*. New York: Wiley.

Cox, A., Rutter, M., Yule, B. & Quinton, D. (1977). Bias resulting from missing information: some epidemiological findings. *British Journal of Preventive Social Medicine*, 31, 131–6.

Cronbach, L. J. (1975). Beyond the two disciplines of scientific psychology. *American Psychologist*, 30, 116–27.

Cronbach, L. J. & Furby, L. (1970). How we should measure 'change' – or should we? *Psychological Bulletin*, 74, 68–80.

Cronbach, L. J. & Gleser, G. C. (1953). Assessing similarity between profiles. *Psychological Bulletin*, 50, 456–73.

Crutchfield, J. P., Farmer, J. D., Packard, N. H. & Shaw, R. S. (1986). Chaos. *Science*,

Edwards, A. L. (1957). Social desirability and personality test construction. In B. M. Boss & I. A. Berg (eds), *Objective approaches to personality assessment*. Princeton NJ: D. van Nostrand.

Ekman, G. (1951). On typological and dimensional systems of reference in describing personality. *Acta Psychologica*, 8, 1–24.

Garrett, H. E. (1946). A developmental theory of intelligence. *American Psychologist*, 1, 372–378.

Gleick, J. (1987). Chaos. *Making a new science*. New York: Viking Press.

Goldstein, H. (1979). *The design and analysis of longitudinal studies: their role in the measurement of change*. London: Academic Press.

Greenwald, A. G., Pratkanis, A. R., Lieppe, M. R. & Baumgardner, M. H. (1986). Under what conditions does theory obstruct research progress? *Psychological Review*, 93, 216–29.

Groves, R. M. (1989). *Survey errors and survey costs*. New York: Wiley.

Harris, C. (ed.) (1963). *Problems in measuring change*. Madison: University of Wisconsin Press.

Janson, C. G. (1990). Retrospective data, undesirable behaviour, and the longitudinal perspective. In D. Magnusson & L. R. Bergman (eds), *Data quality in longitudinal research*, pp. 100–122. Cambridge: Cambridge University Press.

Jöreskog, K. G. (1973). A general method for estimating a linear structural equation system. In A. S. Goldberger and O. D. Duncan (eds), *Structural equation models in the social sciences*, p. 85–112. New York: Seminar Press.

Jöreskog, K. G. (1979). Statistical estimation of structural models in longitudinal developmental investigations. In J. R. Nesselroade & P. B. Baltes (eds), *Longitudinal research in the study of behavior and development*, pp. 303–351. New York: Academic Press.

Jöreskog, K. G. & Sörbom, D. (1989). LISREL 7: *A guide to the program and applications*. SPSS Publications.

Kasprzyk, D., Duncan, G., Kalton, G. & Singh, M. P. (1989). *Panel surveys*. New York: Wiley.

Kliegl, R. & Baltes, P. B. (1987). Theory-guided analysis of development and aging mechanisms through testing-the-limits and research on expertise. In C. Schooler & K. W. Schaie (eds), *Cognitive functioning and social structure over the life course*, pp. 95–119. Norwoord, NJ: Ablex.

Lessler, V. T. & Sirken, M. G. (1985). Laboratory-based research on the cognitive aspects of survey methodology: the goals and methods of the National Center for Health Statistics Study. *Milbank Memorial Fund Quarterly/Health and Society*, 63, No. 3, 565–81.

Lewin, K. (1931). Environmental forces. In C. Murchison (ed.), *A handbook of child psychology*, pp. 590–625. Worcester, MA: Clark University Press.

Lienert, G. A. & Bergman, L. R. (1985). Longisectional interaction structure analysis (LISA) in psychopharmacology and developmental psychopathology. *Neuropsychobiology*, 14, 27–4.

Lord, C. F. M. (1953). On the statistical treatment of football numbers. *American Psychologist*, 8, 750–1.

Magnusson, D. (1988). Individual development from an interactional perspective. A longitudinal study (Vol. 1). In D. Magnusson (ed.), *Paths through life*. Hillsdale, NJ: Erlbaum.

Magnusson, D. & Allen, V. (1983). An interactional paradigm for human development. In D. Magnusson and V. Allen (eds), *Human development: an interactional perspective*. New York: Academic Press.

Magnusson, D. & Bergman, L. R. (1990). (eds). *Data quality in longitudinal research*. Cambridge: Cambridge University Press.

Magnusson, D., Bergman, L. R., Rudinger, G. & Törestad, B. (1991) (eds). *Matching problems and methods in longitudinal research*. Cambridge: Cambridge University Press.

Maxwell, S. E. & Howard, G. S. (1981). Change scores – necessarily anathema? *Educational and Psychological Measurement*, 41, 747–56.

Mednick, S. A., Harway, M. & Finello, K. M. (1984). *Handbook of longitudinal research*. New York: Praeger.

Milligan, G. W. (1981). A review of Monte Carlo tests of cluster analysis. *Multivariate Behavioral Research*, 16, 379–407.

Olsson, U. & Bergman, L. R. (1977). A longitudinal factor model for studying change in ability structure. *Multivariate Behavioral Research*, 12, 221–42.

Poincaré, H. (1946). *The foundations of science*. Lancaster, UK: The Science Press.

Pool, R. (1989). Is it healthy to be chaotic? *Science*, 243.

Rapp, P. E. (1986). Oscillations and chaos in cellular metabolism and physiological systems. In A. V. Holden (ed.), *Chaos*. Princeton: Princeton University Press.

Rogosa, D. & Willett, J. B. (1985). Understanding correlates of change by modeling individual differences in growth. *Psychometrika*, 50, 203–28.

Rovine, M. J. & von Eye, A. (1991). *Applied computational statistics in longitudinal research*. New York: Academic Press.

Rutter, M. (1981). Longitudinal studies: a psychiatric perspective. In S. A. Mednick & A. E. Baert (eds), *Prospective longitudinal research: an empirical basis for the primary prevention of psychosocial disorders*. Oxford: University Press.

Rutter, M. & Pickles, A. (1990). Improving the quality of psychiatric data: classification, cause, and course. In D. Magnusson & L. R. Bergman (eds), *Data quality in longitudinal research*. Cambridge: Cambridge University Press.

Sachs, H. S., Chalmers, T. C. & Smith, H. (1982). Randomized versus historical controls for clinical trials. *American Journal of Medicine*, 72, 233–40.

Saris, W. E. (1988). *Variation in response functions: a source of measurement error in attitude research*. Amsterdam: Sociometric Research Foundation.

Stewart, I. (1989). Does God play dice? *The mathematics of chaos*. London: Penguin Books.

Thorndike, R. L. (1966). Intellectual status and intellectual growth. *Journal of Educational Psychology*, 57, 121–7.

Townsend, J. T. & Ashby, F. G. (1984). Measurement scales and statistics: the misconception misconceived. *Psychological Bulletin*, 96, 394–401.

van Eenwyk, J. R. (1991). Archetypes: the strange attractors of the psyche. *Journal of Analytical Psychology*, 36, 1–25.

Velleman, P. F. & Wilkinson, L. (1993). Nominal, ordinal, interval, and ratio typologies are misleading. *The American statistician*, 47, 65–72.

von Eye, A (1990a). Statistical methods in longitudinal research, vol. 1, *Principles and structuring change*. New York: Academic Press.

von Eye, A. (1990b). Statistical methods in longitudinal research, vol 2, *Time series and categorical longitudinal data*. New York: Academic Press.

Werts, C. E. & Linn, R. L. (1970). A general linear model for studying growth. *Psychological Bulletin*, 73, 17–22.

Index